"What does THAT do?"

Medical technology explained for patients and visitors.

Revised Edition

Laurence J. Street, Author

Kangal Publishing

Kangal Publishing
10333 Royalwood Blvd.
Rosedale, BC, Canada V0X 1X1

The patients described in this book are fictional; any resemblance to any persons living or dead is entirely coincidental.

Contact the author at WDTD@kangalpublishing.biz or at the Kangal Publishing address given above.

ISBN□13: 9781470195021

Dedication

To my family, as always, for their love and support □thank you Sheri, Jordan and Shannon!

And to all my extended family members and friends for their encouragement □especially Frank, who believed in this idea from the start.

Table of Contents

Preface

Going into a hospital for any reason can be a very stressful and sometimes frightening experience. Not only do you have to deal with the illness or injury that brought you there, but you also have to face a tremendous variety of complex, unusual and sometimes downright strange machinery that will be used in the course of your treatment.

I worked as a Biomedical Engineering Technologist in a variety of hospitals for almost thirty years, supporting most of the types of equipment described in this book. Often, while working on something at a patient's bedside, the patient or family members asked me about the equipment around them.

Not everyone is interested in the technology they might see in a hospital, but if you are reading this, you probably are curious about the machines. My aim in this book is to take some of the mystery out of the equipment you will see, and hopefully enable you to feel a little more comfortable and a little more involved in your own care.

Families of patients often feel just as bewildered as the patients themselves. You look at all the tubes and wires connecting your loved one to machines that beep and whirr and have all sorts of knobs and buttons and colorful displays, and you may not know what it all means.

A very wide variety of technological devices is used in the course of treating patients in hospitals. This variety is increasing, and the individual devices are often becoming more complex as well. My goal has been to give a clear and concise description of the principle of operation of each device as well as an outline of the way it is used, so that you can understand both how and why it is being used in your care.

Doctors and nurses are often very busy and may not have the time to explain all the equipment you might see. Patients and families, on the other hand, sometimes seem to have too much time to think about such things.

The table of contents is divided into sections corresponding to various areas of a hospital. Each section includes stories about patients being treated in the area, with descriptions of equipment used in their care. There is also an outline of the functions and layout of a typical department, and then a detailed listing of equipment specific to that area. Since many devices are found throughout the hospital, a special section deals with them in detail. A listing is also given of other equipment that might also be found the same area of the hospital.

After the description of each device, there are three short lists: other names by which the device might be known; equipment used with or related to the device; and the locations where the device is most likely to be found.

Whenever a device is listed in **bold (pp)** in the text, a page reference to the description of that device is included.

Photographs of representative devices are included, though there may be considerable variation between different models. These photographs are mostly of devices "in the field", rather than studio photos, to better give the reader a feel for their appearance while in use. All images, unless otherwise noted, are by the author.

Several appendices are included: Appendix A (p. 340) describes the general structure and function of a typical hospital, with an outline of the various departments within the facility. Appendix B (p. 356) discusses surgery and anesthesia in more detail. Appendix C (p. 373) provides some anatomical drawings for reference, while Appendix D (p. 392) gives normal values for various medical measurements and tests. Appendix E (p. 400) includes a discussion of the heart, ECG waveforms and cardiac arrhythmias. Appendix F (p. 404) and Appendix G (p. 406) provide a bibliography and Internet resources, respectively.

I hope that this book will provide you with some interesting and enlightening reading.

Readers, if you have any questions or comments, or suggestions for expanding or improving this book, please contact the author at WDTD@kangalpublishing.biz

Cast of Characters

Various characters are used throughout the book to illustrate the use of a selection of common devices. Their stories are broken up into the sections of the book that describe the equipment being used in their treatment. Patient stories are highlighted in boxes with lightly shaded backgrounds.

Felipe is 25, a pipe fitter and the victim of an industrial accident in which he suffered broken bones and inhalation of toxic fumes. He is treated in Emergency (p.1), Diagnostic Imaging (p.210), Endoscopy (p.130) and Physical Therapy (p.190).

John is 62, an office manager and smoker who has a heart attack at work. He is treated in Emergency (p. 1), Intensive Care (p.16), Cardio-Respiratory (p.164) and the Surgical Department (p.33).

Elizabeth is 45. She is an artist, overweight and a smoker. Elizabeth has gallstones as well as COPD (chronic obstructive pulmonary disease), and she is treated in Diagnostic Imaging (p.210), the Surgical Department (p.33) and Cardio-Respiratory (p.164).

Angie is a 33-year-old teacher who is pregnant with her third child. In the course of her treatment she is in Diagnostic Imaging (p.210) and Maternity/Nursery (p.72).

Cassie, Angie's newborn baby, spends her hospital time in the nursery of the Maternity Department (p.72).

Martin, 80 years old, retired and suffering from vision impairment caused by cataracts. His cataract surgery is performed in the Eye Clinic (p.111).

Jerry is 66 and is retired on a disability pension due to kidney problems. He has kidney stones and kidney failure and is treated in Diagnostic Imaging (p.210), the Renal Unit (p.119) and the Surgical Department (p.33).

Sundeep, 72, is in the early stages of Alzheimer's Disease and also has found a lump in her breast. She will be treated in Diagnostic Imaging (p.210) and the Surgical Department (p.33)

Chapter 1 – Emergency Department

Emergency Room Description

- Function □ER is the first point of contact for many patients entering the hospital, whether they come on their own, accompanied by family or friends, or via ambulance. Patients are triaged as soon as possible upon entry, a triage nurse separating them into groups. Traditionally, triage was a battlefield process that meant division of patients into three groups: those who need immediate medical intervention; those who can wait for treatment; and those who either do not require treatment or are beyond help. Current hospital □triage□usually breaks down into more than three groups, for example: those with severe trauma or catastrophic illness, who may die in a short period of time if not treated; those with significant trauma or disease and require treatment as soon as possible; those who are in need of significant treatment but are currently stable; those who need some form of more minor medical treatment but can wait; and those who do not require any treatment and can be discharged. Paramedics may perform triage on the scene or in the ambulance prior to arrival to the ER and will communicate their observations to ER staff, along with all other pertinent medical information.

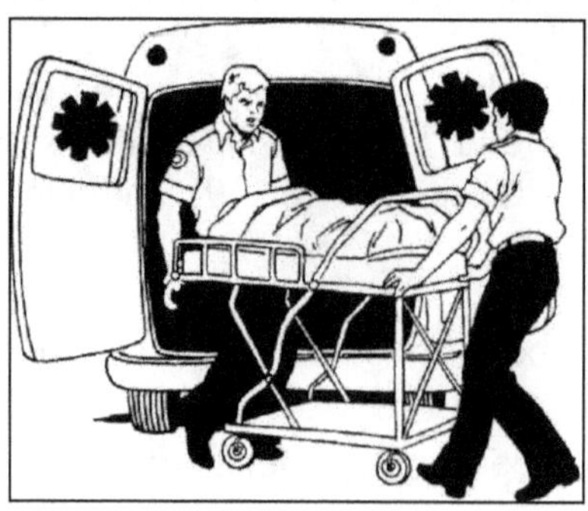

Heart Attack! – John - Emergency

John has just finished climbing the stairs to his office when he feels extreme pressure on his chest, and sharp pain radiating down his left arm. He finds he is very short of breath and is suddenly perspiring and dizzy. He is able to sit on a chair in the outer office and the receptionist asks him if he is all right. He is unable to answer. The receptionist knows the symptoms of heart attacks and calls 911 immediately, then goes to John and helps him lie on the floor, where she covers him with some coats from the coat rack. In minutes, sirens are heard outside and a crew of paramedics arrive. They quickly examine John and ask him a few questions, noting that he is conscious and breathing steadily, though shallowly. They then place an oxygen mask over his mouth and nose and adjust the flow of oxygen. He is loaded onto a stretcher and taken down the elevator and out into the ambulance. Inside the ambulance, John is connected to a portable ***defibrillator-monitor(259)*** *through sticky electrodes placed on each shoulder and on his lower chest. The monitor immediately begins to beep with each heartbeat, and a number shows on the display with the rate, along with a line on the screen showing his ECG activity. One paramedic attaches a small* ***pulse oximeter(320)*** *probe to a finger on one hand and wraps a blood pressure cuff around the upper arm on the other side. Both of these devices are connected to the defibrillator. John feels the* ***non-invasive blood pressure (296)*** *cuff inflating and then deflating, and numbers appear on the screen giving his blood pressure measurements, along with a measure of his blood oxygen level. The other paramedic starts an IV line in John's arm and injects medication into the line along with the regular IV solution. Before the medication can take effect, the ECG display on the defibrillator screen changes pattern and an alarm starts beeping loudly. One paramedic rips open a package of gelled pads and slaps them on John's chest and then grabs the paddles from their holder on the defibrillator.*

Heart Attack! – John continued

The paddles are placed on the pads, the operator presses a button on one paddle and there is a whining noise as the defibrillator charges. When a steady tone sounds indicating the unit is ready, the operator presses buttons on each paddle, producing a clunking sounds and causing John's body to twitch. Paper starts reeling out of the defibrillator's recorder, and the trace on the screen returns to a more normal pattern

When they arrive at the hospital ER, a team meets the ambulance and asks questions as John's stretcher is unloaded and he is moved into the ER and transferred onto a bed. He is quickly disconnected from the defibrillator-monitor and reconnected to a ***bedside monitor (314)*** *with similar ECG electrodes (except a few more of them) and a blood pressure cuff and pulse oximeter sensor. ER staff set about stabilizing John's condition and running his IV line through an* ***IV pump (289).*** *The pump has several channels and, after an examination by one of the ER physicians, a second IV fluid bag is added and run through the pump, joining the first line before it gets to John's arm. After a while, a technologist comes in and takes a 12-lead ECG to add to John 's chart, using a separate set of electrodes.*

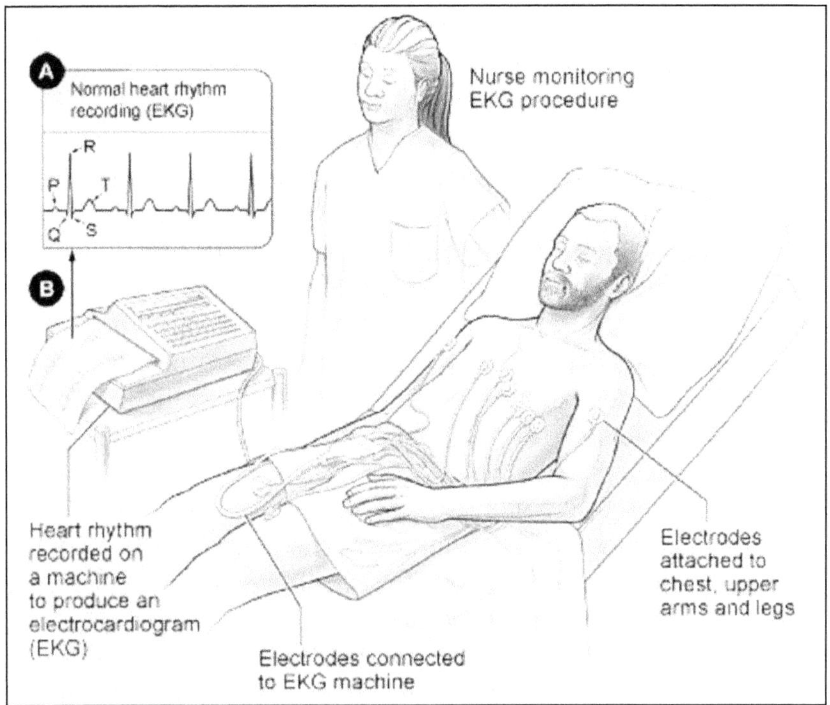

Technologist taking a 12–lead ECG with a patient.
Courtesy of the National Institute of Diabetes and Digestive and Kidney Diseases, National Institutes of Health.

- Layout Emergency Rooms consist of various fairly common areas, as their function is basically universal, differing only in scope. The following areas will be found in almost any ER.
  - Ambulatory entry, where patients come into the ER under their own power or with a friend or family member. This entry is usually near the triage nurse, the admitting clerk, security and the waiting room.
  - Ambulance entry. In a larger ER, there may be multiple ambulance entries. They usually have large, automatic doors and are near the treatment bays that are equipped to handle the most severe cases. There may be an area where multiple gurneys can be stationed along with the paramedic attendants. Paramedics bringing patients to the ER may assist in initial treatments, or there may be a hospital policy preventing them from doing so. The paramedics wait

with the patient until they can be passed over to ER staff, at which time they convey any pertinent information regarding the patient□s history, condition and medications as well as details of any treatment they have administered. Ambulances may be in radio contact with the ER, either directly or through their dispatch office, to allow for as much preparation as possible for the arrival of the patient in the ER.

- Patients not requiring immediate attention as well as anyone accompanying the patient are accommodated in a waiting area. There are usually washroom facilities nearby and vending machines may be provided.
- The triage nurse is stationed near the ambulatory entrance in order to immediately assess patients when they arrive. If possible, the triage nurse will take a brief medical history of the patient.
- Admissions gathers information from the patient or someone accompanying them, regarding their name, their contact information, insurance details if available, family physician name and contact details, and any other information required before the patient can be formally admitted to the hospital. This information is entered into the hospital computer system so that it is available to other areas of the hospital such as the OR, lab or medical wards as required.
- Patients entering Emergency wards may be irrational due to mental illness or substance abuse, or they may be involved in criminal activities that can spill over into the hospital. Security staff is immediately available to help control such situations, and will have special training in dealing with ER cases, including negotiation, physical restraint and communicable disease precautions.
- The ER will have a number of treatment bays, some of which may be specialized for specific types of cases. These may include severe trauma, cardiac arrest, burns, communicable diseases or broken bones. The equipment, supplies, facilities and physical arrangement of the specialized bays have all been optimized for those specific types of cases.

Some but not all treatment bays will have **physiological monitors (314)** to measure and record such parameters as ECG, respiration, blood pressure, **blood oxygen saturation (SpO2) (320)** and temperature. Other less critical bays will have basic equipment for measuring vital signs, and most bays will have equipment for close examination of ears, noses and throats. Some of the bays may be designed for psychiatric patients, and others may have precautions in place for patients with communicable diseases. An area is usually set aside for cast application and removal, though these functions may be performed by a separate cast clinic. Facilities for emergency surgery will be available, again usually in specific bays.

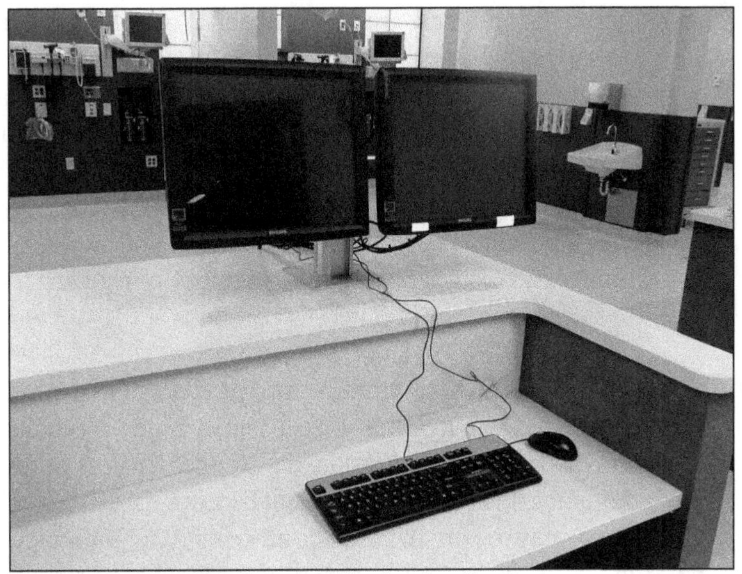

ER Central Monitoring Station.

- The ER nursing station is the core of the department, where staff members can observe the whole area for which they are responsible. Desks are provided for patient charting and examination of records and test results, and computer terminals allow communication in both directions with other areas of the hospital, including the lab for ordering tests and receiving test results. The nursing station may also have special terminals for examining images from the medical imaging department such as **x–rays (241)**, and **CT (214)**, **MRI (229)** or **ultrasound (217)** scans. **Physiological monitors (314)** from each bay so equipped may be connected to a **central station (29)** in the nursing station where specific waveforms and numeric data for each monitored patient can be examined, monitored and recorded. Alarms from the monitors can be checked and adjusted as necessary at the central station as well.

  - Patients will often need to be moved to other parts of the hospital, and it makes the ER function better if these other areas are readily accessible. Medical imaging is often located immediately next to the ER so that patients can have X□ray or other examinations done quickly. The clinical lab is usually nearby as well so that samples can be obtained and delivered easily, and test results made available in a timely manner. Since ER patients often end up being transferred to other areas of the hospital such as the operating rooms or ICU, these areas are usually in relatively close proximity as well.
  - Easily accessible storage areas hold supplies and equipment. These must be checked and replenished as necessary, either as the department consumes them or when their expiry date has passed.

- Staffing □ The primary staff of an ER consists of physicians and nurses. MDs may specialize in emergency medicine, and residents and interns are assigned to the ER on a rotation. Radiologists and various specialist as well as family physicians may be in the ER contributing to patient care at various times. Nurses are also often specialized in emergency medicine, and usually stay assigned to the ER for long periods of time. This is also the case for nursing assistants. Nursing students may rotate through the ER, but usually only for observation. Other staff in the ER may include patient transport personnel; imaging, ECG and laboratory technologists; housekeeping staff; admitting and ward clerks; and other support staff such as biomedical engineering technologists, plant services personnel and Information Systems techs.

- Equipment □ As mentioned above, many of the treatment bays in the ER will have **physiological monitors (314)** mounted in the bay. An ER will likely have one or more **ventilators (334)** available for patients with compromised respiratory functions; **intubation assist units (292)** may be available to help in placing endotracheal tubes for ventilators. **IV pumps (289)** are necessary for medication and fluid delivery, and **defibrillators (259)** must be readily available for treatment of patients with severe cardiac arrhythmias or cardiac arrest. **Fluid warmers (12)** are used to warm IV solutions or blood to near body temperature to help avoid hypothermia in patients who are in critical condition and require relatively large amounts of intravenous fluid administration.

- Supplies □ A wide range of medications, instruments and supplies must be right at hand and well organized, and blood products for transfusion must be accessible at all times. X□ ray equipment may also be stationed within the ER for use as needed. Medical gases including medical air, oxygen and nitrous oxide will be available from outlets in each treatment bay, and wall suction and/or portable suction units will also be easy to access.

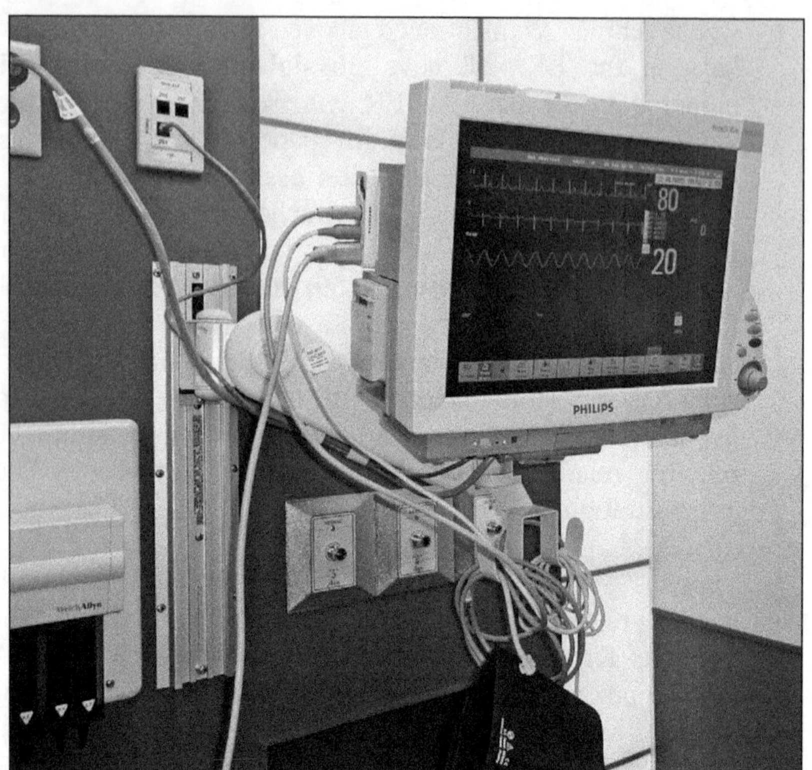

Physiological monitor in an ER treatment bay.

ER Equipment Descriptions

Following are more detailed descriptions of equipment found exclusively or most commonly in this area of the hospital. Equipment that is also found in various other areas of the hospital is described in Chapter 12, p 247.

Devices typically found in Emergency rooms, in addition to the equipment listed in this section, include: **aspirators (250)**, **capnographs (254)**, **ECG machines (270)**, **electronic probe thermometers (279)**, **tympanic thermometers (332)**, **examination lamps (281)**, **gas regulators (285)**, **glucometers (287)**, **intravenous pumps (289)**, **intubation assist devices (292), invasive pressure monitors (294), non–invasive pressure monitors (296), oto/laryngo/ophthalmoscopes (301), physiological monitors (314), point of care blood analysis systems (318), pulse oximeters (320), sphygmomanometers (325), stethoscopes (327), ventilators (334), defibrillators (259), cardiac pacemakers (25), oxygen analyzers (305), cast cutters (256), slit lamps (322)**, and **C–arm units (212)**.

Fluid Warmers

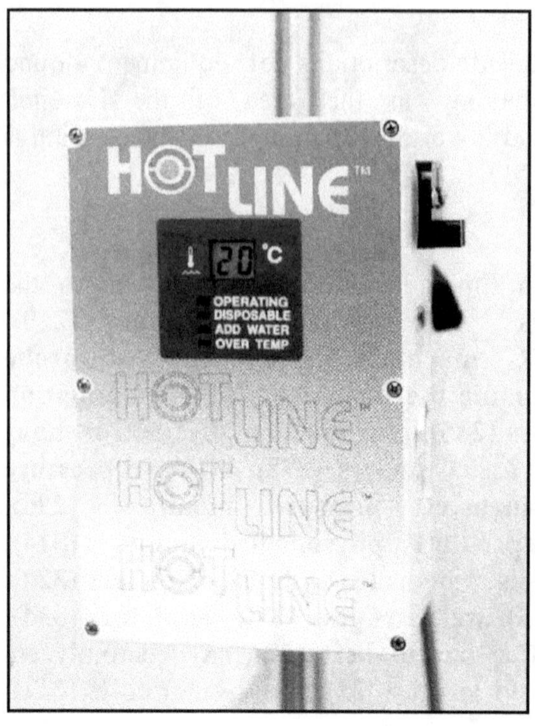

Overview □ Blood must be kept refrigerated to prolong its storage life, but infusing it into a patient at this temperature can cause a serious drop in body temperature, especially if the patient is small and/or hypothermic, or if a large amount of blood is required in a short time.

Function □ A blood warmer is a device that allows blood to be heated to near body temperature before it is infused. This requires careful control, however, as overheating blood can damage it. Blood warming units use either a water bath or metal plate heaters to warm the blood. Since the temperature must be increased substantially in a short time, there must be a large surface area for sufficient heat exchange to take place. In metal plate heaters, the blood passes through a plastic pouch that has a long, back□and□forth passage through it, so the blood has a long distance in which to be warmed. Water bath units have the advantage of quicker heat exchange, often using a double□walled tube, with blood flowing toward the patient in the inside tube and warm water being pumped in the opposite direction in the outer jacket. The opposing flow means that the blood is close to the water temperature when it exits the double□walled section; the total length of tubing within the warmer is much less in this type, which means less wasted blood.

In both types of warmers, the exit of the warmer must be as close to the patient as possible so that it doesn□t cool off too much before reaching the patient. With its somewhat moveable section of double□ walled tube, the water jacket warmer allows for a shorter unheated section of tubing before it reaches the patient.

Both types also usually have a temperature display, as well as a double over□temperature cut□out and alarm system, since overheating the blood can be harmful both to the blood and to the patient.

The section of tubing in the warmer is discarded after use.

These devices may be used together with an IV pump, which would be placed upstream of the warmer so that heat isn□t lost in the pump and associated tubing.

<u>Application</u> □ An intravenous line is established, and the fluid to be delivered is connected to the fluid warmer apparatus. Fluid delivery is begun, and the liquid is warmed as it passes through the device. The short length of tubing between the machine and the patient ensures minimal temperature drop.

<u>AKA</u> □Fluid warmers.

<u>Related devices</u> □**IV pumps (289)**, **hyper/hypothermia units (14)**.

<u>Where found</u> □ emergency rooms, operating rooms, some special care units.

<u>Hyper/Hypothermia Units</u>

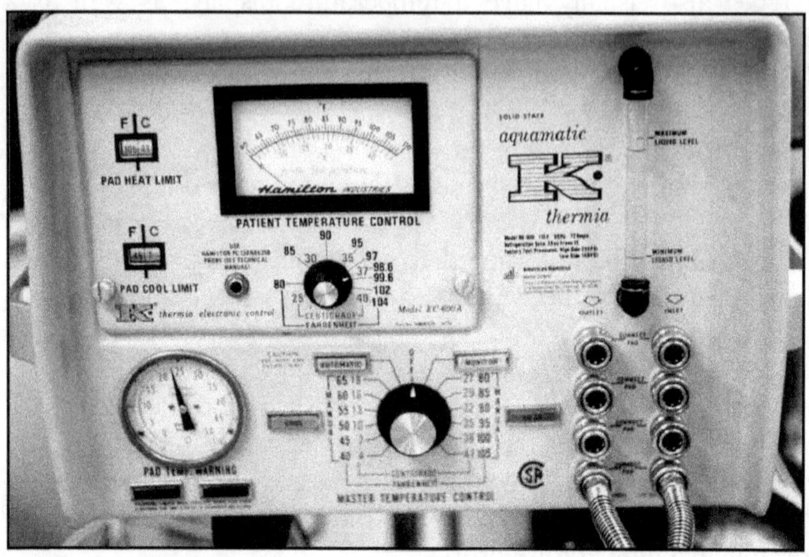

<u>Overview</u> — When a patient's body temperature is significantly higher (hyperthermia) or lower (hypothermia) than normal, it must be returned to the normal range as quickly as possible.

<u>Function</u> — Water immersion provides the fastest heat exchange, either up or down, but this is not always possible or practical. A plastic pad or jacket provides a more flexible and accessible means of delivering heat to or removing heat from the patient.

Some devices perform only one function, either heating or cooling, though some have both functions built into one unit. Warmers, especially air types, are typically much smaller and lighter than cooling units, which require compressors and refrigeration coils. Air has the advantage of quicker heating or cooling, as compared to water, but it also doesn't carry as much heat to or from the patient as water does, though it can flow more rapidly, partially overcoming this disadvantage.

These units normally have a temperature setting control, as well as over and/or under temperature alarms and cut-offs. They may also have a means of displaying patient temperature. The sensor for this must be placed away from the heat exchange pad in order to give an accurate indication of body temperature.

Application □ The heating/cooling pad is placed in direct contact with the patient□s skin, covering as much surface area as possible. Temperature□controlled water or air is then passed rapidly through the pad to warm or cool the patient. Patient temperature and condition must be monitored closely while the unit is being used.

AKA □patient heaters/coolers.

Related devices □**Fluid warmers (12)**.

Where found □ emergency rooms, operating rooms, some special care units.

Chapter 2 – Intensive Care Units

Intensive Care Unit Description

- Function □Intensive care units provide direct critical care to patients. Staffing is usually more than one to one, that is there are more staff members providing care than there are patients. Patients may be admitted to ICU from Emergency after they have been basically stabilized, from the OR following major surgery with the possibility of significant complications, or from general medical or surgical wards when a patient□s condition becomes critical.

- Layout □An ICU consists of a number of patient rooms, each with it□s own **physiological monitor (314)** and special lighting and gas supplies. There is enough room around the bed for several team members should they be required for treatment procedures. Some rooms may have isolation features such as negative air pressure to keep pathogens from escaping from the room and individual hand cleaning stations and mask, gown and glove supplies. A nursing station provides an area for a **central monitoring station (29)**, charting facilities, and areas for staff consultation, plus hospital computer system terminals and diagnostic imaging viewing stations. A large ICU may be divided into two or more sections, each with its own central station. An equipment and supplies storage room will be readily accessible, and since family and friends of the patient are often very worried and want to be nearby as much as possible, most ICUs have their own visitor waiting area.

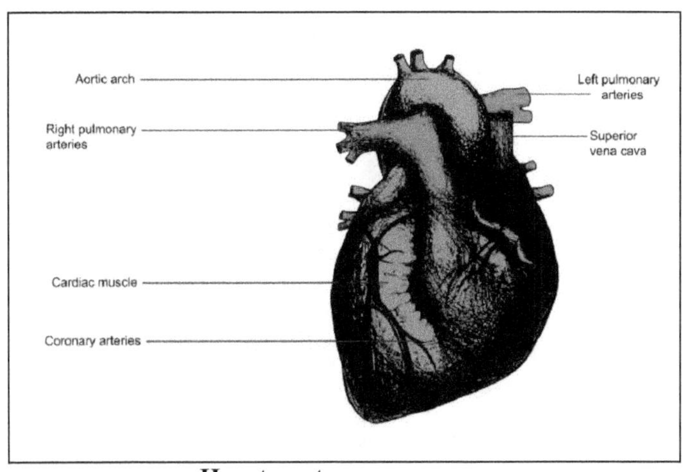

Heart anatomy.
Modified from Shutterstock, Inc, www.shutterstock.com, with permission.

- Staff The primary staffing in any ICU consists of nurses and physicians. Nurses are usually specialized in ICU work, and physicians are generally specialists in an area related to the focus of the particular ICU, though GPs may come to the unit to check on their patients and consult with other staff. Residents will rotate through ICU, but interns and other students will likely only be present for short observation periods. Secondary staffing in an ICU may consist of: imaging technologists, since patients are often too critical to be able to be moved to the imaging department; respiratory technologists, to assist with the application and ongoing support of **ventilators (334)**; dieticians to help assess and meet the special nutritional needs of ICU patients; infection control specialists, since many ICU patients have communicable diseases and otherwise are especially susceptible to infections; biomedical engineering technologists, to troubleshoot any problems with all the high tech equipment in the ICU, and to support the application and most effective use of the equipment; and housekeeping personnel to ensure that the area is kept clean.

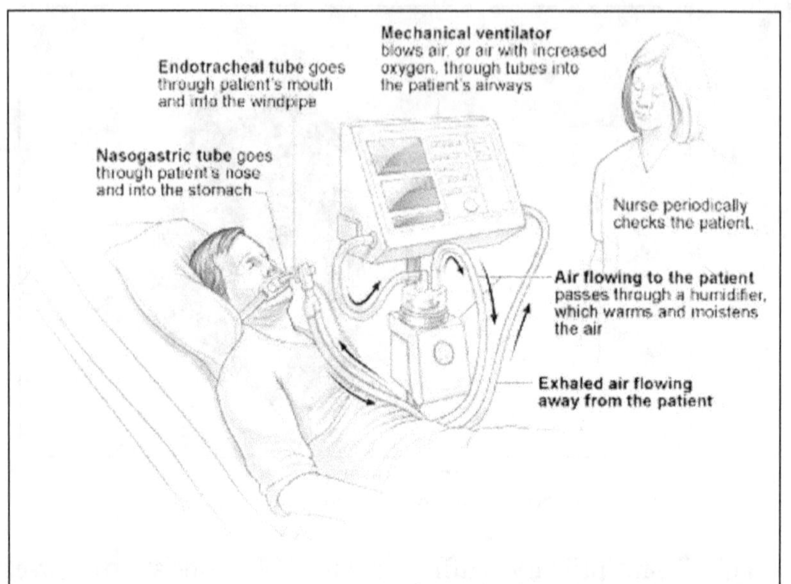

Ventilator set–up, with an endotracheal tube rather than a tracheostomy tube.

Courtesy of the National Institute of Diabetes and Digestive and Kidney Diseases, National Institutes of Health.

Heart Attack! – John – ICU I

John is now relatively stable and comfortable, and is transferred from the ER to the CICU (Cardiac Intensive Care Unit). A module from his monitor in the ER had been switched over to a portable monitor for the move, and now that he is on a bed in the CICU the module is again transferred to the bedside monitor there. This allows all the ECG, blood pressure and pulse oximeter information stored since John came into the ER to be retained for later examination. The ***CICU monitor (314)*** *is also analyzing his ECG waveforms and picking out arrhythmias, sounding an alarm for more serious ones and simply recording other less serious ones that will help in diagnosing his condition. This CICU system allows staff to view information from any other bedside monitor on the monitor they are working with, to help them evaluate potential problems that may or may not require them to go to the other patient.*

<u>Heart Attack! – John continued</u>

From his bed, John can see the nursing station in the middle of the CICU. Several display monitors are on a desk, along with a keyboard and mouse, a dual strip chart recorder and a large laser printer. Together, these components make up the ***central station (29)****. This system collects data from all the* ***bedside monitors (314)*** *in the CICU and displays selected waveforms and numeric information in boxes on the video screens; the boxes give bed numbers and the name of the patient in that bed. Staff can select different information for each patient, and they can zoom in on one particular patient to see a wider range of information. The system stores all patient monitoring data for review and analysis, and can print off letter-sized sheets with selected information, including waveforms, graphs of trends of data such as ECG rates or blood pressure, and system diagnostics. Alarm levels for a variety of parameters including heart rate, respiration, blood oxygen content, blood pressure and certain abnormalities of ECG rhythms (arrhythmias) can all be set for each patient being monitored. The strip chart recorder automatically prints out a long recording of waveforms from bedside monitors if they have detected certain alarms situations. The system has stored older information and a few seconds of this information is also printed out to give staff some idea of what led up to the alarm condition. The strip recording includes date and time, as it may be considered a legal document, and also numeric values for certain relevant parameters such as blood pressure and blood oxygen content.*

Equipment □ICUs have very high concentrations of medical electronics equipment. Each bedside will have a **physiological monitor (314)** that is capable of measuring, displaying and recording such parameters as ECG, respiration, temperature, blood oxygen saturation (SpO2), blood pressure either non□invasively using an automatic arm cuff system or invasively via a catheter inserted into various points in the patient□s circulatory system, exhaled CO2 levels, cardiac output, level of consciousness, and perhaps blood chemistry using a **point–of–care analyzer (318)** built into or interfaced with the main monitor. Information gathered by the monitor is displayed on its video screen in either graphical or numeric format, or both.

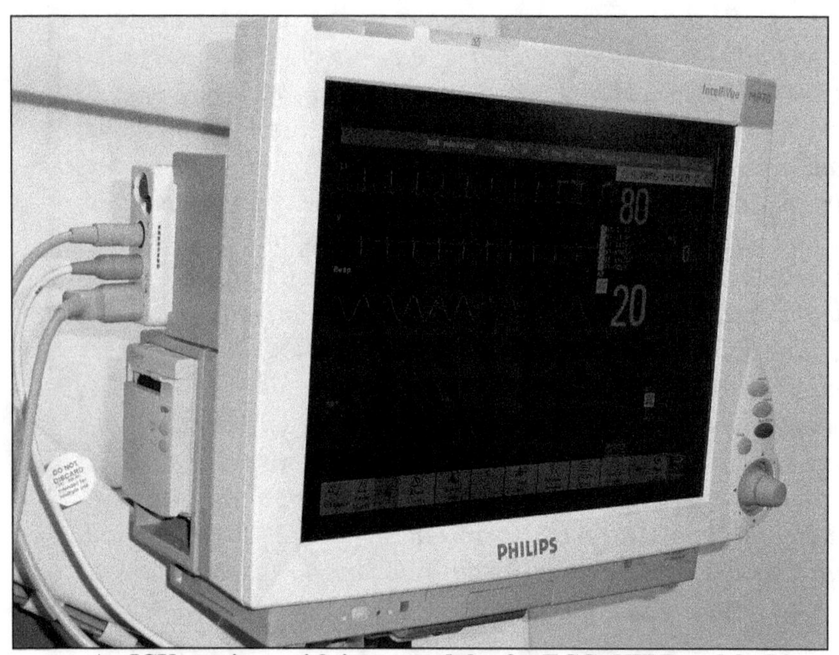

An ICU monitor, with input modules for ECG, NIBP and SpO2 on the upper left side and a strip chart recorder on the lower left.

The bedside monitors will be connected to a **central station (29)** where nurses can watch the waveforms and data from each patient, set and respond to various alarms from the bedside monitors, and record pertinent waveforms or data to form part of the patient chart. Some systems allow information from a second bedside monitor to be displayed on one bedside monitor if a staff member needs to check on the other patient without leaving the side of the first. Systems may also be connected to the hospital computer system and to the Internet, allowing remote viewing of patient monitoring data. ICUs will also have, **defibrillators (259)**, **ventilators (334)**, **intravenous pumps (289)** and **PCA (patient controlled analgesia) pumps (311)** and a variety of other minor equipment. **Portable x–ray (212)** and **ultrasound (217)** machines may be dedicated to the unit. If the particular ICU has patients that need to be monitored but who are able to walk some, they may have a **telemetry system (31)** providing ECG and perhaps SpO2 (blood oxygen level) and non□invasive blood pressure measurements remotely via radio signals from a transmitter pack worn by the patient. Computers form a vital link to the ICU, for sending and receiving lab data, pharmacy orders, service requests, patient charts and admission information, and routine hospital communications.

Heart Attack! – John – ICU II

Despite his optimal medical treatment, John's heart continues to beat erratically, which causes weakness and pain and could lead to another cardiac arrest. Staff connect an ***external cardiac pacemaker (25)*** *to John's chest, and the electrical pulses from this device pass through his chest wall and into his heart, helping to normalize his heartbeat. The pacemaker has several controls on its face, which allow staff to adjust the rate, and strength of the pulses it delivers to John, to match his needs. When John's personal physician gets in to see him, he tells John that he has consulted with a cardiologist and he recommends further tests but thinks that John will need bypass surgery as well as an* ***implantable cardiac pacemaker (25)*** *to ensure his best chance for a return to health.*

When John is relatively stable and feeling better, both he and his doctor want him to be able to move around some, Staff disconnect him from the bedside monitor and connect a ***telemetry transmitter (31)*** *(or telepack) to some of the same ECG electrodes used previously. A pulse oximeter probe is taped to John's finger and is also connected to the telemetry transmitter. The transmitter detects, amplifies and processes the various signals coming from John and transmits them via radio to a receiver in the CICU, which then sends the signals to the central station, where they are handled in much the same way as signals from the* ***bedside monitors (314)****.*

- Special types □ Smaller hospitals often have a just a single ICU that deals with critical patients up to the level of acuity that staff and facilities can handle. Larger hospital will likely have several ICUs specializing in specific types of patients. These specialty ICUs often have their own acronyms and might include cardiac (CICU), cardiac step□down (CSICU), telemetry (TelICU), medical (MICU), neonatal (NICU), paediatric (PICU), burn (BICU), neurological including spinal cord injury (NeuroICU or SICU), psychiatric (PICU), geriatric (GICU), and respiratory (RICU).

ICU Equipment Descriptions

Following are more detailed descriptions of equipment found exclusively or most commonly in this area of the hospital. Equipment that is also found in various other areas of the hospital is described in Chapter 12, p 247.

Devices typically found in these areas, in addition to the equipment listed in this section, include: **aspirators (250)**, **bladder scanners (252), capnographs (254)**, **cardiac output systems (171)**, **ECG machines (270)**, **electric hospital beds (277)**, **electronic probe thermometers (279)**, **tympanic thermometers (332)**, **examination lamps (281)**, **gas regulators (285)**, **glucometers (287)**, **intravenous pumps (289)**, **intubation assist devices (292)**, **invasive pressure monitors (294)**, **non–invasive pressure monitors (296)**, **oto/laryngo/ophthalmoscopes (301)**, **PCA pumps (311)**, **physiological monitors (314)**, **point of care blood analysis systems (318)**, **sphygmomanometers (325)**, **stethoscopes (327)**, **syringe pumps (329)**, **ventilators (334)**, **defibrillators (259)**, **oxygen analyzers (305)**, and **C–arm x–ray units (212)**.

Cardiac Pacemakers

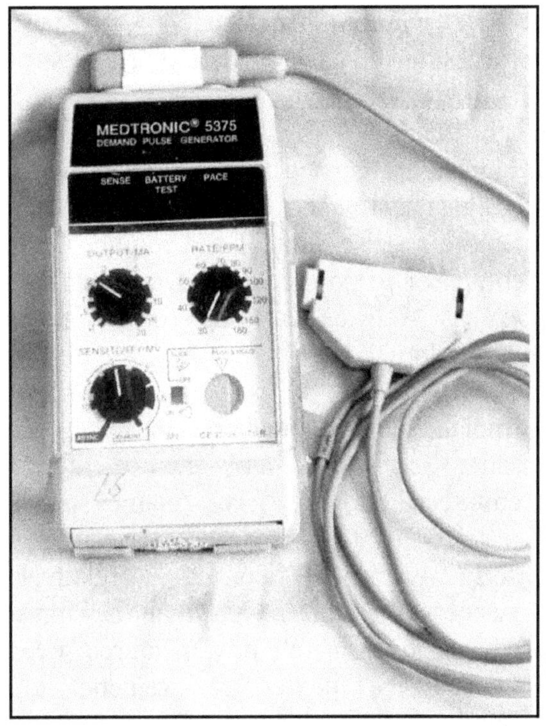

Overview — Cardiac rhythm is normally controlled by a system within the heart, moderated by various parameters such as oxygen demand and levels of hormones such as adrenalin. The natural pacemaker system sends signals to the heart muscle in a pattern that produces coordinated contractions of the various parts of the heart, of a strength and rate appropriate to body state.

Various disease processes can disrupt this natural pacemaker to such a degree that heart contractions are no longer strong enough for the needs of the patient.

Function — In these circumstances, an artificial pacemaker is used to provide proper pacing signals. Pacemakers may be temporary or permanent, and may be external or implanted. External pacemakers can be further divided into invasive and non-invasive types.

External pacemakers are typically used for short-term applications, either until the patient's natural pacemaker can resume normal function or until an implantable pacemaker can be installed, with non-invasive types being used for shorter times than invasive.

Non-invasive external pacemakers use electrodes placed in specific places on the patient's chest to pass electrical signals into the heart. These signals stimulate the heart to beat more effectively, and are usually coordinated with whatever natural cardiac signals are present. They can be adjusted for rate and amplitude, and may either completely control cardiac contractions or act as a □booster□, filling in for missing beats as required. The control signals have to be quite large for enough of the signal to reach the heart, and the signal passes through areas of the body where it isn□t needed. Long□term use of electrodes on the patient□s skin can cause irritation or burns.

Invasive external pacemakers function in a similar way to non□invasive types, except their signals are carried to the heart by wires inserted into the patient□s body and attached directly to the heart. They have the advantage of more precise control and require much less power to effect pacing compared to non□invasive types, but they take much longer to apply, as well as carrying the problems associated with any invasive procedure.

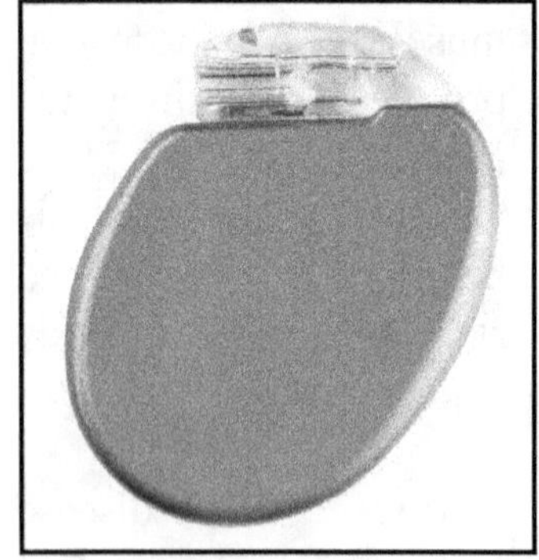

Implantable pacemakers perform the same function as their external counterparts, but have many special restrictions. They are inside the patient□s body and therefore relatively inaccessible. This means that they must have a long□lasting power source; even though the power requirements are small, they may be needed for years. Special battery technology has been developed, and nuclear power sources have been used. The units must have some means of being controlled without physical contact. In earlier devices, and many current ones, rate and signal strength could be adjusted using a powerful magnet placed near the implant site.

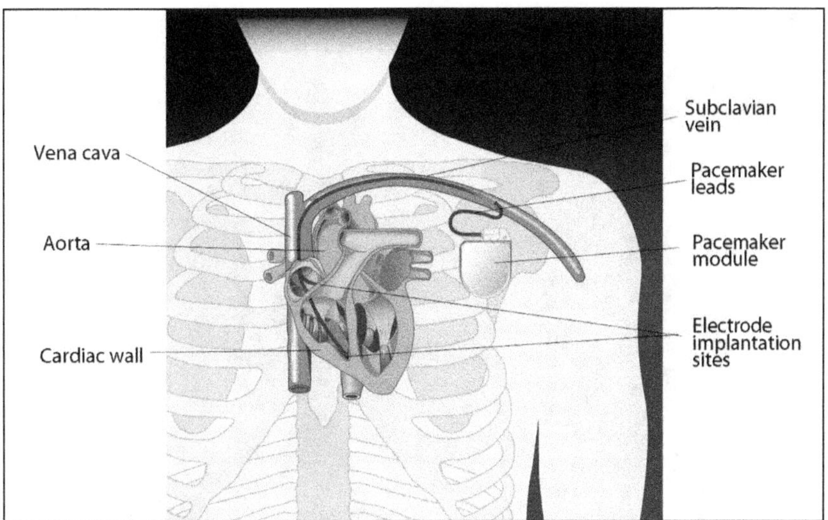

Implanted pacemaker schematic.
(Modified from Shutterstock, Inc, www.shutterstock.com, with permission)

Implantable pacemakers are placed in a □pocket□ formed on the upper left chest of the patient, and the electrode wires are threaded under the skin and into the subclavian vein. They are then guided into the heart using **ultrasound (217)** or **x–rays (212)** and the tips are embedded into heart muscle, where they can provide electrical pulses for pacing.

Newer units may have mechanisms to measure body needs and adjust themselves automatically according to these needs. Implanting a foreign object within the body has its own set of considerations apart from the pacemaking functions, and these factors are an important part of the design criteria as well.

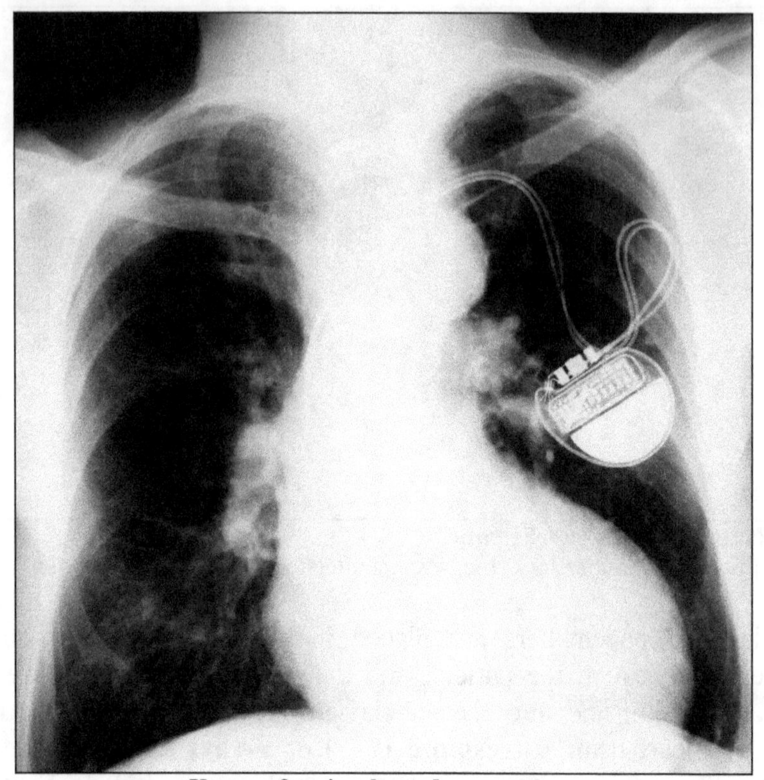

X–ray of an implanted pacemaker.
Modified from Inmagine Corp, www.123rf.com, with permission.

<u>Application</u> Contact is made with the patients heart, either though external or implanted electrodes. Pacing parameters are set by the operator and the unit is started, which thereafter controls the patients cardiac rhythm.

<u>AKA</u> pacers.

<u>Related devices</u> **physiological monitors (314)**, **ECG machines (270)**, **implantable defibrillators (259)**.

<u>Where found</u> cardiac intensive care units, operating rooms, emergency rooms.

Central Stations

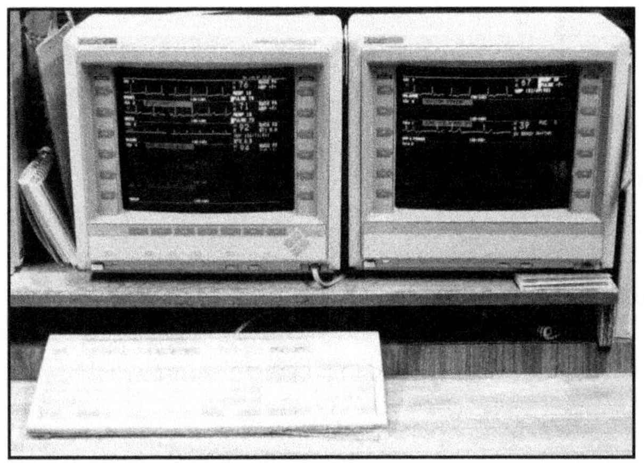

Overview □ In any critical care area, medical staff needs to be able to monitor each patient, but not necessarily from the bedside at all times.

Function □ Physiological monitors and telemetry units are associated with each patient, and send data to a central location where important signals can be displayed. Most central stations display detailed information about a particular patient as necessary, while normally displaying one waveform and numeric values (usually ECG) for all patients simultaneously.

Patient information can be entered (usually with a standard computer□type keyboard) via the central station at admission, and removed on discharge. Staff may be able to adjust alarm levels from the central station, but usually cannot cancel alarms without going to the bedside.

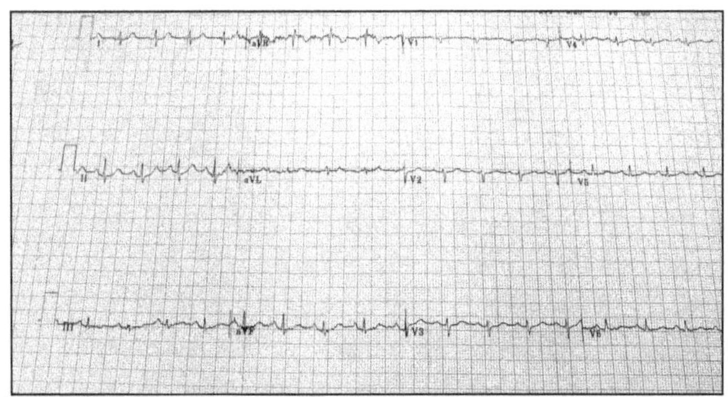

Central station large–format recording of ECG waveforms.

Recordings of information from the various bedsides can usually be made at the central station, either on a strip□chart recorder or on a larger□format recorder or printer (usually used for tables and graphs or more comprehensive reports). Central monitors can be integrated into or connected to patient data recording and analysis systems.

Central monitoring also can give the capability of displaying information from one beside monitor while working at another.

Application Central stations are used as part of a physiological monitoring system.

AKA central monitors, centrals, nursing centrals.

Related devices **physiological monitors (314)**, **telemetry systems (31)**.

Where found intensive and/or critical care areas.

Telemetry Systems

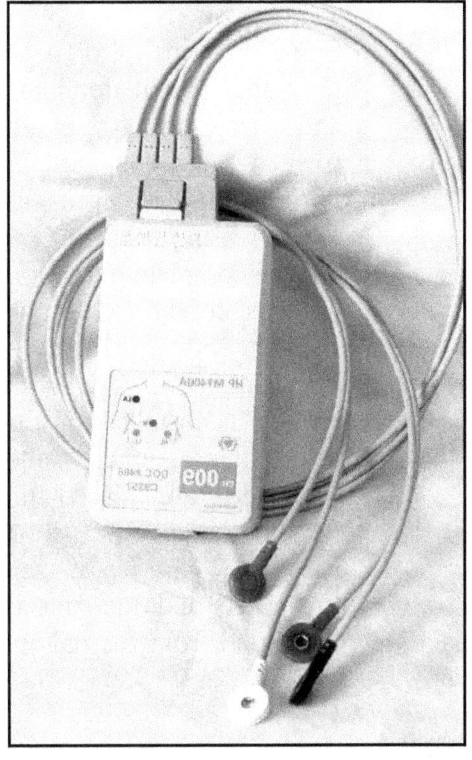

Overview — Cardiac patients are often able to get out of bed and walk around; this may be part of their recovery process, or it may simply be a convenience. In either case, it is important for medical staff to be able to continue monitoring the patient's ECG signals.

Function — Telemetry systems allow patients to be mobile without unwieldy and possibly dangerous long cables.

ECG signals are picked up from the patient's skin by electrodes and wires, just as with regular ECG monitoring. The signals are then amplified and processed, again by similar circuitry as that in a bedside monitor. Within the small module carried by the patient, however, is a radio transmitter that broadcasts signals carrying the ECG information. These signals are picked up by an antenna system and processed to extract the original ECG waveform, which can then be displayed on a central monitor. This monitor can usually display signals from several patients simultaneously, and may be stand-alone or part of central monitoring system that handles information from bedside monitors as well. Recording, trending, patient admission information, and alarms are all handled by the central monitor.

Older telemetries broadcast the ECG information as an analog signal, much like an AM or FM radio station. Newer systems turn the analog signal into a stream of digital information before broadcasting it, which gives better resistance to interference and allows either lower transmitter power (thus prolonging battery life) or else greater range.

Most telemetry transmitters have a nurse call button that the patient can use to signal for assistance or to mark any unusual feelings or symptoms they might have associated with their condition.

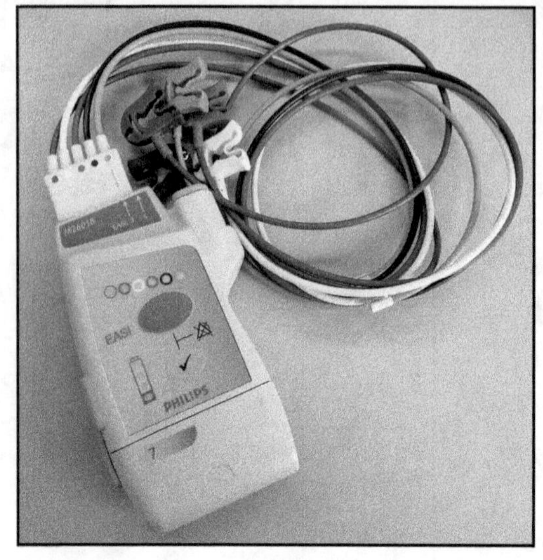

Some systems also have the capability of obtaining and transmitting blood oxygen saturation (SpO2) information as well as ECG, which can help give a more complete picture of patients□condition.

Application □ A fresh battery is installed in the transmitter unit, and electrodes are placed on the patient□s skin. Electrode wires are then attached to the electrodes and to the transmitter, and the unit is placed in a carrying pouch. Signals are transmitted from the patient to the receiver.

AKA □telem, remote monitoring, tele or telly.

Related devices □**physiological monitors (314)**, **central monitors (29)**, **pulse oximeters (320)**.

Where found □cardiac care units, cardiac rehabilitation wards.

Chapter 3 – Surgical Department

Operating Room Description

- Function □Operating rooms are the venues for scheduled and emergency surgical procedures of all kinds. Some larger hospitals may have more than one operating room area, for different areas of specialty within the hospital.

- Layout, overall □The surgical suite of a hospital consists of a number of individual operating rooms, often arranged in a more□or□less circular pattern, with a wide hallway surrounding the rooms. Each room will have many characteristics and components in common but often at least some rooms are specially outfitted for specific types of surgery such as urology, endoscopic procedures, trauma surgery, cardiac surgery, organ transplantation surgery or neurosurgery. A holding area at the entrance to the ORs provides space for patients when the individual room is not quite ready for them, and to allow surgeons, anesthesiologists or other OR staff to speak with the patient before surgery if necessary. This area may also serve as a waiting room for family. The OR office coordinates use of the rooms and performs room and staff scheduling, provides reminder calls for patients, and ensures that OR supplies and equipment are always ready. A sterile supply area is often in the centre of the various operating rooms, to allow easy access to and from each room. A post□anesthesia recovery area will be adjacent to the OR suite, and basic lab and diagnostic imaging facilities will often be included in the area to allow for rapid testing and imaging. Biomedical engineering may have an area in or near the OR suite to provide quick response should there be problems with equipment.

- Layout, individual general OR □ Operating rooms usually have two access doors, a large double door opening to the outside hallway for entry and exit of patient stretchers and a smaller door. Rooms must be spacious enough to allow easy access to all sides of the operating table, to permit potentially five or more staff members to circulate within the room as required, and to allow for all the various devices and supplies that will be used in the course of surgery.

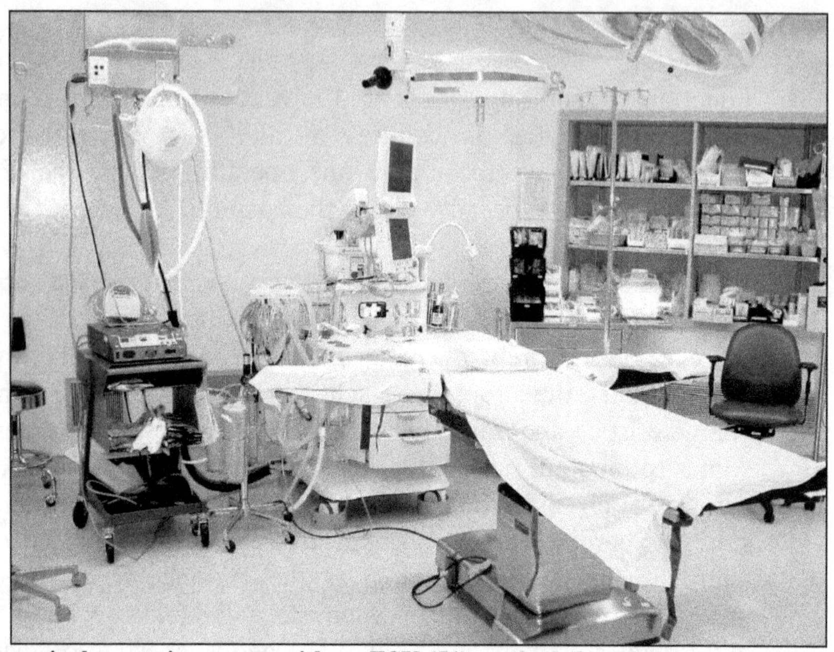

A typical operating room, with an ESU (51) on the left and an anesthetic machine (47) in the center behind the OR table (66).

Equipment may be mounted on wheeled carts that can be moved near the table as required, but it is becoming more and more common for ORs to have special booms suspended from the ceiling, from which most of the critical equipment can be mounted on various arms and platforms. These booms also contain gas supplies, electrical outlets, computer network connections, video interfaces and more. **Anesthetic machines (47)** are usually too heavy and bulky to be mounted on the booms and so are usually freestanding. Diagnostic imaging viewing equipment, either light boxes or high resolution video monitors, are usually stationed on one wall of the room, and a hospital computer terminal may be present, again usually against a wall, out of the way of the main surgical field.

Arriving at the hospital on the day of surgery, Elizabeth fills out a lot of forms and has a quick meeting with the Anesthesiologist for her case, who discusses the procedure (he calls it a laparoscopic cholecystectomy, sometimes abbreviated lap-chole) and asks if she has any questions. He starts an IV line in her arm running through an ***IV pump (289)****, and administers a sedative through the IV line. She is then wheeled into the operating room and transferred onto an* ***operating table (66)****.*

She looks around while the OR staff bustles around in preparation for the surgery, noticing the huge overheard ***surgical lights (64)****, a smaller cart with an* ***electrosurgery machine (51)*** *(or ESU) on it and two larger carts, one holding a variety of* ***laparoscopic equipment (134)*** *with a large video screen on top. The other large cart is the* ***anesthetic machine (47)*** *and has two smaller video screens, various controls and appendages, and a lot of tubing.*

Another drug is injected into the IV line and she soon slips into unconsciousness. If she remained awake (something no one wants), she would see that the Anesthesiologist placed an endotracheal tube into her mouth, guiding it into her trachea with a tiny video ***intubation guidance unit (292)****. Once in place, the endotracheal tube is connected to the breathing circuit of the anesthetic machine. The Doctor adjusts the controls and the machine starts giving a mixture of air, oxygen and an anesthetic gas.*

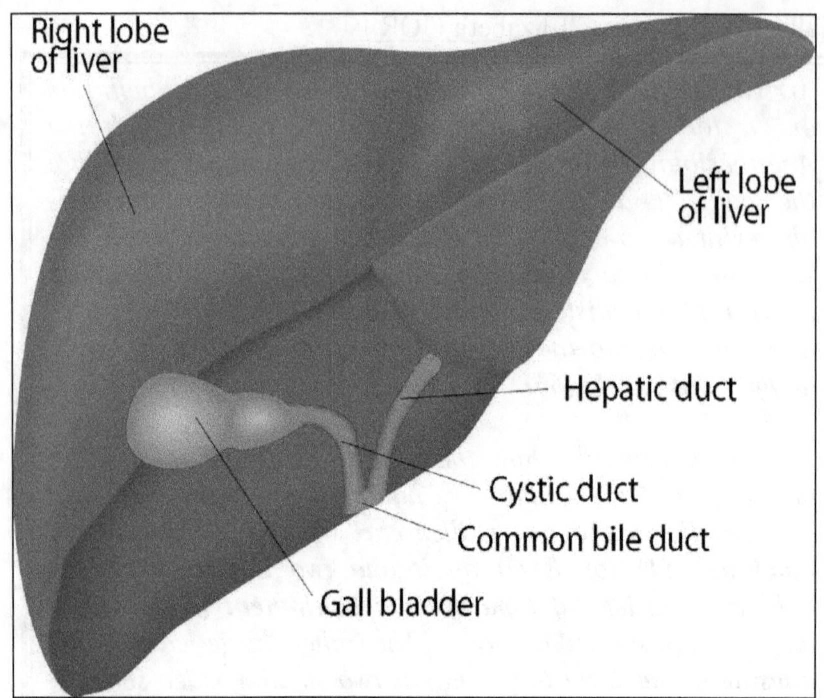

Liver anatomy. The cystic and hepatic ducts combine to form the common bile duct, which drains into the small intestine just below the stomach. Bile is stored temporarily in the gall bladder.

Modified from Shutterstock, Inc, www.shutterstock.com, with permission.

Equipment Operating rooms have the widest variety of equipment and supplies of any area of the hospital.

- The **anesthetic machine (47)** is the central device, providing delivery and monitoring of anesthetic gases and precisely controlled mechanical ventilation of the patient.

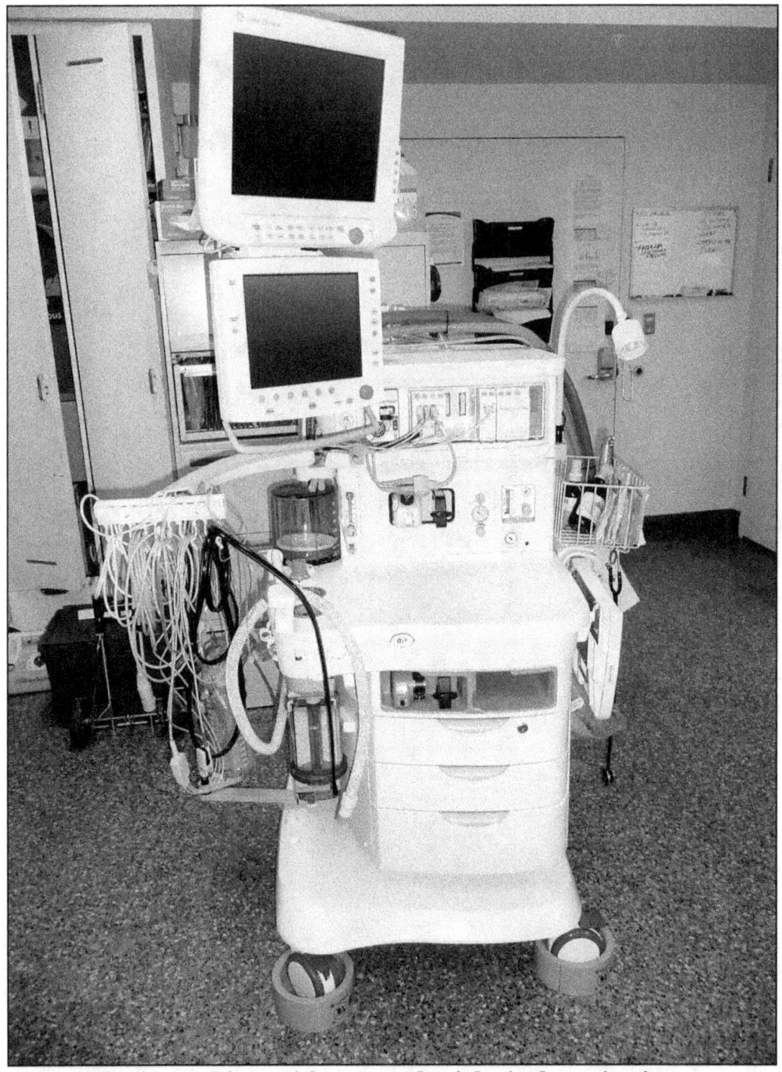

An anesthetic machine, with upper physiological monitoring screen and lower device parameter and gas analysis screen.

- **Physiological monitors (314)** that measure and display a wide variety of vital signs from the patient may be standalone or integrated into the anesthetic machine.
- Much of the actual process of cutting is performed using **electrosurgery machines (51)**, which also provide cauterization and fulguration.

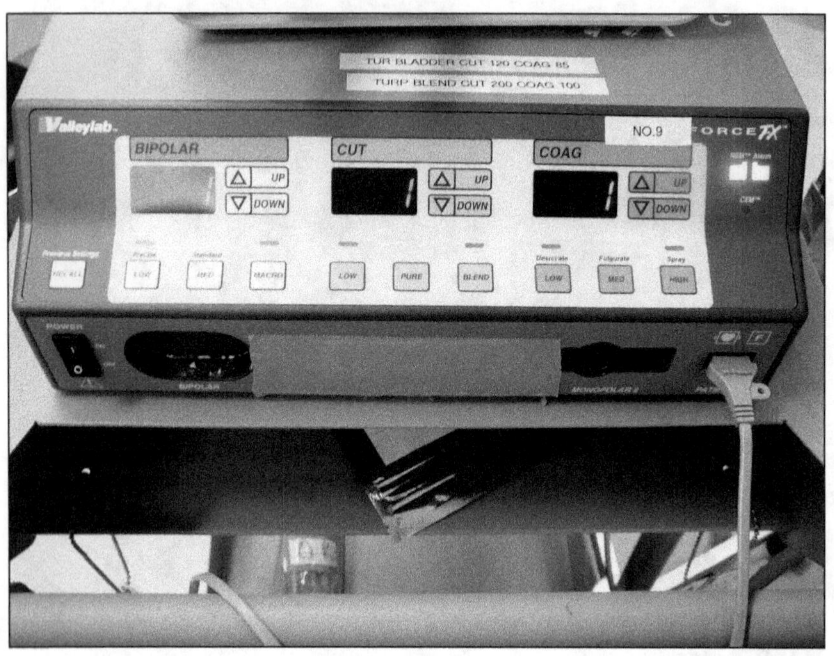

An ESU, showing the different mode controls: Bipolar, Cut and Coag.

Heart Attack! – John – OR I

When John's surgery date arrives, he is prepared in much the same way as Elizabeth *(see p 35)* *and he is connected to an* ***anesthetic machine (47)*** *in the same manner. His surgery is much more extensive, however, with his chest being opened to give access to his heart and a long incision being made in his leg where the vein used in the bypass will be removed. While the surgeon works on connecting the vein to go around the blockages in John's cardiac arteries, his heart must be stopped. This means that a* ***heart-lung machine (57)*** *is used to pump blood through his body and to remove carbon dioxide and add oxygen to the blood. This large machine consists of a special pump that gently but powerfully moves blood without damaging blood cells, and a system of membranes that allow carbon dioxide to pass out of the blood for removal, and the addition of oxygen. The device is operated and closely monitored by a specially trained perfusionist during the surgery.*

John has recovered from his bypass surgery, but there is still an issue of his irregular heart rhythms. He is scheduled for an ***implanted pacemaker (25)*** *to keep his ticker ticking properly. During this procedure, a pocket is created under the skin of his upper chest, and electrode wires are threaded into a vein in his arm and to his heart, where they are guided to the exact location using x-rays. Once at the correct locations they are embedded in the heart muscle, the wires are passed under the skin to the pacemaker itself, and the incisions are closed. The pacemaker has special lithium battery that will provide power for many years, after which the whole pacemaker will be replaced. The functions of the pacemaker can be adjusted using a* ***pacemaker programmer (25)*** *that sends signals magnetically through the skin to control such things as voltage, rate and sensitivity.*

- **Surgical lasers (70)** are used in a somewhat similar manner to electrosurgery machines.

- As both of these types of devices can produce potentially harmful smoke particles in the course of their use, special **smoke evacuator units (51)** are used in conjunction with them.
- The **OR table (66)** gives a solid platform for procedures, and can be moved up, down and sideways as well as being able to tilt lengthwise (pitch) and laterally (roll.) OR tables are controlled by foot pedals.
- Surgical robots are used for some operations, especially delicate procedures on very small structures. Systems can allow the surgeon to control movements of the robotic manipulators on a much smaller scale that they would be able to perform manually. Manipulators can be much smaller than human hands, which means that they can enter areas of the body with much smaller incisions that would be otherwise necessary. Surgical robots used in conjunction with video systems and remote access computers have the potential of allowing surgery to be performed on a patient that is in a location far away from the human surgeon.
- Anesthesiologists use **nerve/muscle stimulators (63)** to aid in evaluating the level of consciousness of the patient.
- **Automatic tourniquets (330)** are used in surgical procedures on limbs, in order to reduce blood flow to the area.
- Endoscopy stacks consist of **light sources (142)**, **insufflators (148)**, **video cameras (144)** and **recorders (146)**, possibly driver units for drills and other power accessories, and one or more video displays. They may be mounted in a standalone cart, or on the OR boom.

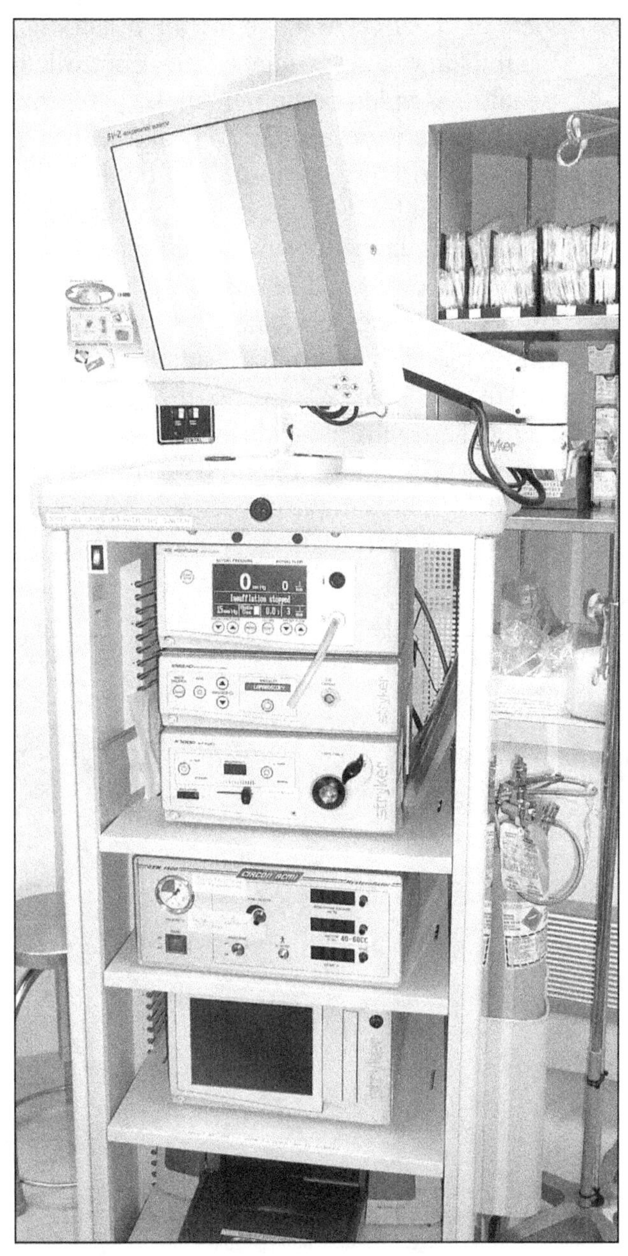

Endoscopy cart with (from top) video display, insufflator, camera console, light source, a specialized insufflator for gynecological surgery and a video storage unit.

- An **operating microscope (68)** is used for microsurgery, including such procedures as cataract removal and lens replacement. These microscopes are quite large and contain their own light source. The viewing head can move in all directions. This plus magnification and focus are controlled by foot□ pedals. A video system may be integrated into the microscope in order to display and record images.

- A variety of surgical tools will be available, including various scalpels, hemostats, forceps, suturing and stapling equipment, saws, drills, hammers, wrenches and screwdrivers. The range of tools varies with the procedure being performed.
- Gas supplies are on the wall of the room or more commonly on the OR boom, and include oxygen, medical air, nitrous oxide and vacuum.
- Certain hardware required may be required for surgery, for example the components of an artificial hip or knee, screws, nails, pins and plates.

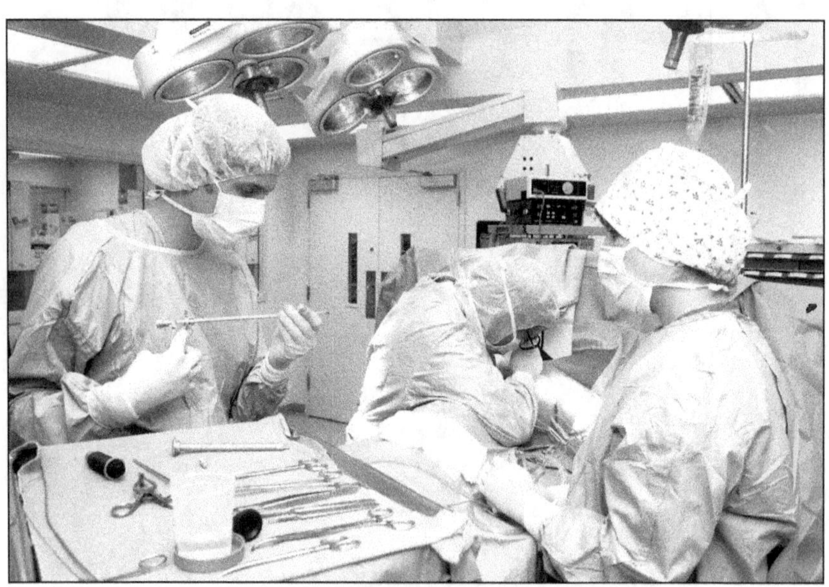

Preparing for a laparoscopic surgical procedure.
Public domain image, from the National Cancer Institute Archives.

- Drugs and IV solutions as well as a range of other surgical supplies such as sponges and dressings, will be on a tray or readily available from the central sterile supply room.
- **Defibrillators (259)** will be immediately accessible in case of cardiac emergency.
- Patient body temperature may be subject to rapid fluctuations during surgery, and so **warming/cooling units (14)** are available, often with both functions integrated into one device.
- Many hospitals have a system called **PACS (232)** (picture archiving and communication system) that allows central storage and remote display of any diagnostic images that have been produced for patients in the hospital. A large, high-resolution PACS video display will be available in the OR, though this function may be integrated into a general-purpose video system.
- A hospital information computer terminal will be in the room or nearby, to allow access to patient demographic information, medication history and test results. As with PACS, the hospital computer system may be integrated into a general-purpose unit.
- Particularly in teaching hospitals, ORs may be equipped with high-resolution observation and recording video equipment, allowing students or remote specialists to observe procedures.
- Last but not least, a stereo is an integral part of most operating rooms, as many surgeons prefer to work with music in the background.

Kidney Complications – Jerry – OR

Finally, even hemodialysis is not enough to keep Jerry going. He is very fortunate to be able have a kidney transplant, which restores kidney function to normal with the new kidney and frees him from the restrictions of dialysis. A transplant carries its own set of requirements for continued success but the freedom it provides Jerry is far more than worth it to him. He joins celebrities such as Gary Coleman, Steven "Cojo" Cojocaru, Natalie Cole, George Lopez and Neil Simon, all of whom have had kidney transplants.

- Lighting A variety of equipment meets the specific lighting requirements of surgery. Large, bright **overhead surgical lights (64)** can be moved around and focused on particular areas, and designers attempt to minimize heat production while providing bright light with consistent color characteristics.

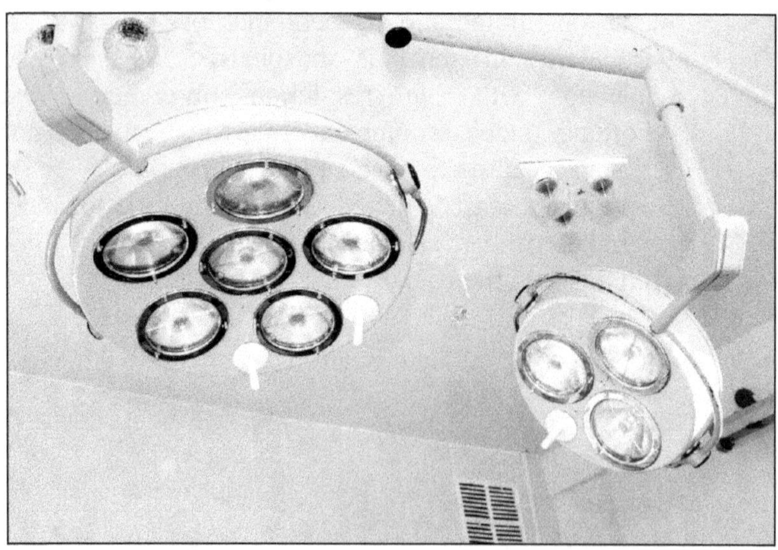

OR lights.
(Modified from Shutterstock, Inc, www.shutterstock.com, with permission)

Surgeons may utilize headlights to illuminate the specific area on which they are working. **Fiber optic light sources (142)** are used in a variety of situations because they provide good light quality with minimal heat and can be directed through small, flexible channels to difficult to access locations. ORs are usually equipped with hand held **laryngoscopes (301)** and **ophthalmoscopes (301)**, which have built□in illumination.

- Displays □ A variety of **video displays (147)** may be found in operating rooms, though there is a trend towards integrating the displays of various components. Displays may include video from **endoscopes (135)**, **operating microscopes (68)**, **PACS (232)**, patient record and lab result information, **physiological monitoring (314)**, and **anesthesia monitoring (47)** and control. Video feeds may be provided to multiple large wall mounted screens within the room, or to screens in various teaching and observation areas within the hospital.

- Staff □ The surgical team is described in detail Appendix B, p. 356.

- Specialized OR types □ Suites may be specially equipped and set up for specific types of surgery, including ophthalmologic procedures, orthopedics, Cesarean sections, dental surgery or urology.

OR Equipment Descriptions

Following are more detailed descriptions of equipment found exclusively or most commonly in this area of the hospital. Equipment that is also found in various other areas of the hospital is described in Chapter 12, p 247.

Devices typically found in Operating Rooms, in addition to the equipment listed in this section, include: **aspirators (250)**, **capnographs (254)**, **electronic probe thermometers (279)**, **gas regulators (285)**, **intravenous pumps (289)**, **intubation assist devices (292)**, **invasive pressure monitors (294)**, **non–invasive pressure monitors (296)**, **physiological monitors (314)**, **point of care blood analysis systems (318)**, **pulse oximeters (320)**, **stethoscopes (327)**, **syringe pumps (329)**, **defibrillators (259)**, **lithotriptors (157)**, **automatic tourniquets (330)**, **PACS (232)** and **C–arm units (212)**.

Anesthetic Machines

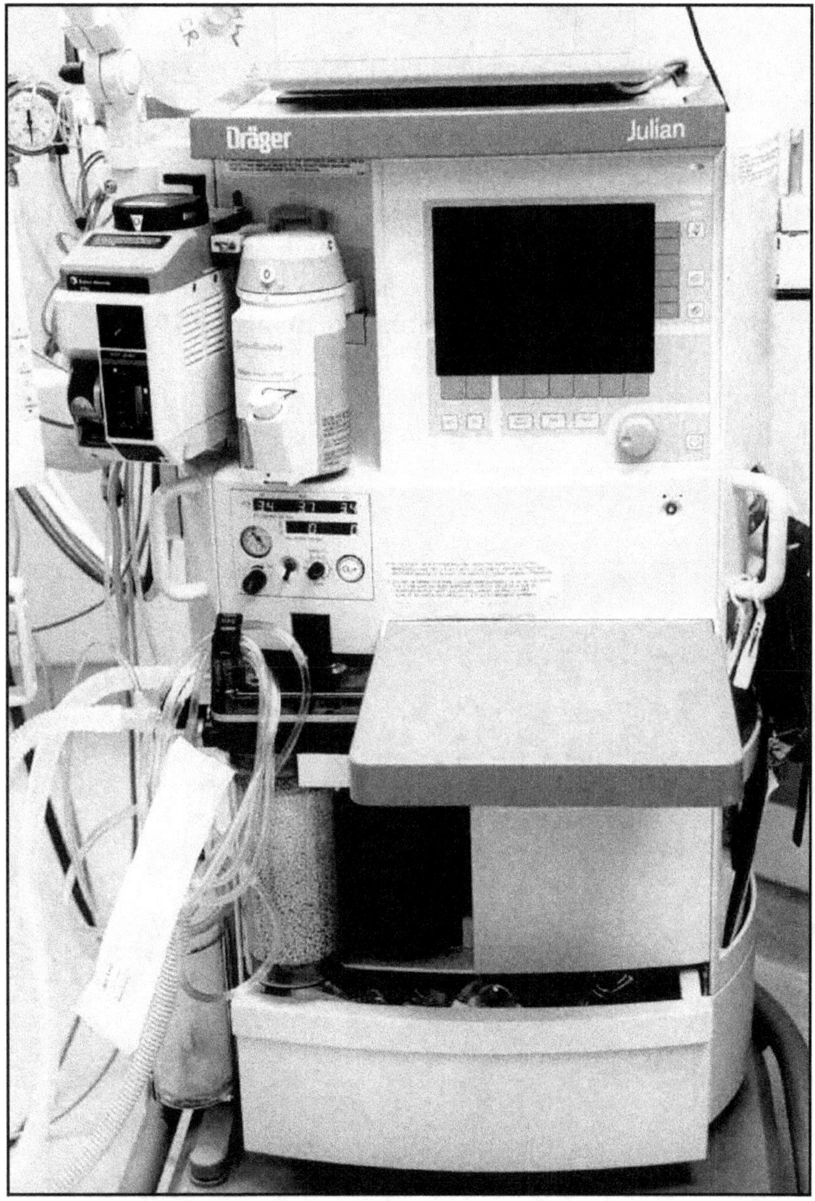

Overview □During surgery, there are a number of important considerations for the well□being of the patient, many of which are addressed by the attending anesthesiologist using an anesthetic machine.

Primary among these considerations is the elimination of the sensation of pain, which is accomplished by the administration of one or more gases that render the patient unconscious.

Function □The anesthetic machine provides a source for these gases, regulates their pressure and flow, mixes them with oxygen, adds humidification if required, and delivers the final mixture to the patient. Since the levels of the various components are critical, machines often have systems to measure and display percentages and flow rates, with associated alarms for high or low levels. This function may also be performed by an auxiliary unit, either stand□alone or integrated into a **multi–parameter monitor (314)**.

Hypothermia is a common reaction during surgery, and so air provided to the patient may be heated; in this case, humidification is especially important to prevent drying of airway tissues.

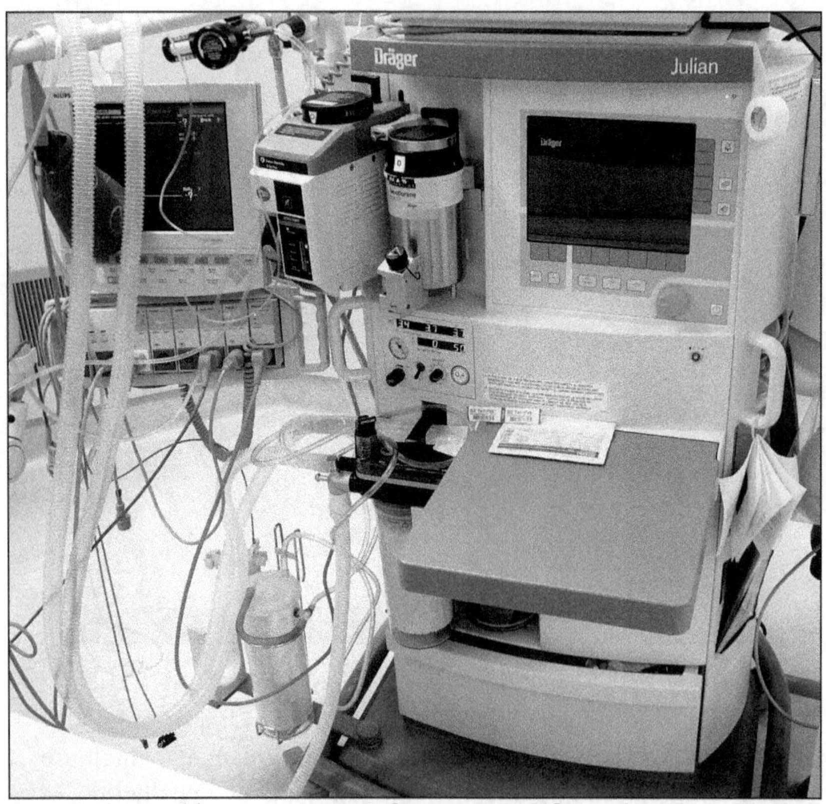

Anesthetic machine components, from upper left: patient breathing circuit (two vertical tubes), physiological monitor (314) with parameter modules underneath, anesthetic agent vaporizers, control screen.

Some surgical procedures require that the patient's muscles be immobilized to prevent unwanted contractions in response to either the physical trauma of surgery or to the electrical stimulation of electrosurgery units. Drugs to accomplish this are administered, but they paralyze breathing muscles as well, which means that the anesthetic machine must be able to provide artificial ventilation at a controlled rate and volume. This ventilation is delivered via an endotracheal tube, which in these situations also carries the anesthetic gases.

Galling Gall Stones – Elizabeth – OR II

Yet another drug is fed into the IV and this causes Elizabeth's muscles to be paralyzed so that there is no undesirable twitching during surgery. She is now dependent on the machine to breathe for her, and the doctor keeps a close eye on all her vital signs, which are displayed on one of the two video screens of the anesthetic machine. The other screen shows the function and settings of the machine itself, along with measurements of oxygen, carbon dioxide and anesthetic gas concentrations. Exhaled breaths pass through an absorber cartridge that removes most of the carbon dioxide while allowing air, oxygen and the anesthetic gas to pass through so that they can be recycled into the patient. A vacuum system removes any excess gases so that the OR staff are not exposed.

The anesthetic machine measures Elizabeth's ***ECG (400), blood oxygen concentration (SpO2) (320), temperature (279) and level of consciousness (276)****. Surgery often lowers body temperature but overheating can also occur, so a* ***hyper/hypothermia unit (14)*** *is used to adjust temperature as necessary.*

Anesthetic machines must also provide access to monitoring of vital signs such as ECG, blood pressure, temperature, blood oxygen saturation, and expired CO2 levels. These functions may be built into the anesthetic machine itself, or the machine may simply be a platform on which an independent physiological monitor is mounted.

Application □ Anesthetic machines are operated by physicians specialized in anesthesiology. They administer intravenous medications as required, and then connect the patient to the anesthetic machine breathing circuit. After adjusting the appropriate parameters such as gas mixture ratios, gas flow rates, and patient breathing rate, the gas flow is initiated. Patient condition is closely monitored at all times to maintain adequate levels of anesthesia □ enough but not too much.

AKA □anesthetic units.

Related devices □ **physiological monitors (314)**, **electrosurgery units (51)**, **ventilators (334)**, **nerve/muscle stimulators (63)**, **level of consciousness monitors (276)**.

Where found □operating rooms.

Electrosurgery Units (ESU)

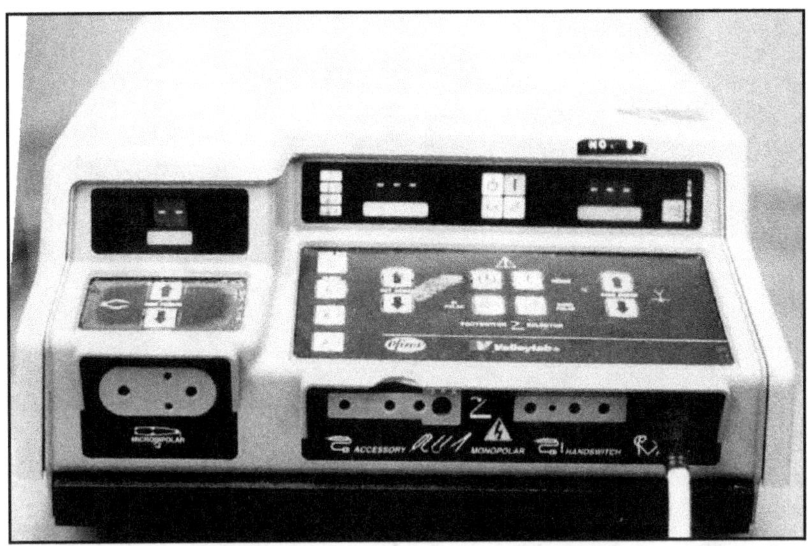

Overview □ One of the problems encountered in surgery is bleeding from the many blood vessels of various sizes that are severed while incisions are being made. This is more prevalent in some types of tissue, and results in not only an increased loss of blood for the patient, but also decreased visibility for the surgeon and support staff.

Function □ Electrosurgery units help to solve the problem of excess bleeding by using high intensity electrical signals to perform cutting procedures. A pencil□type probe with a blade on the end (which comes in a variety of shapes for different circumstances) applies the electricity to the cutting point, while a large conductive grounding pad placed on a fleshy part of the patient provides a return circuit.

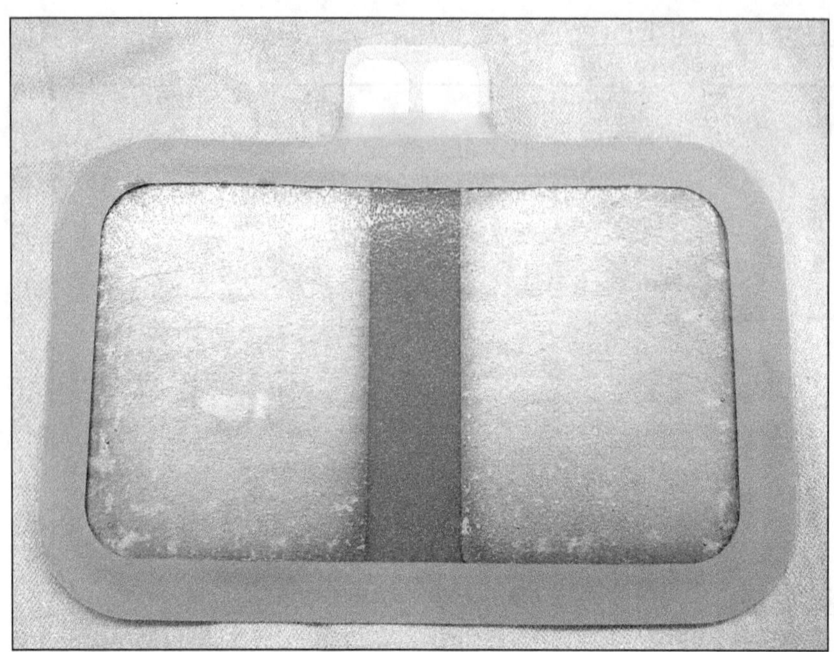

Gelled ESU return electrode pad. The two sections are used in a circuit to ensure adequate contact with the patient.

Power levels are adjusted for different procedures. The electrical energy vaporizes the tissue immediately around blade, and there is enough energy spreading into nearby tissues to heat them to a point where many of the smaller blood vessels are sealed off (cauterized). Larger vessels must still be tied off, but much of the excess bleeding experienced with scalpel incisions is avoided.

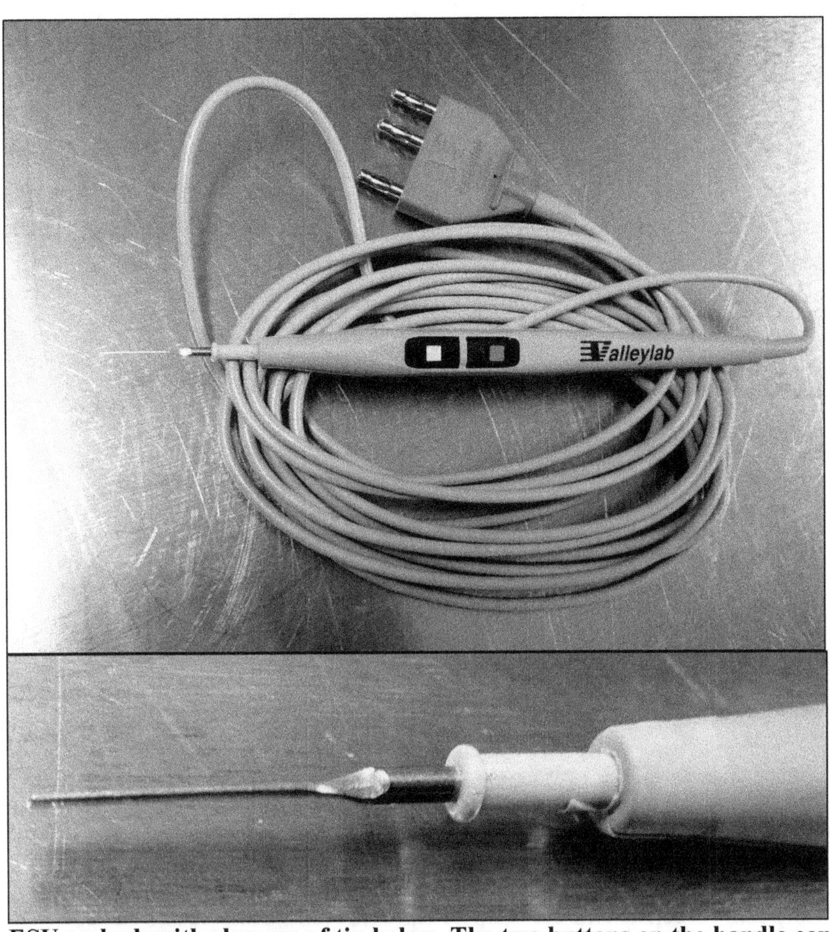

ESU scalpel, with close up of tip below. The two buttons on the handle control either CUT or COAG modes.

In some circumstances, a very localized effect is needed, such as when performing tubal sterilizations. In such instances, a special electrode is used which passes current directly from one side of the probe to the other, passing through the tissue to be cauterized. This function is called "bipolar" operation, as opposed to the more normal "monopolar" operation using a surgical pencil and separate ground pad.

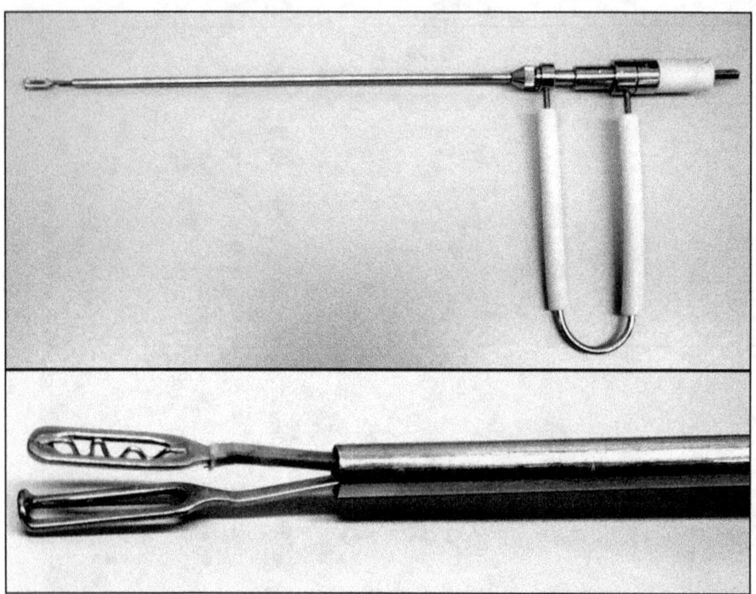

ESU bipolar forceps, with close up of tip below. Current passes between the two parts of the tip to cauterize (or if enough current is applied, cut) the tissue in between.

Experimentation has shown that different shapes of electrical signals produce different effects — more concentrated cutting, more general cauterization, or a blending of each.

Some electrosurgery units utilize a highly charged beam of gas (usually argon) to perform the cutting and cauterization, instead of a metal blade.

In some circumstances, only cauterization is needed, and simpler devices which use the same principles as full-function electrosurgery units but which only provide cauterization are used. Simple cauterization generally requires less power and less precise control than cutting, so these units are usually smaller and less expensive.

Application □Electrosurgery units are operated by setting the desired power level and applying the blade to the target tissue, then activating the current by depressing a foot switch or using a hand switch located on the operating tool. Specialized attachments such as loops and small forceps are used for laparoscopic surgery. Special attention must be paid in set up to ensure that the return electrode (ground pad) is placed on a fleshy area of the patient, well away from the surgical site. Because of the nature of the high frequency energy involved, power can flow out of the patient□s body through alternate pathways if the grounding pad is improperly placed or if it comes loose. These alternate pathways can cause burns to patients and/or staff, so alarms circuits are used which measure the degree of contact of the ground pad, and prevent operation of the unit if they are not within certain limits. A value that is too low can mean that saline or blood has made a path from the incision site to the ground pad, which can result in extreme burns or even fires.

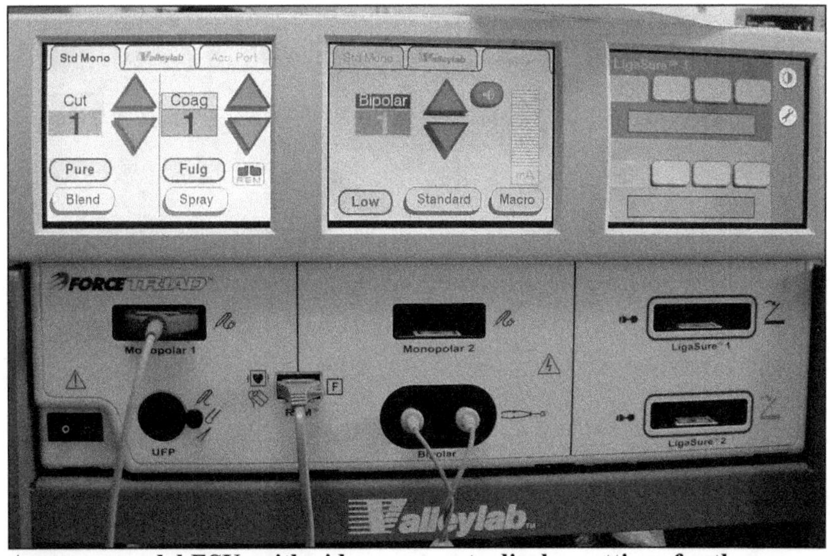

A newer–model ESU, with video screens to display settings for three separate channels.

There is concern that particles of smoke produced by electrosurgery units may contain active virus particles and/or toxins. To help alleviate this problem, most operating rooms are equipped with smoke evacuator units that are used in conjunction with electrosurgery units.

AKA □ ESUs, electrocautery units, cauteries, Bovies (after an early manufacturer).

Related devices □**surgical lasers (70)**.

Where found □operating rooms, outpatient surgery clinics.

Heart□lung machines

Overview □During some cardiac surgery, the patient□s heart must be stopped so that surgeons can perform their work. Blood flow and oxygenation must be continued for this time, which may be several hours, and heart□lung machines perform this function.

The first successful use of a heart□lung machine in human surgery was in 1953 in Philadelphia, using a machine developed by John Gibbon.

Because they are used for relatively short terms in high□acuity environments, there is no need for these units to be small or portable.

Function □ The majority of total blood flow is drawn from the patient□s venous system, usually the superior vena cava or the right atrium. It is then pumped into a membrane system that allows the escape of carbon dioxide from the blood and the intake of oxygen to the blood. The blood is then pumped into the aortic arch where it continues to circulate through the patient□s body. The heart and lungs are bypassed, and the heart can be made to stop to allow surgical procedures to take place.

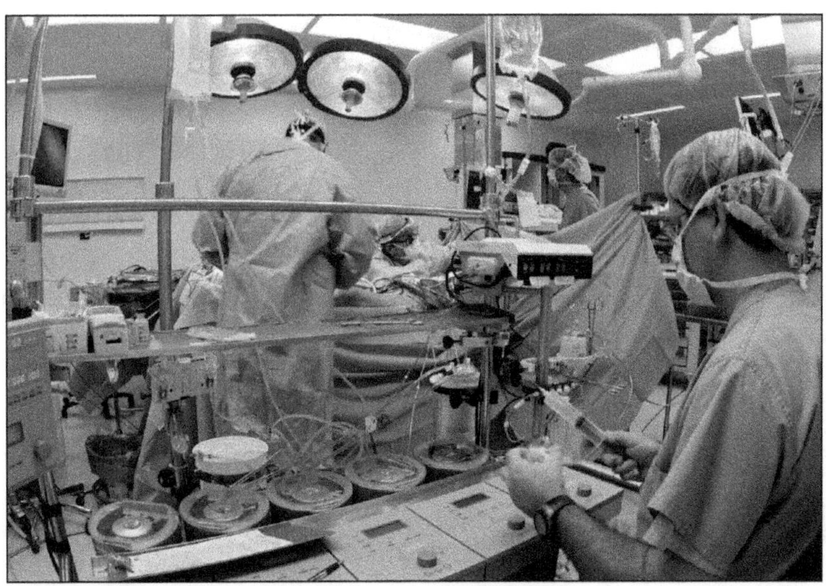

A heart lung machine, operated by a perfusionist.
Modified from Shutterstock, Inc, www.shutterstock.com, with permission

A number of factors must be considered in the design of heart□lung machines:

- The system must have adequate and adjustable pumping capacity to maintain appropriate blood flow through the patient.

- The gas exchange system must be sufficiently effective in both removing carbon dioxide to keep blood levels below harmful levels, and in adding oxygen to simulate normal ventilation. Membranes are made of materials such as polypropylene or silicone.

- Pumping systems must cause minimal mechanical damage to blood cells. Pumps may be of the roller peristaltic type, or of a centrifugal type in which rotation of blood within the pump head produces flow. Centrifugal pumps tend to cause less damage to cells.

- An anti□clotting agent, usually heparin, must be added to the blood to prevent clots forming in the system and passing to the patient. This agent must be neutralized immediately following surgery so that normal clotting can take place.

- Temperature of the blood must be controllable in order maintain, raise or lower patient body temperature as required by specific circumstances. It may be advantageous to induce hypothermia in order to minimize tissue damage during certain procedures.

Application □ Heart lung machines are operated by perfusionists, specially trained technologists who monitor and control system functions working in coordination with anesthetists, surgeons and the rest of the surgical team.

AKA □none

Related devices □**ventilators (334).**

Where found □operating rooms

Laparoscopy Systems

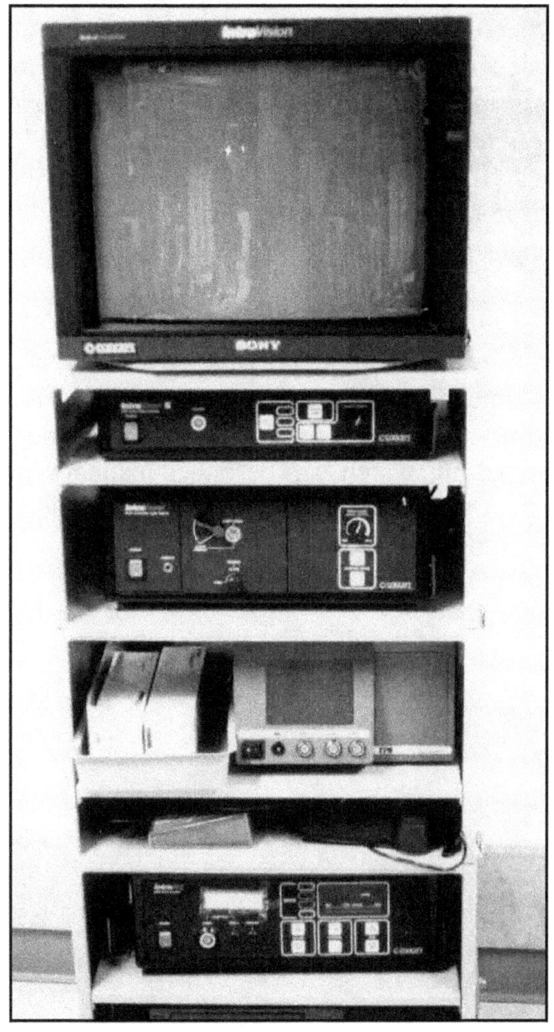

Overview □ Traditional abdominal surgery is traumatic for the patient. Large incisions are a direct shock to the system. They require a high degree of anesthetization, which is itself hard on body systems, and healing times and risks of infection are both significant. The large scars left are a cosmetic problem for some patients, as well.

Function □ Laparoscopic surgery reduces these negative aspects of surgery by reducing the incision size from ten to thirty centimeters or more, to as little as one or two centimeters. This is made possible mainly by advances in fiber optic technology; optical cables provide a flexible pathway for illumination and also for conveying images of the surgical target to the surgeon.

In order for the surgeon to be able to see the target, the abdomen must be filled with gas (insufflated). This requires a **gas control system (148)** that regulates and measures flow rates, delivered volumes and sometimes inflation times. To provide a constant degree of inflation, the gas supply must be able to sense and control the gas pressure within the abdomen.

Some simple procedures are done with a simple lens and eyepiece, which allows the surgeon to directly observe the internal structures and instruments. Most procedures, however, are visualized by an **electronic camera (144)** pick-up attached to fiber optic cables. The camera feeds an electronics module that conditions the signal and sends it to one or more high-resolution color **video monitors (147)**, which the surgeon observes. This allows other personnel to see the progress of the operation for teaching purposes and to allow more effective assistance. Images are often recorded for future examination.

Because color is sometimes critical in identifying structures and diseased tissues, both the illumination and display components of the system must have high color accuracy. **Light sources (142)** must provide high intensity illumination, which can be either manually or automatically controlled; light levels may interact with the video system, as well, to provide optimum values.

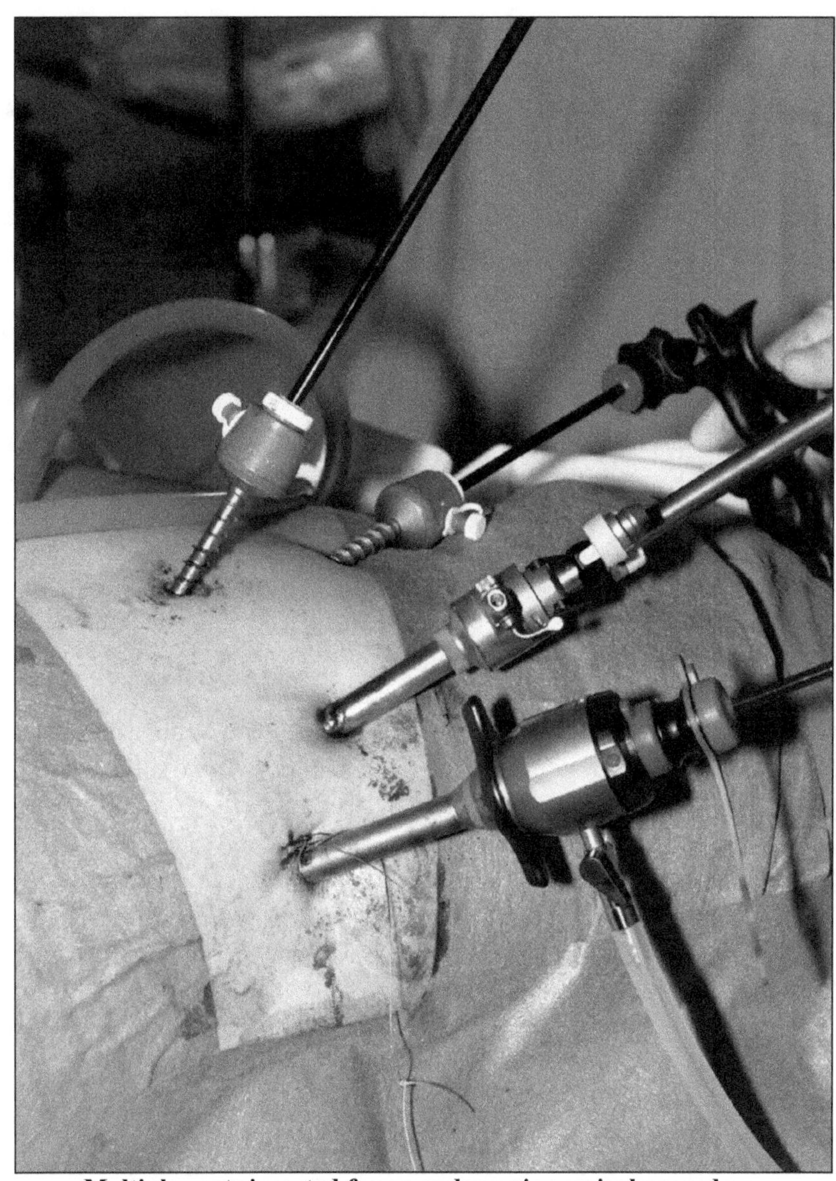

Multiple ports inserted for an endoscopic surgical procedure.

Modified from Shutterstock, Inc, www.shutterstock.com, with permission.

A channel in the access tubing allows insertion of the actual surgical instruments; these may be mechanical cutting or dissection devices, specially□designed **electrosurgery (51)** probes, or attachments to break up kidney stones or gallstones.

Sometimes one tube is used for observing the site while another provides access for surgical instruments.

Suction must also be available, for removing excess fluids from the site and for aspirating excised tissues.

Application □ The patient is sedated or anesthetized as necessary for the specific procedure, and then a small incision through the layers of the abdominal wall is made to allow insertion of the tube or tubes. The abdomen is insufflated, and the surgical site located and cleared as much as possible. The surgery is performed and the area is checked, then the gas is removed, followed by the tubes. The incision is then closed.

AKA □ lap systems, lap□chole systems (an abbreviation for laparoscopic cholecystectomy □ gall bladder removal), lap□gyne systems (for laparoscopic gynecologic procedures)

Related devices □ **ESUs (51)**, **gas regulators (285)**, **lithotriptors (157)**.

Where found □ operating rooms.

Nerve/Muscle Stimulators

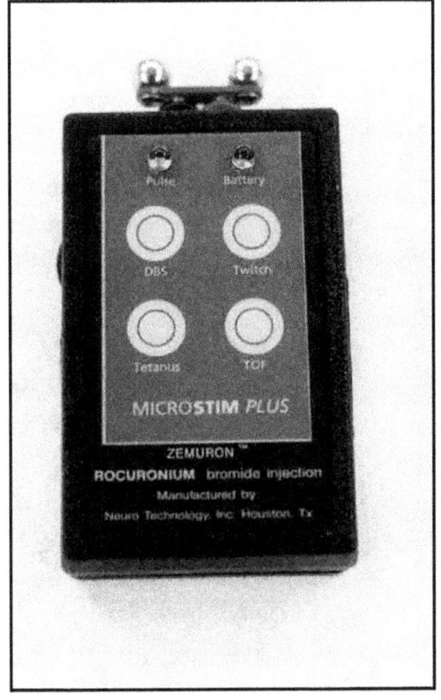

Overview □ Some surgical procedures, such as those using **electrosurgery units (51)**, can cause a patient□s muscles to contract sharply. This can cause problems for both staff and patient, and a muscle□paralyzing agent is administered to prevent this from happening. Before surgery commences, the anesthetist must determine whether muscle paralysis has been effective. Also, patients must be monitored to ensure that excessive doses of the paralyzing agent are not given. Since the patient is unconscious at these times, a means for testing the depth of paralysis is required.

Function □ Muscle stimulators allow anesthetists to test for depth of muscle paralysis. Electrodes (which may be like ECG electrodes, or simple conductive rubber pads or metal ball terminals) deliver signals to the skin, where they are transmitted to underlying muscle. The intensity of signal required to produce a given response is a measure of the degree of paralysis. Controls on the unit allow for varying intensity, signal shape, and signal frequency.

Application □ Electrodes are placed in a convenient location, usually on a limb near smaller muscle groups. When the patient is anesthetized, signals are applied to the electrodes, and the depth of muscle paralysis is determined. Tests are repeated frequently during surgery; if paralysis is too great, the flow of paralyzing agent is reduced, and vice versa.

AKA □ stimulators.

Related devices □ **Electrosurgery units (51)**, **Transcutaneous Electrical Nerve Stimulators (TENS) (203).**

Where found □ Operating rooms.

Operating Room Lights

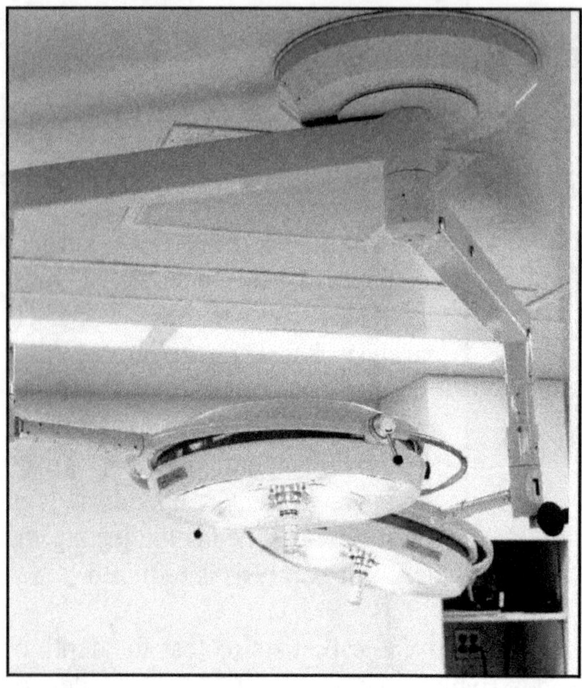

Overview □ It is imperative that surgeons and support staff have a clear view of the operating field.

Function □ OR lights must supply illumination that is adjustable for both intensity and direction, evenly distributed so that all areas are illuminated evenly, and with a proper degree of □whiteness□ so that the colors of anatomical structures and tissues are natural.

OR lights are ceiling□mounted, with articulating arms to allow for a variety of positions. They generally have either a single, high□intensity bulb whose light is reflected from a large, carefully□shaped mirror, or a number of bulbs in a single housing, each with its own reflective area, to provide the even illumination required. Two or more lights may be mounted in the operating theater for increased illumination and placement flexibility.

Because intensity levels are high, a part of the design of OR lights is to reduce infrared heat, which could cause discomfort for staff and possible tissue drying for the patient. Mounting the light at a suitable distance from the OR table and using special coatings on glass surfaces minimizes heat effects.

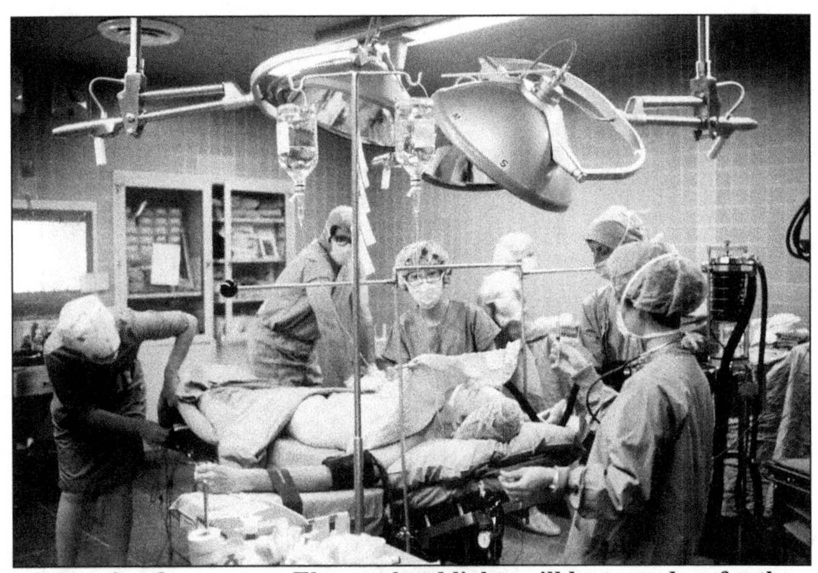

Preparing for surgery. The overhead lights will be turned on for the procedure.
Public domain image, from the National Cancer Institute Archives.

Application The lights are turned on and adjusted for optimal illumination.

AKA surgical lights.

Related devices **OR tables (66)**.

Where found operating rooms, some emergency rooms.

Operating Room Tables

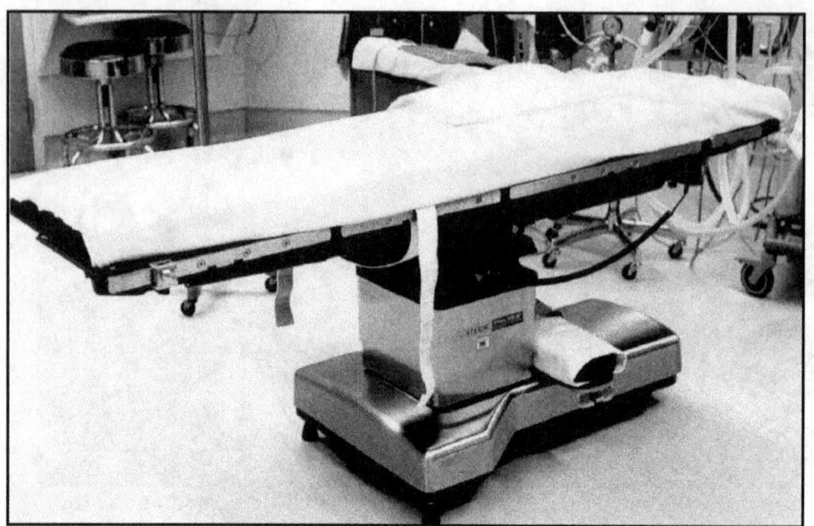

Overview During surgery, the patient must be in a stable, convenient and adjustable position. There must be room for a number of people to have access, and there has to be provision for taking x rays during the procedure.

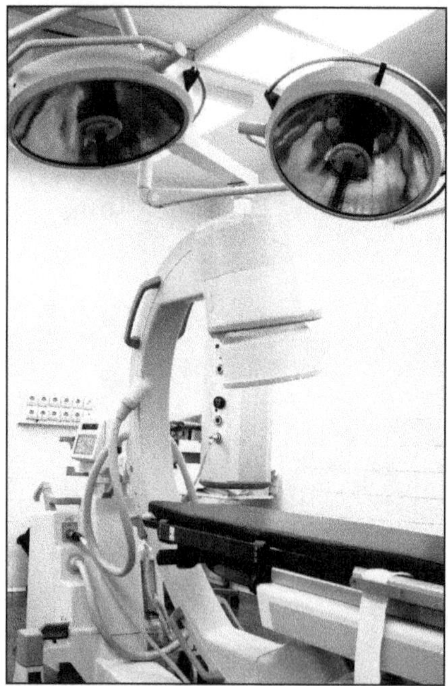

A C–Arm x–ray unit (212) built in to an OR table.

Function – OR tables are designed to move easily in three directions, as well as to be adjustable for head-to-foot and side-to-side angle. They are driven by either electric motors or hydraulics, though hydraulics is preferred because it is usually smoother, quieter and safer (especially in regards to electrical shock hazards) when compared to electrically-operated versions.

Movements are controlled by a footswitch or by hand controls, and there are locking mechanisms to hold the selected position solidly. An under-table chamber allows for insertion of x-ray film cassettes; some tables have a fluoroscope pick-up in the base, and some may have facilities for rapid repeat exposures of x-rays.

Application – Patient position is chosen to optimize access and comfort for the surgeon(s) and assistants. Certain surgical procedures and/or patient conditions may require the head of the table to be tilted up or down. The surgeon may perform adjustments, or they may be done by an assistant; position may be modified during the course of a procedure as well.

AKA – OR tables, surgical tables.

Related devices – **Electric hospital beds (277).**

Where found – operating rooms.

<u>Operating Microscopes (OPMI)</u>

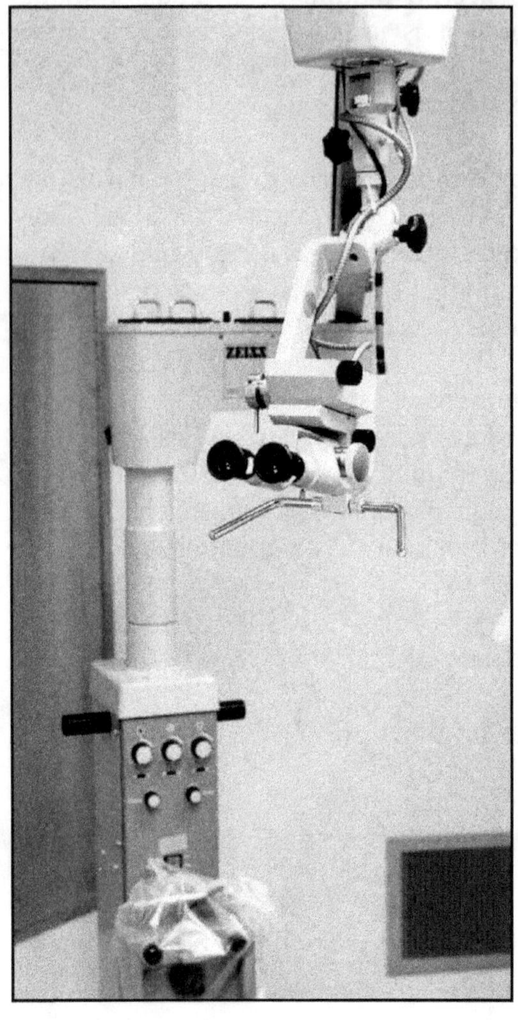

<u>Overview</u> □ Certain surgical procedures involve very small structures, which require magnification to visualize and work on.

<u>Function</u> □ Operating microscopes are one type of device used to provide this magnification. To be effective, they must meet a variety of design considerations.

Primarily, they must provide an effective view of the surgical site. This requires high□quality optics in a binocular arrangement (to give a three□dimensional image), with variable levels of magnification and high□ quality spot illumination.

For practicality, the surgeon and/or support personnel must be able to position the viewing head accurately, and it must remain stable during use. This requires a ceiling mount (in rooms that are dedicated to this type of procedure) or a heavy, wheeled floor mount. The head is attached to the mount with a relatively long arm that is multi□articulated to allow a range of positions. Vertical positioning and focusing are usually performed using a footswitch; other functions such as angle, horizontal position, and magnification may be powered or manual.

To accommodate the variety of positions needed, light is usually delivered to the viewing area via a flexible fiber□optic cable. This also has the advantage of reducing the amount of heat delivered to the site. Colored filters may be supplied, which help to highlight certain aspects of anatomy.

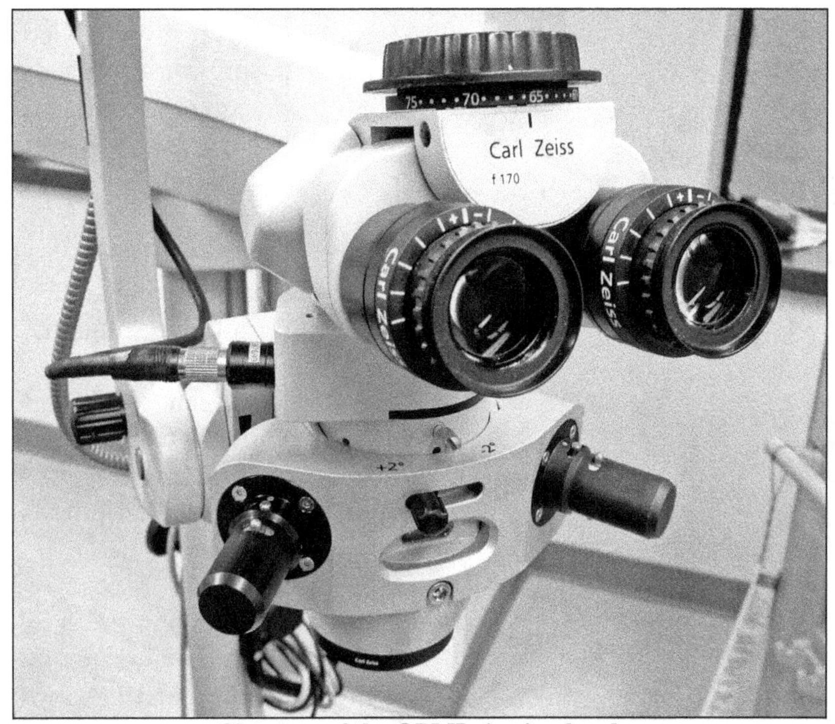

Close–up of the OPMI viewing head.

Operating microscopes may be equipped with dual viewing heads (looking through a single objective) for use by a student or assistant. They may also have a video camera so that the image seen by the surgeon can be displayed in a large video monitor, and possibly recorded for future reference.

Application The surgeon views the surgical site through the microscope, adjusting position, focus, lighting, and magnification as necessary.

AKA OpMi, OR scopes, operating scopes/microscopes.

Related devices **OR lights (64)**, **phacoemulsifiers (115)**.

Where found operating rooms, specialized outpatient clinics, some emergency rooms.

Surgical Lasers

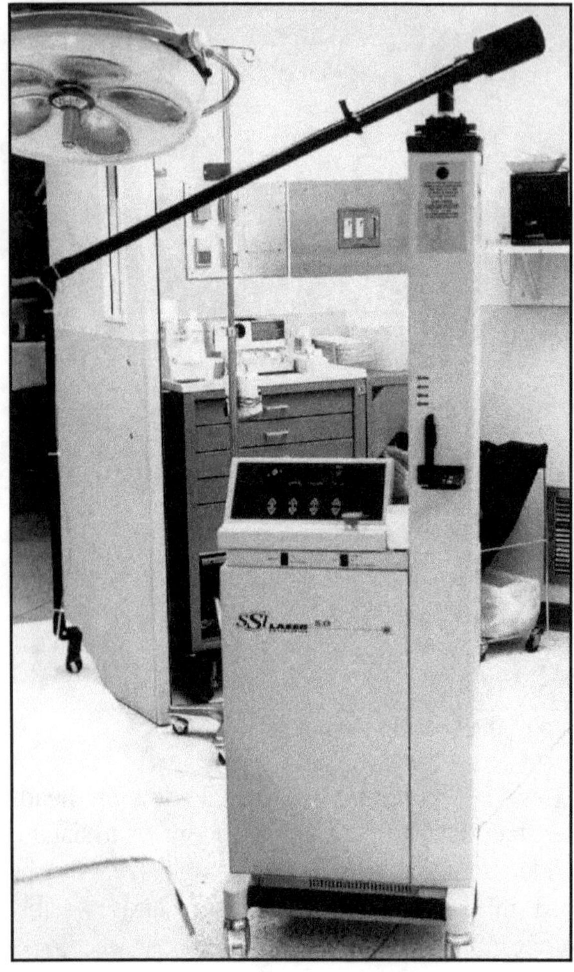

Overview □ Certain surgical procedures require that tissues be vaporized in order to achieve the desired results, such as removal of skin abnormalities or cutting through tissue. Coagulation of tissues adjacent to the cutting site may also be desirable, or coagulation may be the goal.

Function □ Surgical lasers utilize very pure and controlled light beams to heat tissue. Depending on the width and power of the beam, this heating may be extreme, vaporizing the tissue, or less so, in which case cauterization is produced. The laser beam may be controlled so that the depth of its effect is very precise, allowing removal of skin blemishes or tattoos.

A power supply and optical system develop the laser beam. Its characteristics are determined in part by the material used to generate the laser light. Some such materials are CO_2, Holmium, Neodymium/Yttrium/Argon (Nd:YAG), and Erbium YAG. The laser beam is directed by a series of mirrors to the target area.

A low-powered laser beam, utilizing the same pathway as the treatment beam, may be used to point the system at the correct location before applying power. Control circuitry allows for adjustment of beam power and duration of treatment.

In order to properly visualize the target area, and to observe the effects of the laser beam, a microscope system may be used.

Application – The surgeon utilizes a hand-held probe to direct the laser beam, applying power by depressing a footswitch until the desired effect has been achieved.

Because laser beams may cause damage to the retina, either through direct exposure or by reflection, all personnel in the area must use proper eye protection, and adequate signs must be posted in the vicinity to warn that lasers are in use.

There is concern that disease agents such as viruses may be present in the smoke produced by laser surgery. To guard against possible infections caused by these agents, a smoke evacuator system is used to remove and filter out most of the smoke from the surgical site.

AKA – (none).

Related devices – **electrosurgery units (51)**.

Where found – operating rooms, outpatient clinics, doctor's treatment rooms.

Chapter 4 – Maternity Department

Maternity Department Description

- Function □ Maternity provides care for women during their pregnancy, delivery and immediate postnatal period. Counselling and education is available regarding prenatal nutrition and health, birthing alternatives, birthing preparation, infant care, lactation, fertility and family planning. Complications of pregnancy due to maternal or fetal medical issues are dealt with, and testing such as fetal monitoring and non□stress procedures are available. Many hospitals have designed or renovated their maternity units to be more comfortable and home□like for patients.

<u>*The Pregnant Woman – Angie – Maternity/Nursery I*</u>

Angie is a 33-year-old woman who is nearing the due date of her first pregnancy. She was fine for the first few months, with very little morning sickness, but then she developed gestational diabetes, a form of diabetes that is usually limited to the time of pregnancy but can have serious consequences for both mother and fetus. Under the supervision of her Obstetrician, she is keeping the condition under control by eating a well-balanced diet with reduced consumption of sugars and refined carbs. She also monitors her blood-sugar levels with a ***glucometer (287)*** *to make sure she stays within healthy limits. The glucometer is a tiny device, and all she has to do is prick her finger with a disposable lancet, place a drop of blood on a test strip, and insert the strip in the meter. Five seconds later, the reading shows on the LCD screen. Angie knows what the normal or safe values should be, and she adjusts her diet to compensate for any changes in her blood glucose levels.*

- Layout □ Patient rooms in Maternity are for expectant mothers who may require pre□delivery medical care due to complications of pregnancy and for new mothers for recovery following birth. Some mothers in good health may leave the hospital the same day as they gave birth or within a day or two, while others may have medical issues that necessitate longer stays. Hospitals often have facilities that allow the newborn to stay in the same room as the mother until discharge, while others have separate nurseries for all babies. Infants requiring special care will stay in the nursery, either in a bassinette or in an **infant incubator (100)**. Special facilities such as **birthing beds (89)** will be available in the department, sometimes in special labor□delivery rooms and sometimes in the regular patient rooms.

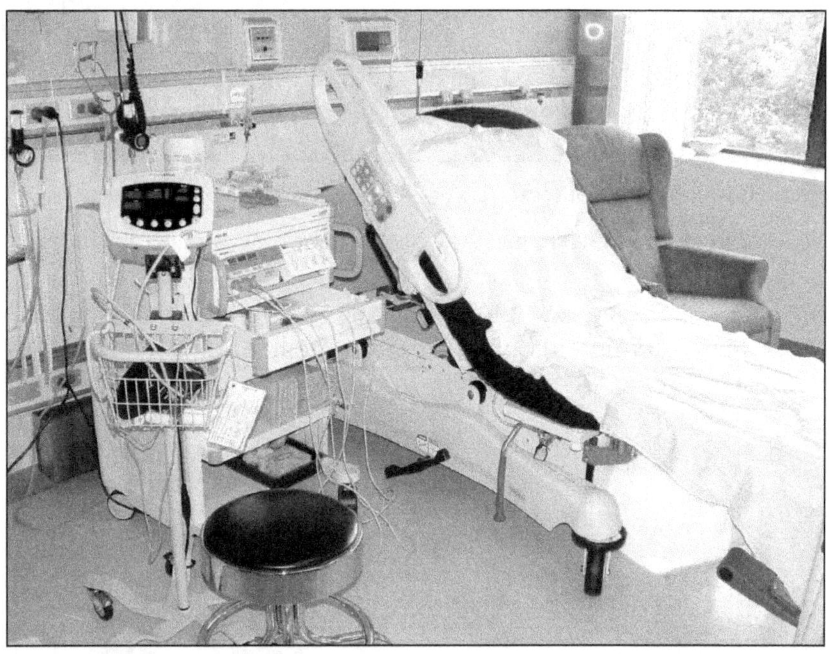

A typical labor–delivery room. Equipment includes the vital signs monitor on the stand, a fetal monitor on the cart and the specialized labor–delivery bed with patient or staff adjustable positions and a removable section at the foot to allow staff access to assist in delivery.

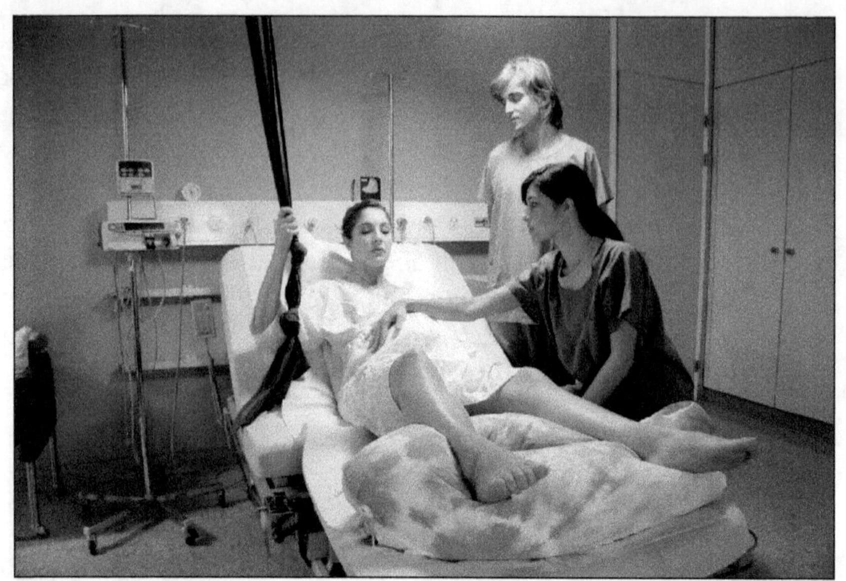

A patient in labor.

(Modified from Shutterstock, Inc, www.shutterstock.com, with permission)

An operating room for Cesarean section births may be part of the Maternity unit, with the same facilities as a regular OR.

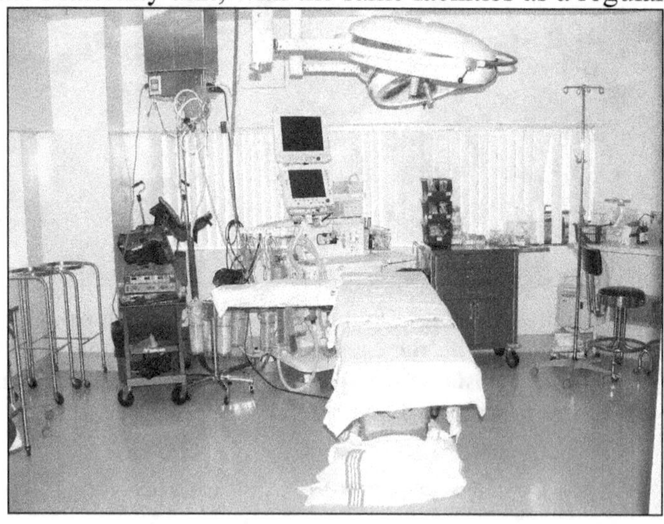

An operating room specialized for Cesarian sections. It includes and electrosurgery machine on the left, an anesthetic machine at the back, a surgical table and overhead surgical lights.

A nursery will be in close proximity to the patient rooms, with the traditional viewing windows.

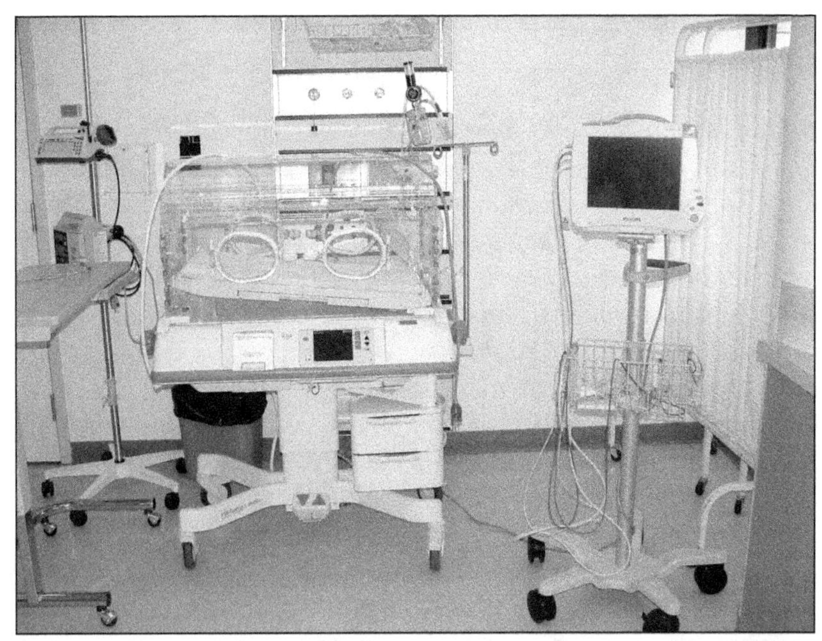

Part of a nursery with an infant incubator and mobile physiological monitor.

Rooms may be available for procedures such as non‑stress testing and other examinations. A nursing station will have facilities for charting and other such routine nursing procedures, and may have a **central station (29)** for either **fetal monitor (95)** data or neonatal **physiological monitoring (314)** information, or both. A small kitchen is usually present for fresh food preparation for pre and post‑delivery mothers, fathers and birth coaches, as well as a lounge for those involved in the birthing process. The lounge may double as a visitor waiting room, or the two may be separate. If the hospital has a neonatal intensive care unit, it is usually in close proximity to Maternity, if not an integral part of the area. Some maternity units have special facilities, such as pools for water births.

The Pregnant Woman – Angie – Maternity/Nursery II

Angie is visiting the outpatient clinic of her hospital's Maternity Department. Women are often checked during the later part of their pregnancy as a mater of course, but with Angie's gestational diabetes, her Doctor is keeping a closer watch than normal. She is familiar with the non-stress test routine so the nurses don't have to explain the process to her. Since gestational diabetes is often accompanied by high blood pressure, a nurse takes Angie's pressure using a vital signs monitor (a unit that combiners ***an electronic probe thermometer (279)****, a* ***pulse oximeter (320)*** *and a* ***non-invasive blood pressure monitor (296)****.) Angie has worn a loose top and her comfiest pants, so when she gets onto the examining bed she can pull the top up and the waistband of her pants down so her pregnant belly is exposed. A* ***fetal monitor (95)*** *is positioned right next to the bed. A nurse sits next to the bed, turns the machine on, and helps Angie slip an elastic belt under her back and around her belly, and shift onto her side. The nurse then takes an ultrasound probe about the size of a computer mouse from a drawer under the monitor and squirts some warm, clear gel on one side of the probe. She places the probe on Angie's abdomen and moves it around until a swishing sound starts coming form the monitor's speaker. This sound is produced when ultrasonic signals from the probe are reflected back from the baby's heart and are picked up by the probe.* **160** *flashes on the digital display of the monitor, which Angie knows is the baby's heart rate. The nurse presses a button to start the recorder part of the monitor, and a sheet of graph paper starts to slowly feed out of the machine. One part of the graph has a line that corresponds to the baby's heart rate, producing a changing line over time as the rate goes up and down. The nurse then hands Angie a cord with a button on the end and reminds her to press the button whenever she feels the baby move.*

The Pregnant Woman – Angie – continued

There are magazines and a CD player with headphones on a table beside the bed, but Angie has a novel with her, so she settles down to read while the test continues, pressing the button to make a mark on the graph paper whenever the baby moves. The nurse pops in every once in a while to adjust the probe to get the best signal, and when the test is finished, she wipes the excess gel from Angie's skin and helps her up so she can get ready to go home.

- Staff □ Maternity is primarily staffed by nurses. Physicians may or may not be present for vaginal deliveries, though any complications usually mean a family physician, resident or gynecologist will be involved. Surgeons perform C□sections. Professional labor coaches or midwives are often available, as well as social workers, dieticians and lactation advisors. Housekeeping staff is vital for maintaining order and cleanliness, especially following birth.

- Equipment □ **Fetal monitors (95)** allow the measurement of fetal heart rate and the relative strength of labor contractions. They may also include **pulse oximetry (320)** and **non–invasive blood pressure (296)** measurement.

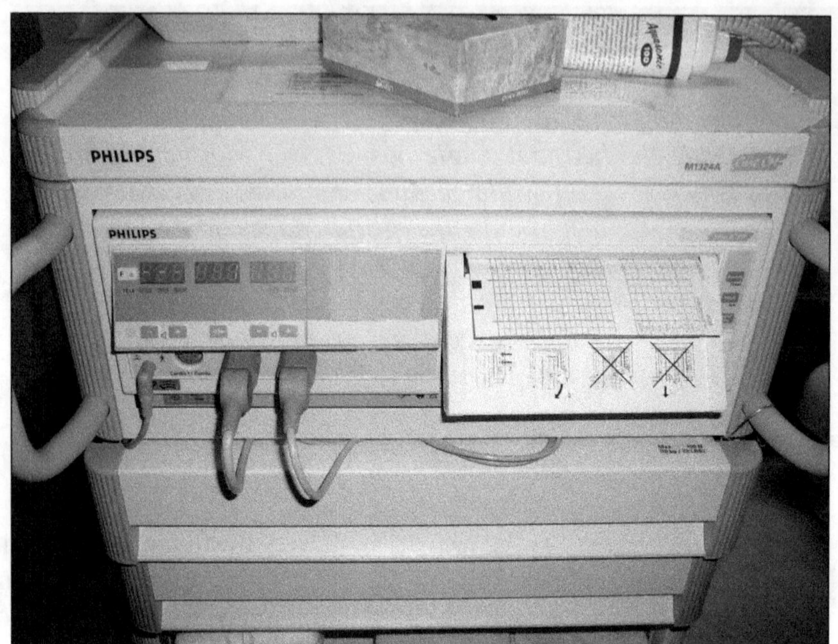

A fetal monitor.

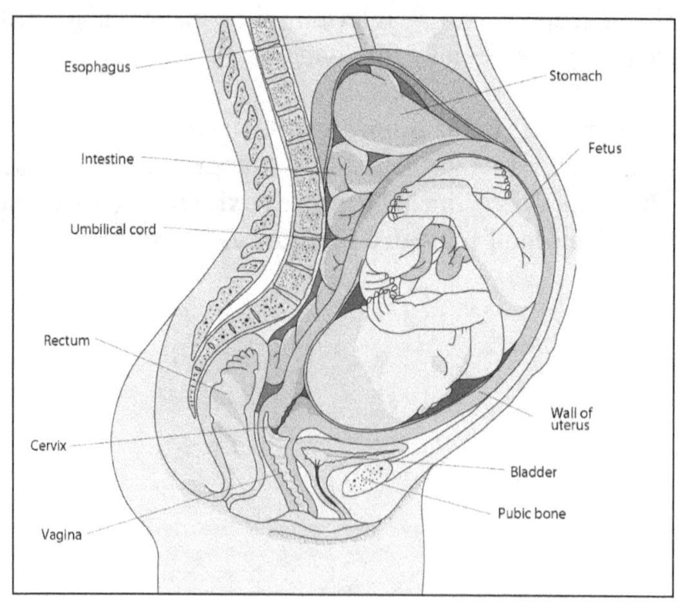

Anatomy of pregnancy… close to full term.
Modified from Shutterstock, Inc, www.shutterstock.com, with permission.

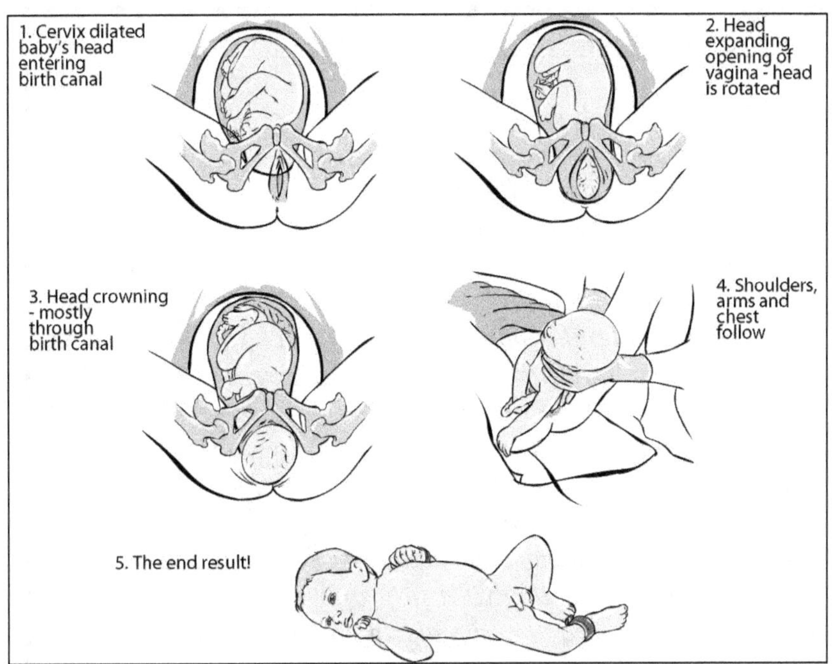

The birth process.

Modified from Shutterstock, Inc, www.shutterstock.com, with permission.

The Pregnant Woman – Angie – Maternity/Nursery III

Angie goes into labor at 3 am and her husband brings her to the hospital at 5. Because she was classified as "high risk" due to her gestational diabetes (which, among other things, often results in the baby being heavier than usual), she is connected to the ***fetal monitor (95)*** *as soon as she is settled. Women in labor often find it helpful to walk around some, so the staff used a* ***fetal monitor telemetry pack (31)*** *with Angie so that she can move about while the pack sends information via radio signals back to the monitor. The same ultrasound probe is connected as in her previous non-stress test, and another transducer is added. This tocotransducer is strapped around her abdomen and detects the rigidity of the surface, which increases during contractions. This gives the monitor a signal that can be analyzed to graph the relative strength of contractions, and the signals are recorded on the same paper as the baby's heart rate, so staff can see if there is any serious reduction in the heart rate corresponding to contractions, or to any other factors. Angie is experiencing considerable pain during contractions, so she is offered the use of a* ***nitrous oxide unit (109)****, consisting of a mask that fits over her nose and mouth, connected to a supply of nitrous oxide and oxygen. This accomplishes two goals: it helps ease some of the pain for Angie, and it also boosts her blood oxygen levels. This last factor was important, as staff had noted a worrisome drop in the baby's heart rate during contractions. A nurse brings in a vital signs monitor and set it to measure Angie's* ***blood pressure non-invasively (296)*** *every five minutes using an inflatable cuff around her upper arm. She also fits Angie's finger with a* ***pulse oximeter (320)*** *probe from the same monitor, which gives a display of her blood oxygen level as a percentage of maximum (SpO2) as well as a relative measure of how well blood is flowing through her finger (perfusion). Finally, her labor pays off and she and her husband are thrilled when their new baby girl finally makes an appearance and starts crying.*

The Newborn Baby – Cassie – Maternity/Nursery

After a quick cuddle with Mom and Dad, the new baby seems to be having a little trouble breathing, so she is placed in an ***infant care unit (105)*** *to make sure she's OK. The unit has gentle suction to clear airways and a tiny oxygen mask in case that is needed. There is a bright overhead light and infrared heating elements to keep baby warm and well illuminated. The unit also has an* ***APGAR timer (86)****, which gives a signal at pre-determined times so the baby's condition can be evaluated.*

APGAR Score - Following birth, the status of the infant may be evaluated at specific time intervals using the APGAR scoring method. Though named after its originator, Dr. Virginia Apgar, the term has been developed into an acronym for the five factors that are considered. Each factor is rated as either 0, 1 or 2 and the total gives a good indication of overall infant condition. The five factors are: A □activity, or muscle tone; P □ pulse presence and rate; G □ grimace, or reflex response; A □ appearance, mainly skin color; and R □ respiration quality. The total APGAR score can range from 0 to 10.

Baby Cassie is back with Angie, and all is well for the first day, but then Cassie develops jaundice and she is placed in an ***infant incubator (100)*** *for a while to stabilize her physically and allow for jaundice treatment using a* ***bilirubin therapy light (87)****. While she is in the incubator, her Mom uses a* ***breast pump (91)*** *to help collect her breast milk so that Cassie can continue to receive this special nourishment. The incubator has clear double walls and several access doors, and temperature and humidity are controlled. The incubator temperature can be set by staff to keep the inside air constant, or it can use a temperature probe taped to Cassie's skin to provide more or less heat depending on her body temperature. The bed of the incubator can be tilted to help make breathing easier, and oxygen can be added as well.*

The Newborn Baby – Cassie - continued

Too much or to little oxygen can cause problems, so the unit has an ***oxygen monitor (305)****. Nurses set the oxygen level desired and the system adds just enough oxygen to maintain that level. The fans that circulate warmed, humidified air are very quiet to protect Cassie's sensitive hearing. The clear top of the incubator allows ultraviolet light from* ***the bilirubin therapy light (87)*** *to fall on Cassie's skin, which can be mostly exposed in the warm incubator. Soon she is back to normal color and good health and is back with Mom and Dad.*

Some units connect a number of fetal monitors to a **central station (29)**, and they may also be equipped with **telemetry (31)** so that mother in labor can move around more freely. Hand□held **ultrasonic fetal heart detectors (93)** allow for quick checks of fetal status. Special devices, sometimes called **infant resuscitators (105)**, with radiant heating elements, lights, oxygen and suction, **APGAR timers (86)** and facilities for x□rays are available for newborns who are having some degree of difficulty following birth. **Infant incubators (100)** in the nursery area have Plexiglas walls that allow easy observation of the child inside while maintaining controlled levels of temperature, humidity and oxygen.

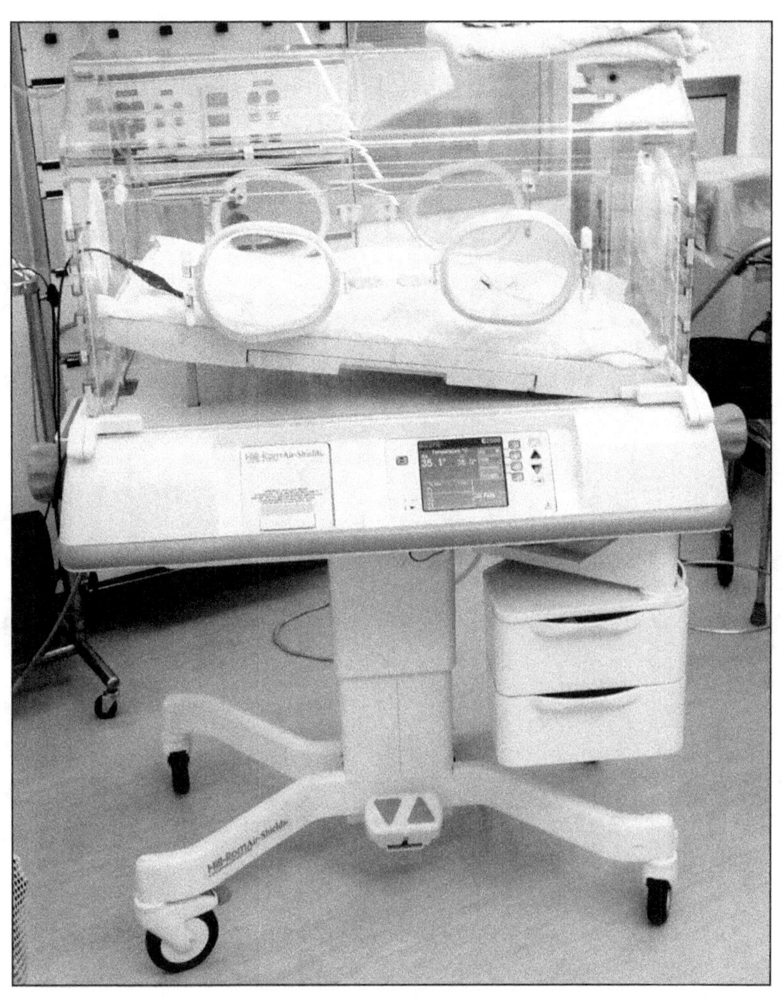

An infant incubator.

The incubators have access ports to allow for changing diapers or performing other procedures without allowing and significant amount of outside air into the unit. Some newborns have an excess of bilirubin in their system, and **UV therapy lamps (87)**, often referred to as bililights or phototherapy units, help to break down the bilirubin in the infant's skin. Bililights may consist of overhead or side mounted lamp fixtures, or they may utilize fiber optic technology to deliver UV light to the inside of a blanket placed around the baby. **Breast pumps (91)** are available for mothers who cannot directly breastfeed their babies but wish to provide them with their own breast milk. Special **birthing beds (89)** are equipped with electrical controls to adjust bed position in many configurations, as well as built□in stirrups to aid in birthing, and a removable centre foot section to allow access by the delivering physician or midwife.

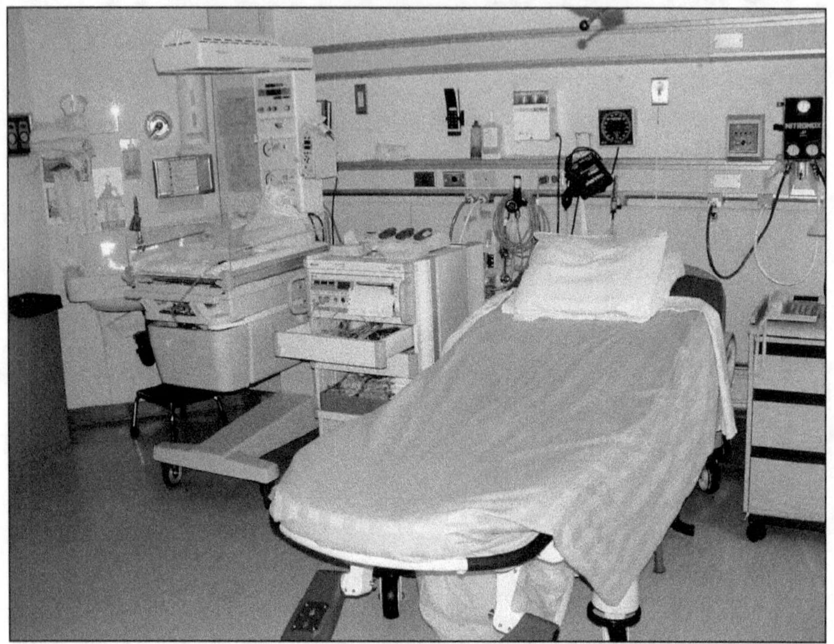

Another view of a labor–delivery room.

Security is often a special concern in maternity units, especially the nursery, and so security systems are often in place. These may consist of limited access doors, alarms, video camera and tags worn by babies that allow remote tracking. Such tags may trigger automatic alarms if they pass beyond certain boundaries.

Maternity Equipment Descriptions

Following are more detailed descriptions of equipment found exclusively or most commonly in this area of the hospital. Equipment that is also found in various other areas of the hospital is described in Chapter 12, p 247.

Devices typically found in maternity wards, in addition to the equipment listed in this section, include: **anesthetic machines (47)**, **aspirators (250)**, **defibrillators (259)** **electronic probe thermometers (279)**, **tympanic thermometers (332)**, **examination lamps (281)**, **gas regulators (285)**, **glucometers (287)**, **intravenous pumps (289)**, **non–invasive pressure monitors (296)**, **oxygen analyzers (305)**, **physiological monitors (314)**, **patient–controlled analgesia pumps (311)**, **point of care blood analysis systems (318)**, **pulse oximeters (320)**, **sphygmomanometers (325)** and **stethoscopes (327)**.

APGAR Timers

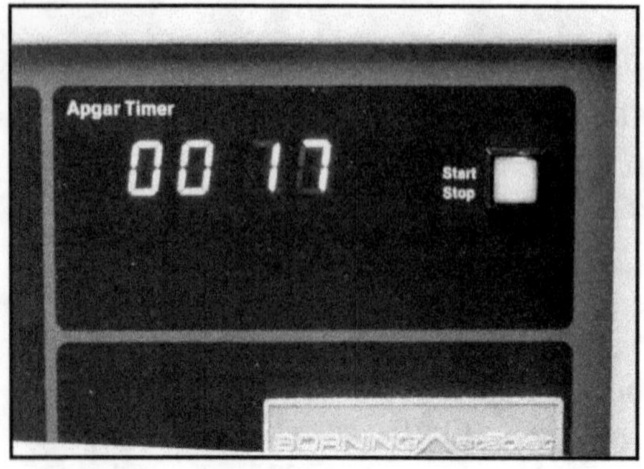

Overview □ The condition of newborns can be somewhat difficult to assess. To help in this, Dr. Virginia Apgar developed a set of tests to be performed at specific intervals postpartum, the results of which give a quantitative evaluation of health.

Function □ An Apgar timer is simply a device that prominently indicates the times for doing the tests, either audibly or visibly or both. It may be stand□alone or integrated into an infant resuscitation unit.

The observations are made at one, five, and ten minutes after birth, and the tests can be listed using the name Apgar as a Mnemonic: Appearance (color); Pulse (heartbeat); Grimace (reflex); Activity (muscle tone); and Respiration (breathing). Each parameter is rated as 0, 1, or 2 (with 2 being highest) and the scores are added to give a total score at each time. A score of seven or more (out of a possible ten) indicates that the baby is in good condition.

Application □ The timer is started when the infant is under observation. The specified parameters are observed and recorded at the times indicated, and the scores are totalled for each time.

AKA □(none).

Related devices □**infant resuscitators (105)**.

Where found □labor and delivery rooms.

Bilirubin Therapy Systems

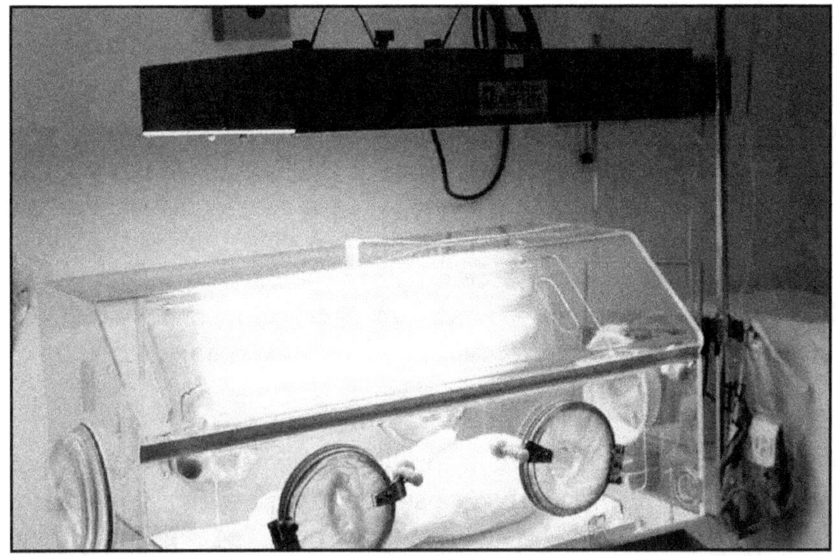

Overview Newborns sometimes have an excess of bilirubin in their system, which causes a jaundiced appearance (yellowish skin.) It is desirable to reduce these levels, and the simplest method of doing so is to expose the skin to ultraviolet (UV) light, which causes the bilirubin to break down.

Function Bilirubin therapy systems are simply light sources that produce ultraviolet light of the optimum wavelength and intensity. Too much exposure can cause burns, while too little is ineffective. Some systems use overhead fluorescent lamps that are designed to emit the correct type and amount of UV light. Several factors affect the amount of exposure the baby receives, such as the skin surface available, material such as the Plexiglas of an **incubator (100)** between the light source and the infant, the distance between the light and the baby, and the age and condition of the bulbs. Because of these variables, it is important that the UV levels *at the baby's skin* be measured at the start of treatment, and at intervals if the treatment time is prolonged. In order to prevent excessive exposure, it is also desirable that a timer mechanism be used to either cut off the UV light after a predetermined time or to remind staff to turn the light off. Overhead systems often have a tape measure built in to aid in placing the light at the correct distance from the baby. Since the lights produce some heat, and also because much of the baby's skin is exposed to facilitate treatment, it is important to monitor the baby□s body temperature during treatment.

Another type of bilirubin therapy system avoids some of the problems associated with overhead lamp types. This method uses a □blanket□ of material in which fiber optic strands are embedded. These strands carry UV light from a central source and distribute it evenly, so that the baby□s skin is exposed to a consistent illumination wherever it is covered by the blanket. The factors of distance and of intervening materials are eliminated, and the light sources used tend to be more stable than fluorescent bulbs. The blanket system is also smaller and less cumbersome than an overheard lamp system. Of course, output levels must be checked regularly and exposure times limited.

Application □ After determining the desired exposure, the lamps or blanket are put into the correct position, treatment time is selected, and the light turned on. The infant must be observed regularly during treatment.

AKA □bililights, UV lights.

Related devices □ **infant incubators (100)**, **electronic probe thermometers (279)**.

Where found □nurseries, pediatric wards.

Birthing Beds

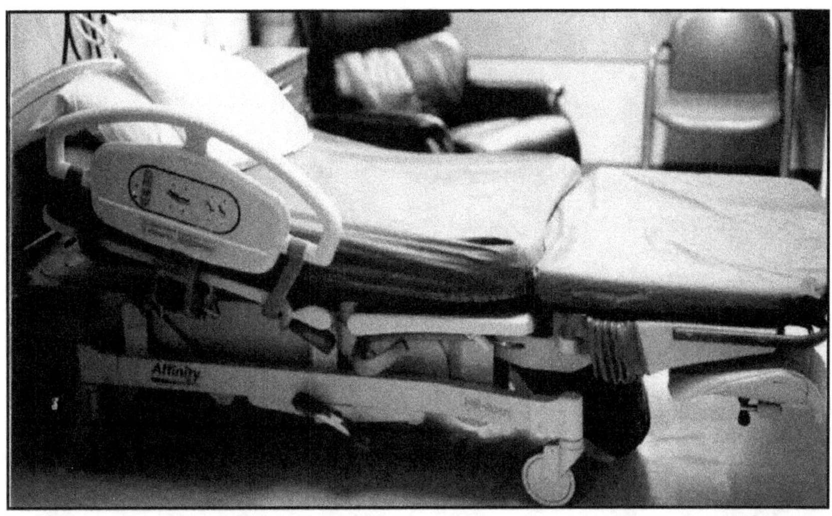

Overview □During the process of labor and birth, it is important that the mother is as comfortable as possible, and that she be able to get into a good position for delivery. It is also important that the attending health care personnel are able to access the mother and baby both before and during delivery. Birthing beds are designed to meet these needs.

Function □Birthing beds consist of a comfortable, flexible mattress, and a frame and mechanism that allow for a variety of maternal positions. Controls activate motors that raise or lower the whole bed, the head, the feet, and the hips independently (within ergonomic limits); these controls are usually placed both on a pendant or stalk so that the patient or a bedside attendant can use them, and at the foot of the bed for attendant control. Sometimes duplicate controls are on the bed rails on either side of the mattress.

Beds usually have a removable section at the foot to allow caregivers to get close to the birth canal in order to assist in delivery. They generally have channels for optional placement of stirrups, if they will be useful in birthing. As with most hospital beds, the whole unit is on wheels, which can be locked to prevent movement if necessary. Rails on either side of the bed can be raised or lowered, often in multiple positions, to help prevent the patient from falling out of bed.

The mattress is covered with an impermeable material to aid in cleaning.

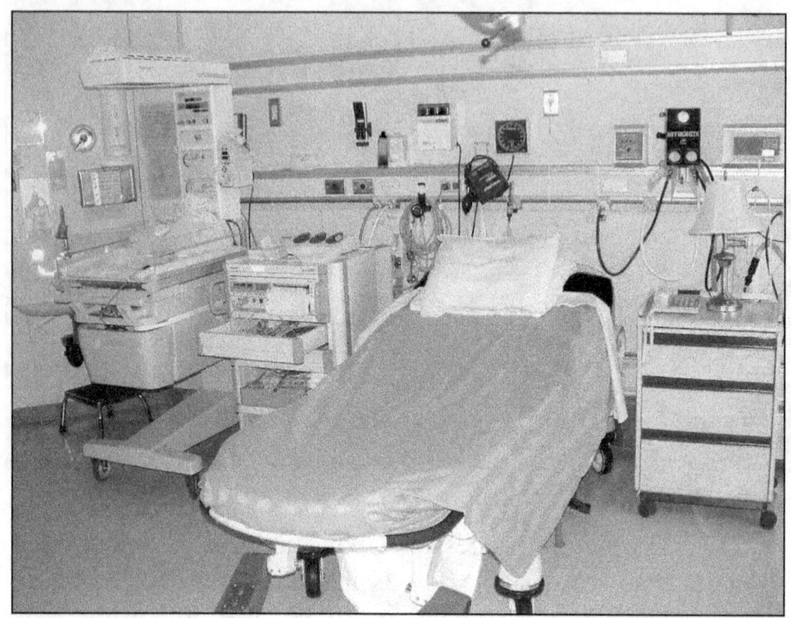

A birthing bed, with fetal monitor (95) to the near left and infant resuscitator (105) to the far left.

<u>Application</u> □ Patients are made comfortable in the bed and shown how to operate the controls. Adjustments are made by the patient, a companion, or a caregiver to suit the needs of the patient. When delivery time approaches, the section at the foot of the bed may be removed to allow attendants access to assist in delivery.

<u>AKA</u> □(none).

<u>Related devices</u> □**electric hospital beds (277)**.

<u>Where found</u> □maternity ward.

Breast Pumps

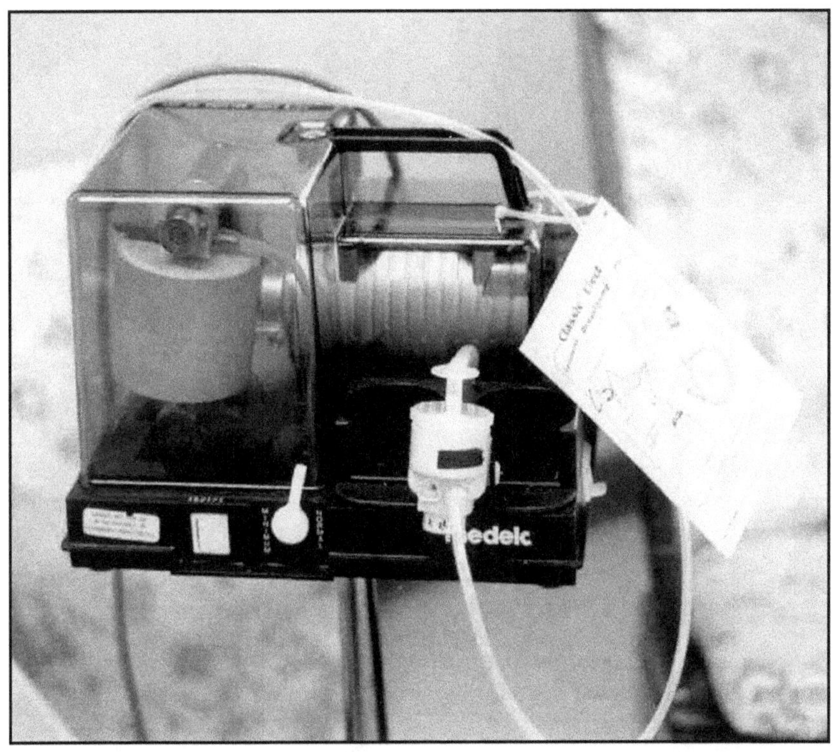

Overview — In certain circumstances, infants may need mother's milk at times when it isn't possible for the mother to nurse, such as when the infant is in an intensive care incubator.

Function — Breast pumps provide a means of extracting mother's milk so that it can be stored for later use.

These range from simple devices consisting of a suction bulb attached to a collecting cup and reservoir, to somewhat more complex units with electrical pumps. The electric-powered versions usually have controls to vary the rate and/or intensity of suction. Suction levels are limited so that undue discomfort to the mother is avoided. A rhythmic action, with periods of suction alternating with no suction seems to work best, as this simulates a baby nursing. The collecting cup and reservoir are similar in all systems, with a cup designed to give a comfortable but snug fit to the mother□s breast and a reservoir that allows the user to see exactly how much milk has been collected.

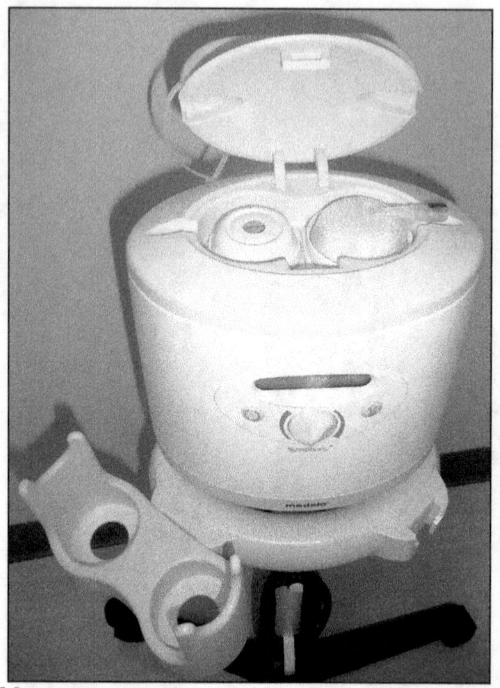

A newer model breast pump. A cartridge fits in the top and is actuated by pistons. Milk is collected in containers that fit into the bracket on the left.

Application □ The collecting cup is applied to the mother□s breast, positioned so that the drainage channel is over the nipple, and the pumping action is initiated. With adjustable units, the rate and intensity are modified to give a balance between comfort and optimal milk extraction. Milk that is not to be used immediately is refrigerated.

AKA □(none).

Related devices □**infant incubators (100)**.

Where found □infant nurseries.

Doppler Fetal Heart Detectors

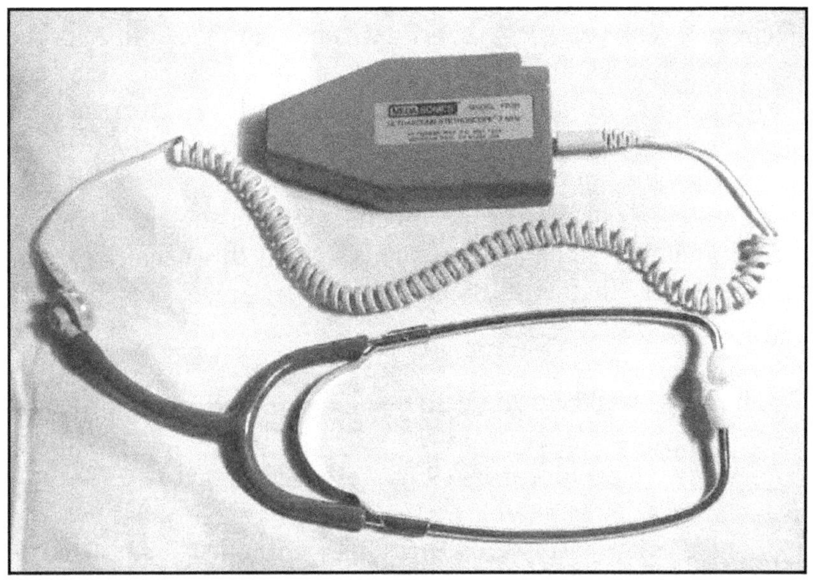

Overview □ An important part of prenatal care involves determining the strength and rate of the fetus□heartbeat. This can be done with a stethoscope, but the sounds are often faint, especially earlier in pregnancy, and can be obscured by other sounds from within the mother□s abdomen. Doppler probes are more effective for this purpose.

Function □ These probes utilize the Doppler Principle, which is that sound waves from a moving source are changed in frequency when the source is moving toward or away from the observer. In this case, sound waves are produced by an ultrasonic probe placed on the mother□s abdomen and reflected from the baby□s heart. When part of the heart tissue is moving away from the probe, the reflected wave frequency decreases; when moving toward the probe, the frequency increases. The reflected signals are picked up by the probe, and processed in such a way as to produce a sound. The sound is played on a speaker or headphones, and the heart rate and strength can be determined. Some units include a digital readout of heart rate.

Application □ A probe is selected, and ultrasound gel is applied to the face, which is then placed in contact with the mother's abdomen.

Power is applied and adjusted as necessary, and the operator scans the beam to locate the fetal heart. When the appropriate signal is heard, position is optimized and the fetal heart□beat is evaluated.

This technique can be very sensitive, and can pick up a fetal heartbeat very early in pregnancy. It requires some skill and patience, however, as the target, especially early in term, can be difficult to locate.

It is possible to focus the probe on the mother□s aortic artery, in which case a similar sound is produced; though this usually gives a much lower rate than the fetal heart, care must be take to differentiate the two.

AKA □doptones, fetal heart detectors.

Related devices □**fetal monitors (95)**, **stethoscopes (327)**.

Where found □ maternity wards, maternity outpatient clinics, home visit medical kits.

Fetal Monitors

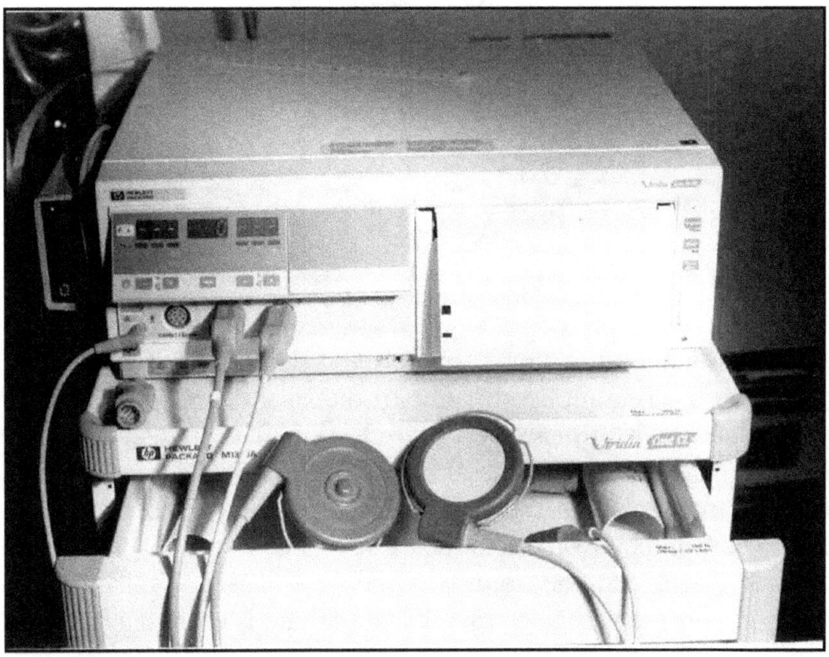

Overview □ The time of labor and delivery is critical for the baby, and it can be very useful to be able to monitor its condition, particularly its heart rate. This can be done on a short□term basis with a **stethoscope (327)** or **Doppler unit (93)**, but for longer□term monitoring, a fetal monitor is preferred. Fetal monitors can also measure and record other parameters.

Function □ Fetal heart rate is picked up in one of two ways. Most commonly, a special transducer is placed on the mother□s abdomen. This transducer has several crystals, which produce a beam of ultrasound.

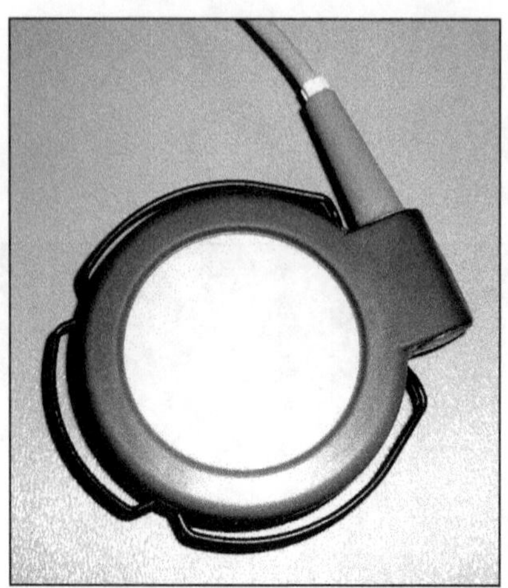

Fetal monitor ultrasound transducer.

The beam is focused at approximately the depth of the fetal heart. When it hits the beating heart, some of the signal is bounced back to the transducer, which picks up this reflection. The frequency of the reflected signal varies as the fetal heart moves in its beating, and this change in frequency can be processed and analyzed to produce a signal corresponding to the fetal heart beat. The rate is displayed as a numerical value, and the sound of the beat is also available at a speaker so that the caregiver can hear if the rate is changing, or if the beam is no longer focused on the baby's heart. The signal is also recorded on a graph chart, which allows caregivers to see trends in the rate over time. In order to allow maximum transmission of the ultrasonic signal, a gel is placed between the transducer and the mother's skin. The transducer is usually held in place by an adjustable elastic belt.

The ultrasound transducer is quick and easy to apply and can give very valuable information. However, it can lose the signal through movements of either the fetus or the mother.

The second method of picking up the fetal heart rate is through an electrode. A curved section of fine silver wire is inserted through the vagina and pierces the surface of the fetal scalp. A second plate electrode on the mother's skin provides a reference, and electronic circuitry can pick up the electrical signals of the baby's heart. This ECG signal is somewhat more stable that that from an ultrasonic transducer, but it requires that the fetus be in the head-down position and that dilation is sufficient to allow placement. The electrical ECG signal can also provide certain information not available with the ultrasound signal. The ECG signal is used to display a numerical value and tone, as well as record on a chart, just as with the ultrasound signal.

Another function of the fetal monitor is to measure the relative strength of uterine contractions. This is important since the fetus is most likely to be distressed during contractions. The uterine contractions are measured by a transducer disk (called a tocograph, or TOCO, transducer) that presses a central tab against the mother's abdomen. During a contraction, the muscles in the uterus become much harder, and the disk is pushed back into the transducer. These variations are measured and processed to produce a graph of relative contraction strength, which is displayed as a numerical value on the monitor, and is also graphed on the same chart as the fetal heart rate. This allows a good correlation to be made between contractions and any possible fetal distress.

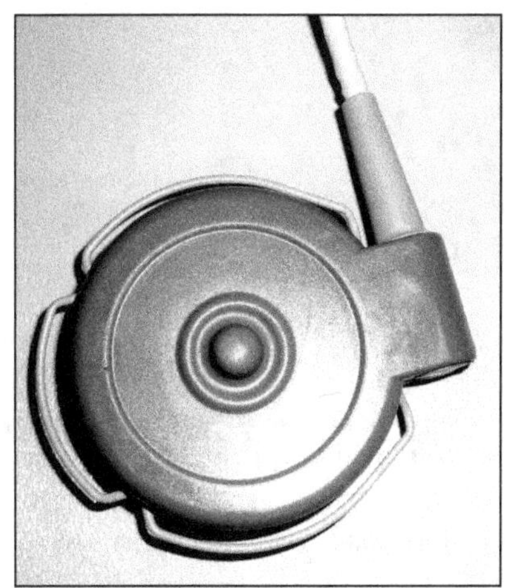

Fetal monitor toco transducer.

Some fetal monitors also measure maternal blood oxygen saturation (SpO2), as low oxygen levels can be very harmful to the fetus.
Another option for a monitor is the ability to handle twins; this simply requires a second, independent ultrasound portion, one for each fetus. Graphs are both on the same chart.

Some fetal monitoring systems have telemetry, with which the transducers are plugged into a small, battery-powered transmitter. The transmitter sends the signals back to the monitor; this has the benefit of allowing the mother to walk around.

Application □Ultrasound gel is applied to the ultrasound transducer, positioned to give the best fetal heart signal; if a scalp electrode is used instead of ultrasound, the electrode lead is inserted via the mother's vagina and attached to the fetal scalp. In either method, once a suitable signal is obtained, the transducer and cables are secured. The TOCO transducer is then applied and secured, and electronically zeroed while between contractions. If the unit has SpO2 capability, this transducer is usually placed on the mother's finger. All signals are checked and adjusted as necessary, and the chart recorder is started.

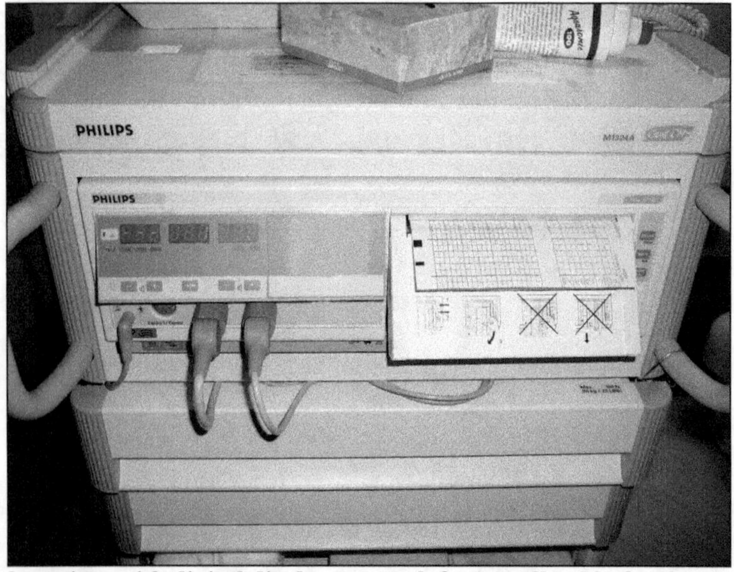

Fetal monitor with digital displays at top left, a small cable for the patient marker button at lower left beside the two larger cables for ultrasound and toco. The chart recorder is on the right.

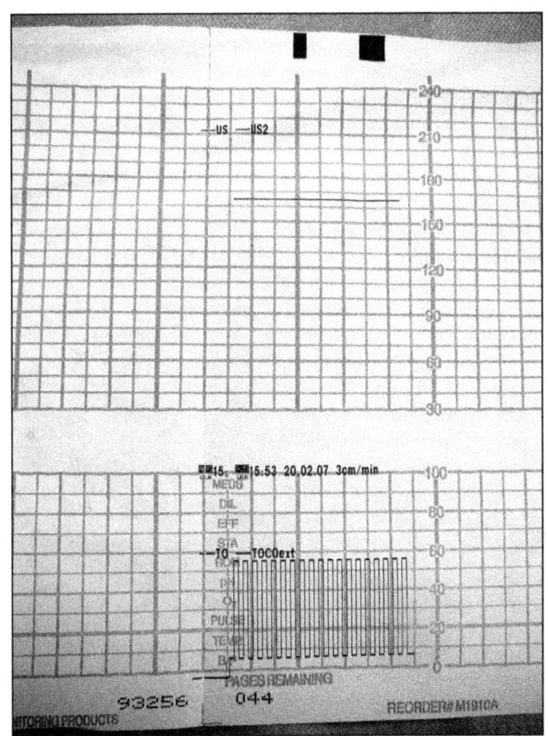

Fetal monitor chart recording, with fetal ECG rate on the top portion and relative contraction strength (toco) on the bottom.

<u>AKA</u> □(none).

<u>Related devices</u> □ **pulse oximeters (320)**, **ECG machines (270)**, **Doppler units (93)**, **stethoscopes (327)**.

<u>Where found</u> □maternity wards.

Infant Incubators

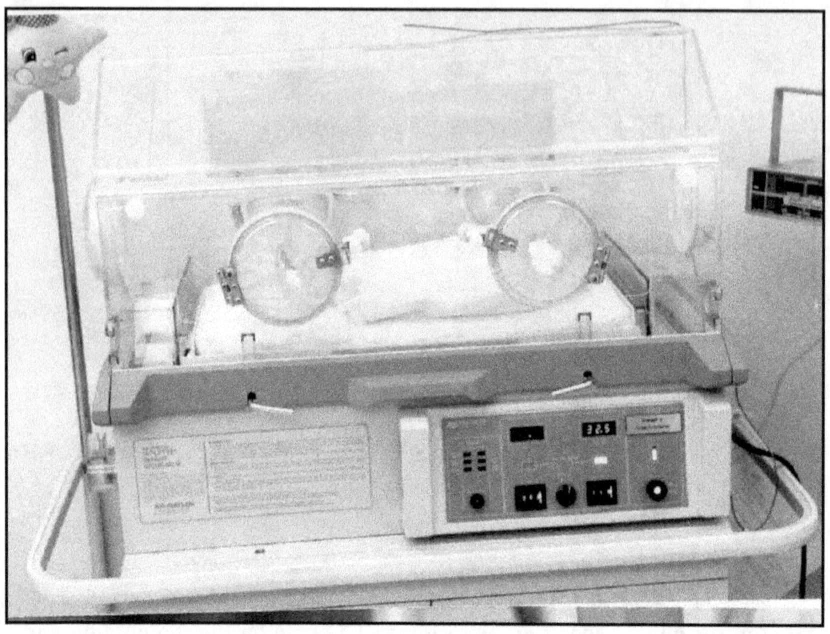

Overview □ Newborns, especially if they are premature, need an environment in which factors such as temperature and humidity are controlled, and in which they are easily observable. Caregivers must be able to access the infant to change diapers, administer medication, feed, and simply provide physical contact, preferably without disturbing the controlled environment.

Function □Infant incubators are made up of a clear plastic chamber, electronic and mechanical systems to monitor and control the environment, and a stand to bring the chamber up to a comfortable working height. The stand is usually on lockable wheels and has storage compartments for diapers and other supplies.

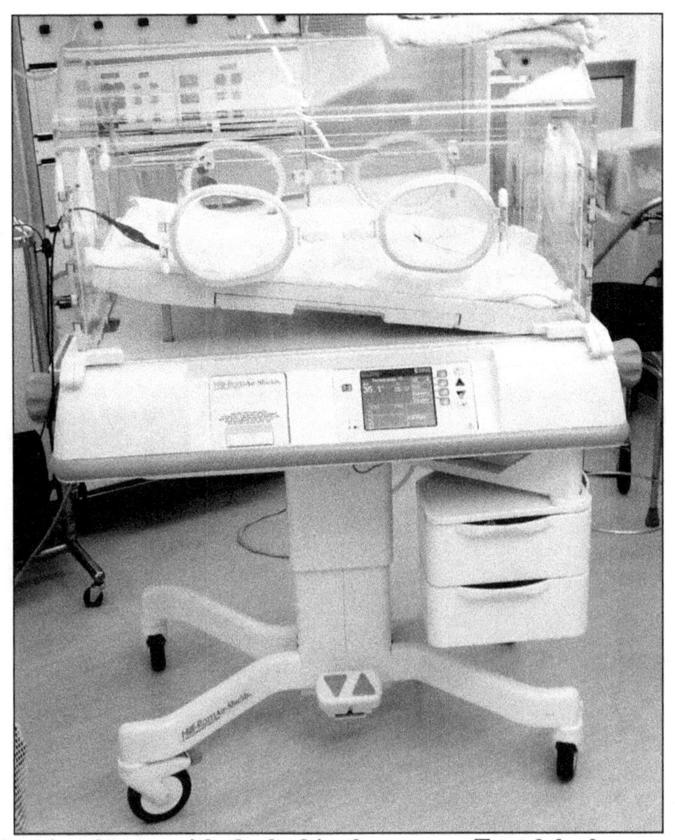

An infant incubator, with the bed in the reverse Trendelenburg position.

The plastic chamber is designed to give maximum visibility from various angles while providing reasonable insulation from exterior conditions and access to the infant. There is a larger hatch for moving the infant in and out of the incubator when necessary, and also several "portholes" with flexible sleeves to allow caregivers to reach in to the baby, with minimal air leakage. The portholes are usually covered by a clear door when not in use. The outer wall of the chamber may be double layered to provide better insulation and also to control air flow; warm air may be directed between the outer layers and distributed into the interior at several points for more even heating. The chamber material must be strong enough for safety, but it must also be very clear for visibility, and allow penetration of ultraviolet rays for **bilirubin therapy (87)**, if that is needed.

Temperature is the most critical environmental parameter to be controlled in an incubator. Newborns are often unstable in their internal temperature control; being small, and often having little body fat, their temperature can change quickly. It is important, though, for caregivers to be able to see as much of the infant's skin as possible, to watch for changes in color and texture, which may indicate problems. Skin surface exposure is also important for bilirubin therapy.

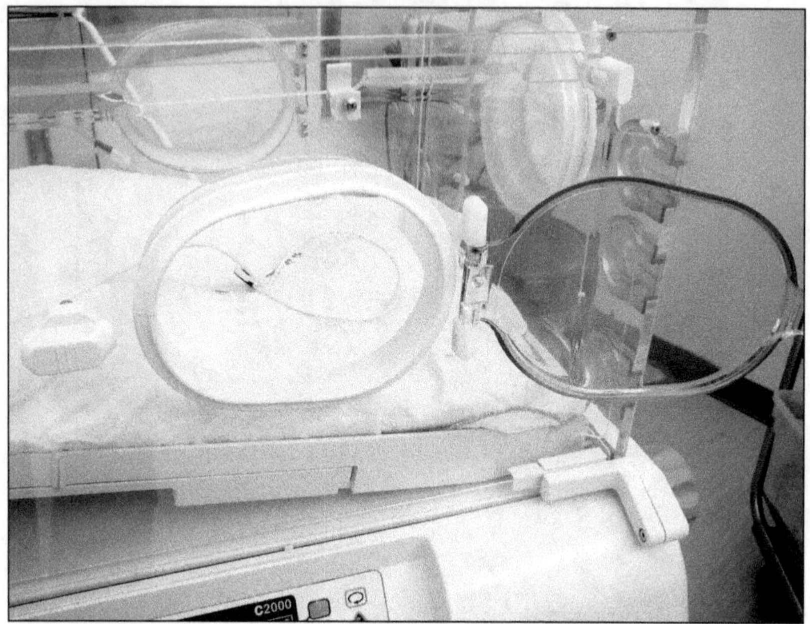

Incubator access door. A pulse oximeter (320) probe is visible through the door.

Temperature may be controlled in one of two ways. Most commonly, a sensor measures air temperature; then, the output of the internal heater is adjusted after comparing the measured temperature to the desired temperature set by the caregiver. This sensor may be built into the unit, at some point in the airflow, or it may be a plug□in type with the actual temperature pickup suspended in the air above the infant.

The second method of temperature control involves placing a **temperature sensor (279)** directly on the baby□s skin. Again, this measurement is compared to the desired temperature set by the caregiver, and heat output is adjusted accordingly. To be effective, this method requires that the sensor be placed carefully; limb temperatures may vary considerably from torso temperature; the sensor must not be covered, and it must not interfere with treatments. Additionally, the adhesive used may irritate the baby□s skin, and the sensor and wire may hinder removal of the baby for feeding, bathing, cuddling, or treatment outside the incubator. Given these considerations, incubators may not have skin temperature monitoring/control.

Temperature measurements are displayed on a front panel, which also shows the settings for desired temperature. There are alarms for over and under temperature, and usually a redundant high temperature alarm set somewhat above the primary high temperature alarm. Alarms are usually visual and audible.

Humidity control is usually simple, with a supply of sterile distilled water being placed in the airflow so that some of it can evaporate. Care must be taken to keep the water reservoir clean, as bacteria or fungi may grow in it, with potentially harmful effects.

Air must be filtered to remove as much dust as possible, and these filters must be changed regularly.

Incubators normally have a port by which oxygen can be added to the interior air. Since oxygen levels must be high enough to be effective but not so high as to cause problems with infant retinal development, the oxygen concentration in the incubator should be **monitored (305)** and alarmed.

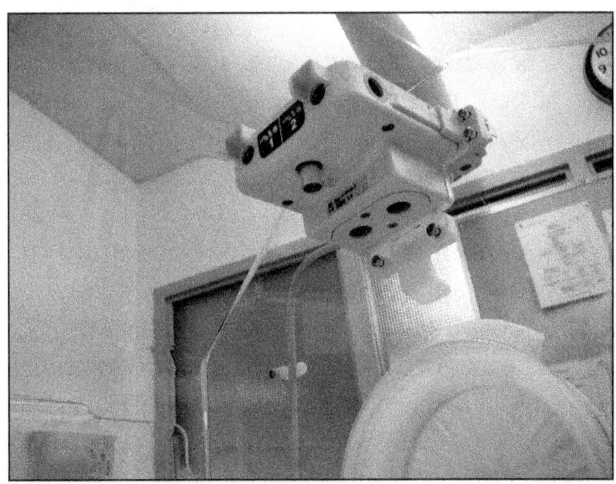

Dual oxygen sensors (305) inside the incubator, viewed from below.

It is important that air be well circulated within the incubator to maintain even and controlled heat. A fan, usually located near the heating element, accomplishes this. Because of the many hard surfaces within the incubator chamber, and because infants have sensitive hearing, fan noise must be designed to be as low as possible. Also, since proper air flow is critical, most incubators have some kind of detector that will initiate an alarm if air flow is lower than normal.

Some units have a built□in **scale (108)** so that the infant□s weight can be tracked.

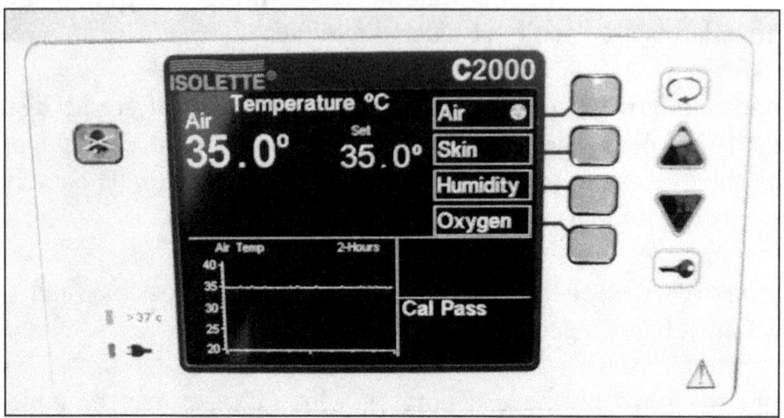

Incubator control and display panel.

Finally, since incubator function is critical, most have a power failure alarm, so that staff can respond appropriately if power is interrupted.

Application □ When the unit has warmed to the desired temperature, the infant is placed in the incubator in a safe and comfortable position, usually with only a diaper on. Oxygen is adjusted if needed (and an **oxygen analyzer (305)** is used to check concentration levels) and humidity checked. If the unit is to be used in the infant skin temperature control mode, a sensor is placed on the baby's skin and connected to the appropriate socket. If ultraviolet therapy lights are to be used, they are placed at the appropriate height and checked for output. Ports and doors are closed to allow conditions to stabilize.

AKA □ incubators, care□ettes.

Related devices □ **oxygen analyzers (305)**, **infant resuscitators (105)**, **bilirubin therapy units (87)**.

Where found □ maternity wards, nurseries, pediatric wards.

Infant Resuscitators

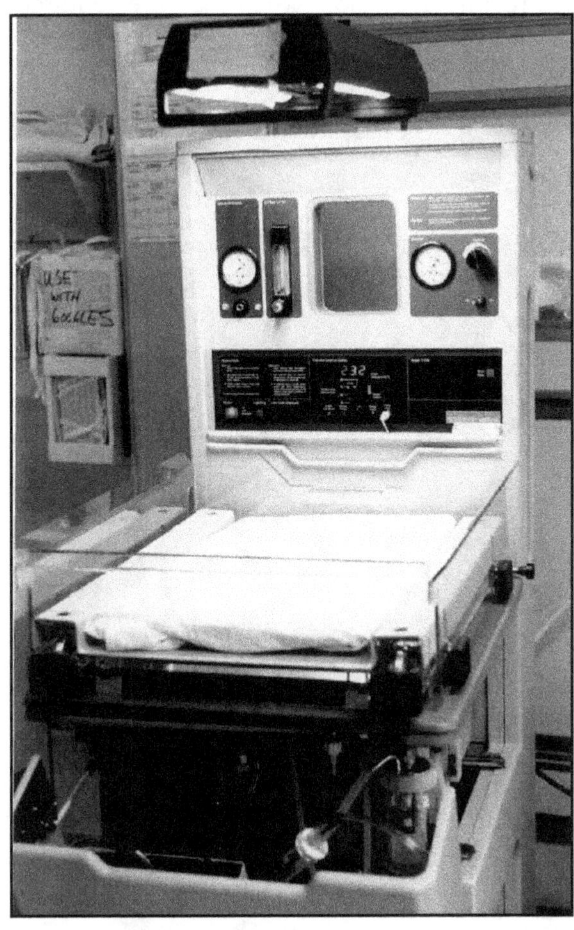

Overview □The immediate postpartum period is critical for infants at risk, and effective aids to intervention must be directly available and easily applied. Infant resuscitators were developed to meet this need.

Function □Infant resuscitators consist of various components integrated into a single unit. There is a bed surface for the baby at a comfortable working height; this area usually has sidewalls, generally made of a clear plastic material for increased ease of observation, and to keep the baby in place. The sidewalls can be lowered or swung down for access, and are often marked in centimeters for approximate measurements of the infant. The bed surface usually has a chamber underneath to hold x□ray film cassettes. This means that the surface must be made of materials that are transparent to x□rays.

An overhead module provides bright lighting and radiant heating. The heating can often be controlled by a **sensor (279)** on the baby□s skin, so that a relatively constant body temperature is maintained even though most or all of the baby□s body is uncovered. The overhead module is on a pivot so it can be swung out of the way when x□ray or other apparatus is being used.

The system has both **oxygen and suction (285)** available to be used on the baby if needed; they are located so that they are out of the way when not needed, but readily accessible when they are required. There are indicators associated with these functions to show pressures and flow rates.

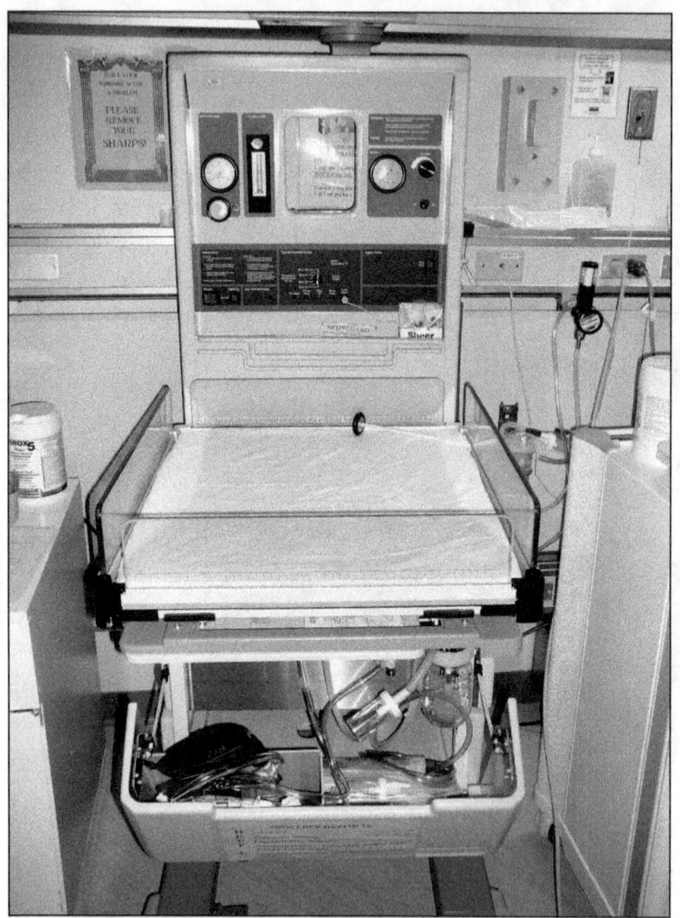

Another model of resuscitator.

As part of the evaluation of the infant's condition, an APGAR test is usually performed: a set of observations performed at specific intervals. A **timer (86)** with visual and audible timing signals is often built into the resuscitator.

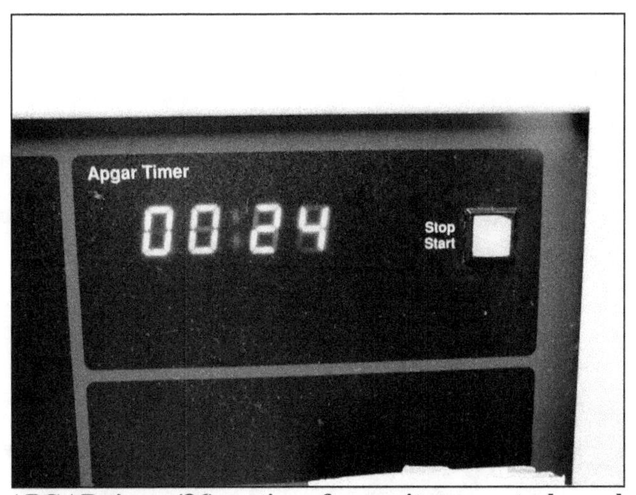

APGAR timer (86) section of resuscitator control panel.

Application The infant is placed on the resuscitator mattress and care is administered as required.

AKA neonatal intensive care unit, NIC, Kreiselman (after an early manufacturer).

Related devices **infant incubators (100)**, **Apgar timers (86), gas regulators (285), aspirators (250), mobile C–arm x–ray units (212).**

Where found labor/delivery areas.

Infant Scales

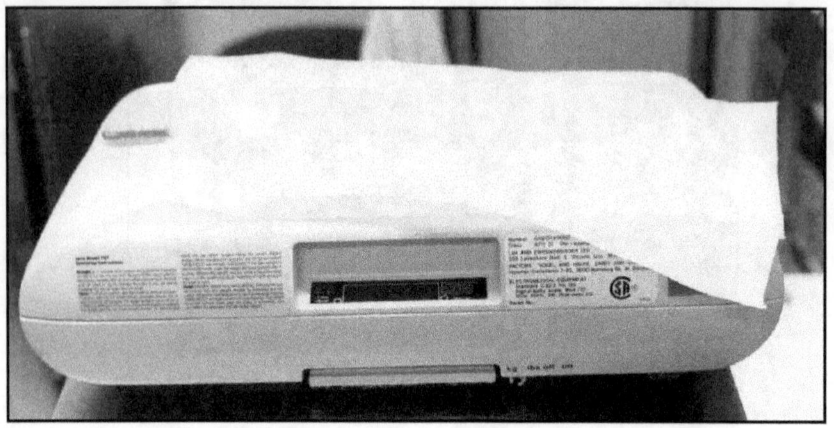

Overview □ It is vital to keep track of the weight of newborns in order to monitor their progress. Infant scales are basically simple scales but with a few important differences.

Function □ Because babies might be moving vigorously, the scale must have sides to keep the baby in place. The scale, whether mechanical or electronic, must have some capacity to even out variations in readings caused by movements. There must be a □tare□ provision to allow for subtraction of the weight of diapers or blankets, and ideally, there should be a □hold□ function to lock in a measurement when it is stable so it can be recorded later. Electronic scales usually have a switch to change between grams and pounds/ounces, and a large digital read□out.

Infant scales may be built in to **infant incubators (100)**.

Application □ The infant is placed safely on the scale□s weighing compartment. When a stable measurement is obtained, the value is recorded.

AKA □(none).

Related devices □**Infant incubators (100)**.

Where found □ nurseries, pediatric wards, emergency rooms, outpatient clinics.

Nitrous Oxide Units

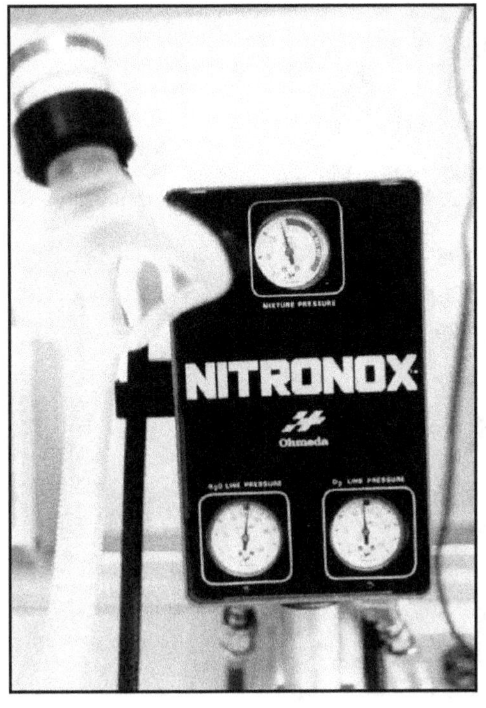

Overview – Nitrous oxide ("laughing gas") is sometimes administered to patients who are experiencing relatively short-term pain, such as during minor surgery, dental procedures, or childbirth.

Function – Devices to provide safe and effective doses are generally simple, consisting of a source (either a central supply with a wall outlet, or a portable high-pressure tank), a **regulator (285)** and gauge, a mixer to add air or oxygen to the nitrous oxide gas, a flow meter, a hose to carry the mixture to the patient, a mask to fit over the patient's nose and mouth, and a valve to open the line and deliver a dose to the patient. The valve may be manually operated, by either the patient or a caregiver, or it may be a "demand" type that opens every time the patient breathes in.

Safety mechanisms include an alarm that sounds if either the nitrous oxide or air/oxygen pressures fall too low, and over-pressure valves to guard against failures that might deliver excessively high pressures to the patient.

Application – When required, a mask is placed over the patient's nose and mouth. Oxygen and nitrous pressures are checked, and the main valve is opened. Depending on the design, the patient may receive a dose continuously, at each breath, or when a button is pressed. Patients must be monitored carefully when using nitrous oxide to avoid over-exposure and to check for possible side effects.

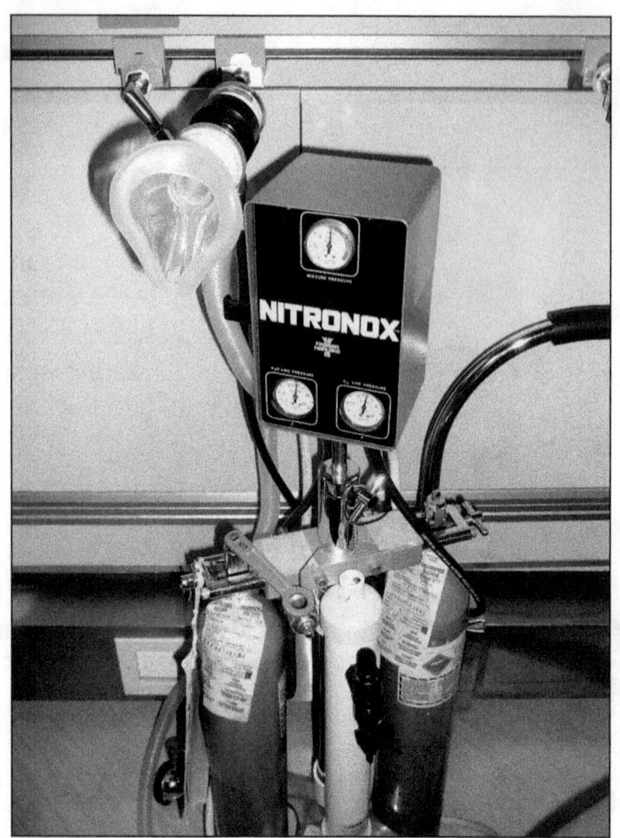

Nitrous oxide unit on stand.

AKA □Nitronox (after a common model), nitrous.

Related devices □**anesthetic machines (47), gas regulators (285)**.

Where found □labor/delivery areas, outpatient clinics, dental clinics.

Chapter 5 – Eye Clinic

- Function □ Provides treatment for patients with ophthalmic (eye) conditions such as cataracts, detached retinas and macular degeneration.

- Layout □ Clinics generally have a relatively large waiting area, as many procedures done in the unit are performed on an outpatient basis, and as they usually affect the patient□s vision, a family member or friend needs to accompany the patient when they are discharged. One or more relatively small procedure rooms are nearby, as is a nursing station and offices. The waiting area may double as a recovery area for patients to rest after procedures until they are ready to go home.

- Staff □ The eye clinic is staffed by one or more ophthalmologists, pre□and post□procedure nurses, nurses to assist the ophthalmologists with procedures, an admitting clerk and other support staff.

- Equipment □**Non–invasive blood pressure monitors (296), pulse oximeters (320), operating microscopes (68), ophthalmic lasers (299)** and **phacoemulsifiers (115)**.

The Eyes Have It – Martin – Eye Clinic

Martin has been having difficulty with his vision for some time, so he is not surprised when, following examinations including one with a ***slit-lamp unit (322)****, his Ophthalmologist informs him that he has cataracts, a cloudiness of the lenses in his eyes. Once a sentence for a long decline into blindness, cataracts are now routinely treated and good vision restored. Martin is scheduled for lens replacement surgery on a day-care basis.*

The Eyes Have It – Martin – continued

On the day of his procedure, a nurse establishes an IV line, and a saline solution is administered under the control on an ***IV pump (289)****. A* ***non-invasive blood pressure (296)*** *cuff is fitted to his upper left arm, and a* ***pulse oximeter (320)*** *probe is attached to a fingertip on his right hand. These are both connected to a small* ***vital signs monitor (338)*** *that is mounted on a wheeled stand.*

His signs normal, Martin is taken into the procedure room where he is positioned on a firm table. A sedative has been injected into the IV line to help him relax, though he remains conscious. Glancing around the room, he can see a large device with articulated arms and various attachments. This is the ***operating microscope (68)*** *that the surgeon will look through while performing the procedure.*

Nearby is a large console with a video screen on top and a tall pole with a fluid container at the top. The ***phacoemulsifier machine (115)*** *will be used to break up and remove the old lens so that a new, plastic one can be inserted. There is also a large video monitor mounted on the wall with a video recorder underneath. The monitor will display the images that the doctor sees through the operating microscope.*

Once Martin is in position, the surgeon moves the microscope head so he has a view of the eye to be operated on, and he uses a foot switch to adjust focus, magnification, illumination and fine positioning. He uses a scalpel to make a very small incision in the side of Martin's eye and inserts the phaco probe. The tip of the probe produces ultrasonic vibrations which, when in contact with the lens, cause the hardened material to break up into small particles.

The Eyes Have It – Martin – continued

Channels in the phaco tip both suction out the particles and also inject special fluid to maintain proper pressure with the eye. The phaco machine performs all of these functions under control of another footswitch. Once all of the old lens material has been removed, the surgeon inserts a rolled-up plastic lens into Martin's eye and lets it unfurl, making sure it is in the correct position. The phaco tip is then withdrawn from the eye, the whole procedure only having taken fifteen minutes.

Due to the small size of the incision and the nature of the tissue involved, no sutures are needed and the incision heals quickly. Martin must wear an eye shield when he sleeps and place drops in his eyes for a few weeks following surgery. He is advised to avoid various activities that could place strain on the surgical area, but after a week or so he can resume normal activities, with much improved vision.

Feeling much more confident about the whole process, Martin looks forward to having the other eye done in a few weeks.

Eye Clinic Equipment Descriptions

Following are more detailed descriptions of equipment found exclusively or most commonly in this area of the hospital. Equipment that is also found in various other areas of the hospital is described in Chapter 12, p 247.

Phacoemulsifiers

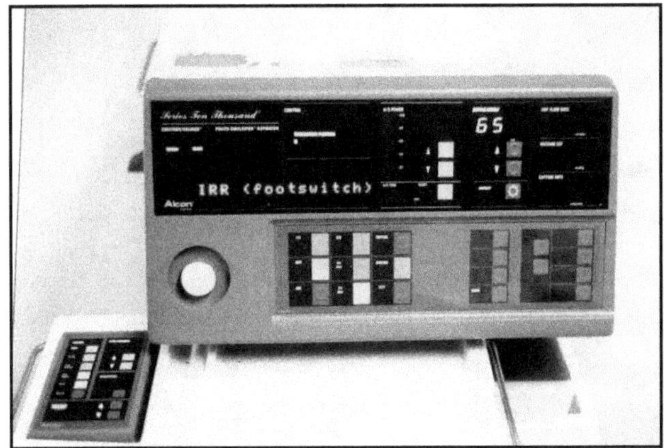

Overview □ Cataract surgery is performed often, and the techniques of removing the clouded natural lens from the eye and replacing it with an artificial one are finely tuned. One aspect of the procedure, that of removing the old lens, is aided by a specialized device called a phacoemulsifier.

A primary objective in surgery is to minimize trauma, and to this end, incisions are kept as small as possible. This is especially true for ophthalmic surgery, but the ideal incision size does not allow for removal of the lens in one piece during cataract surgery.

Function □ The phacoemulsifier aids in this step by breaking the lens material into very small pieces (emulsifying it) and extracting the resulting product. A fine tip delivers very□high□frequency vibrations that break up the solid lens material; a parallel duct then applies suction to the area, removing the lens particles, while a second duct supplies irrigation fluid as required. Some units utilize a specially□ tuned laser beam to break up the lens.

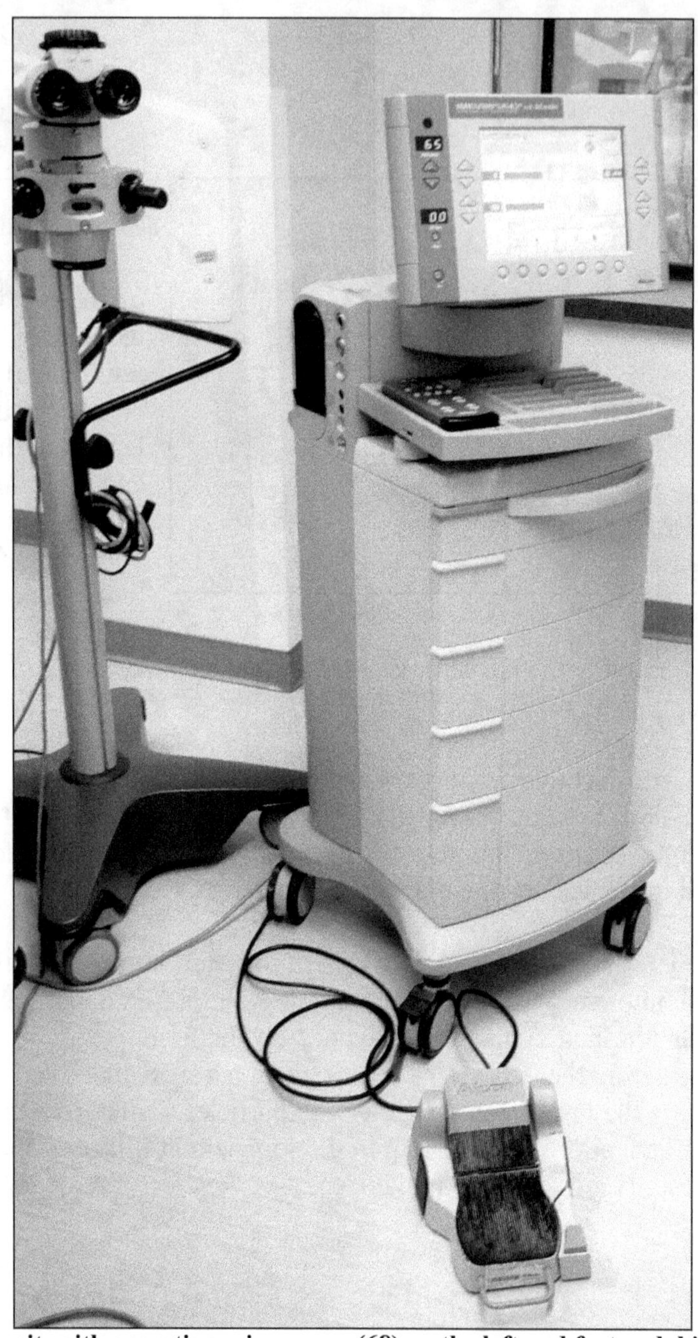

Phaco unit, with operating microscope (68) on the left and foot pedal in front.

The unit requires controls for the various steps (these controls can usually be operated by a foot pedal assembly, leaving the surgeon's hands free), as well as displays showing suction and infusion levels.

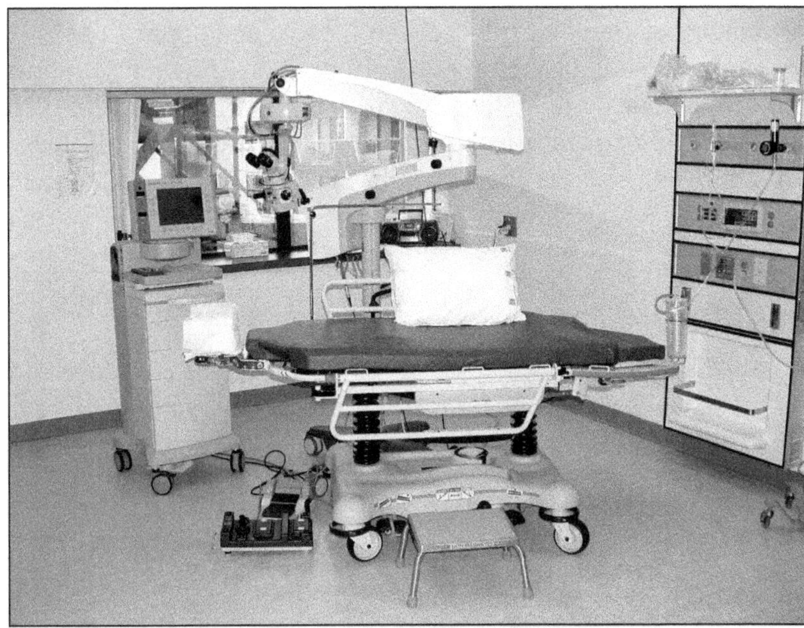

Eye clinic OR, phacoemulsifier (115) on the left and operating microscope (68) behind the OR table (66).

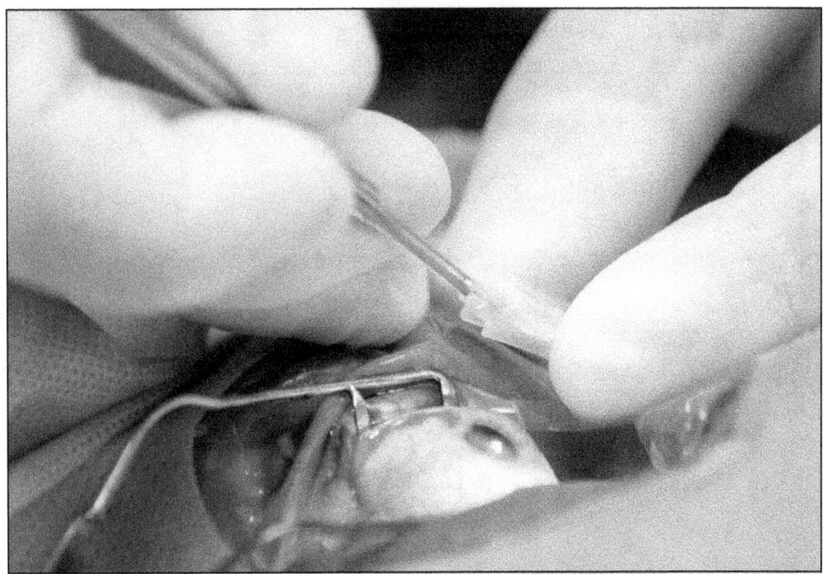

A surgeon prepares to insert an intraocular lens into the eye of a patient.
Modified from Shutterstock, Inc, www.shutterstock.com, with permission.

Application Patients are sedated, but usually conscious during these procedures. Once the surgeon has established an appropriate incision, viewing through an **operating microscope (68)**, the phacoemulsifier tip is introduced into the eye and applied to the lens. The lens material is broken up and removed by the system. Some of the clear material within the eye may need to be replaced if it is carried away along with lens particles. Once the entire old lens has been removed, the surgeon can begin installing the replacement plastic lens.

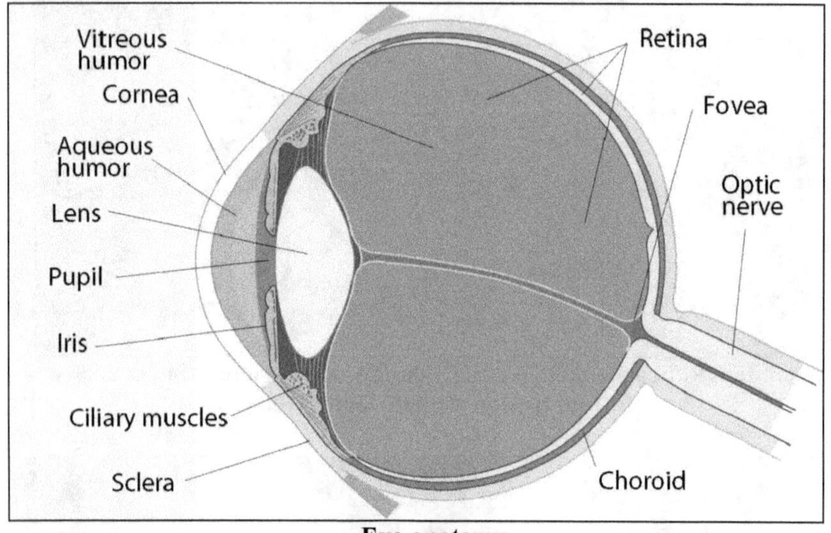

Eye anatomy.

Modified from Shutterstock, Inc, www.shutterstock.com, with permission.

AKA phaco machines.

Related devices **operating microscopes (68)**, **ophthalmic lasers (299)**.

Where found operating rooms, specialized outpatient surgery units or clinics.

- Function □ Patients with kidney disease come to renal units for counselling, dietary advice and dialysis. Two basic forms of dialysis treatment are provided, **peritoneal dialysis (128)** (PD), for patients with less severe kidney function impairment and **hemodialysis (123)**, for patients with severe impairment to complete kidney failure.

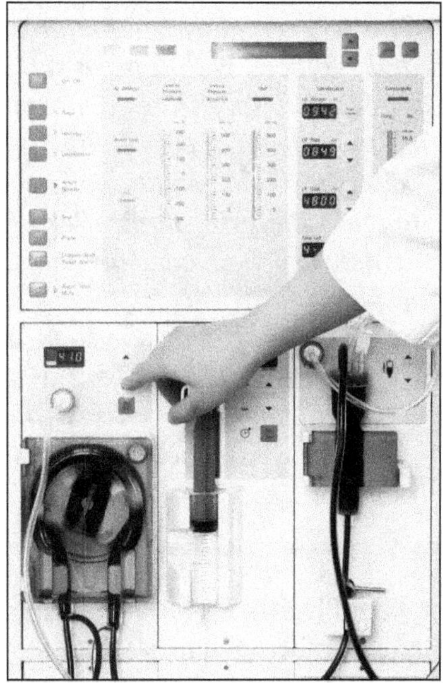

Hemodialysis machine.

(Modified from Shutterstock, Inc, www.shutterstock.com, with permission)

- Both are performed on an outpatient basis, though peritoneal dialysis can often be performed by the patient or a family member away from the hospital. Peritoneal dialysis involves the infusion of a dialysate solution into the abdominal (or peritoneal) cavity of the patient. In continuous ambulatory PD, the solution remains in place for several hours as the patient is free to go about daily living activities. At a later time, the solution, which has absorbed impurities, is then drained, the cavity is flushed and a new batch of solution is infused.

Kidney Complications – Jerry – Renal Unit II

Despite the successful removal of his kidney stones, Jerry is still having kidney problems and tests show that his kidney function is dropping to dangerously low levels, so that toxins and excess fluids normally removed by his kidneys are still circulating in his body, causing a variety of negative symptoms. His nephrologist recommends he start on peritoneal dialysis, a procedure in which special solutions are fed into his abdominal, or peritoneal, cavity, when Jerry is sleeping. The solutions remain for an hour or so, and are then drained out and replaced with a fresh set. The solutions are in contact with all the tissues in his abdomen, where they absorb some of the toxins and excess fluids that his kidneys are no longer processing. The solutions are administered through a ***peritoneal dialysis controller (128)****, which measures the fluid delivery and controls the fill and drain cycle times. In the morning, a set of fluid is left in Jerry's abdomen to work all day, and is drained out at the start of the next evening's process. The fluids are delivered and drained through a catheter that passes though Jerry's abdominal wall, and he must be very careful to avoid infections at the insertion site.*

- With automated PD, the solution is infused and exchanged automatically a number of times while the patient is sleeping at night. Hemodialysis requires that a port be in place to connect equipment to the circulatory system of the patient. Blood is taken from the port and passed through a hemodialysis machine that removes impurities, and is then returned to the patient. This process takes several hours and must be repeated several times per week. Because of the size and complexity of hemodialysis machines, the treatment is manly performed in clinics, though some patients may be able to afford to purchase and maintain a unit in their home. Renal units may include equipment for treating kidney stones.

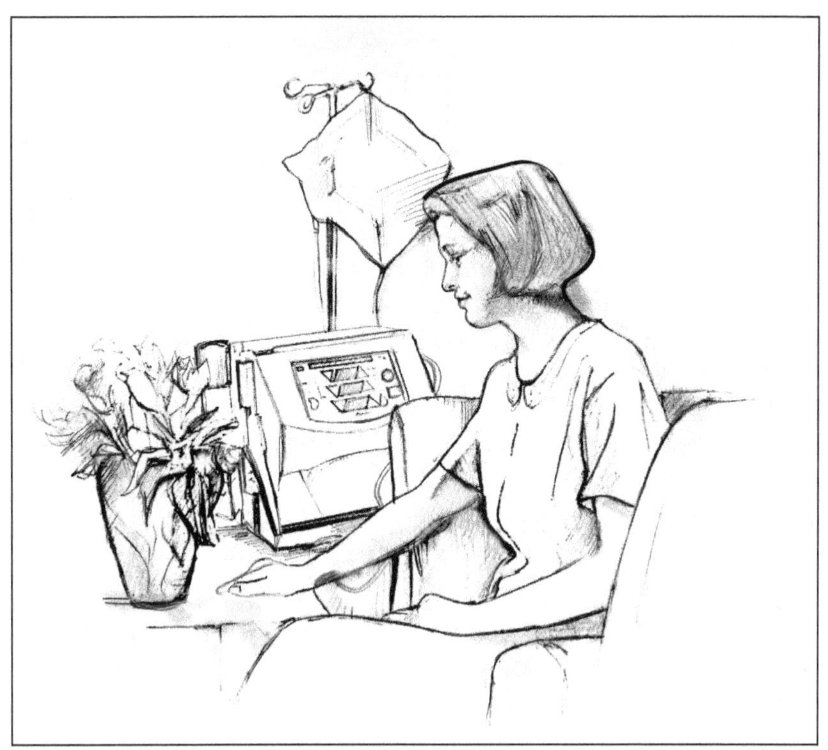

A patient undergoing peritoneal dialysis, with the controller and fluid bags on a stand beside the chair.

Courtesy of the National Institute of Diabetes and Digestive and Kidney Diseases, National Institutes of Health.

- Layout Since patients are required to be in the renal unit for extended periods with little movement, the units are usually designed to be otherwise pleasant, with comfortable beds, relaxing décor and music or television available. A nursing station allows staff to monitor patients and perform record keeping and other duties, while significant areas must be available for equipment storage and maintenance.

- Staff The renal unit is staffed by nurses and renal technologists, with biomedical engineering technologists present to perform equipment repair and maintenance.

- Equipment The **hemodialysis (123)** and **peritoneal dialysis (128)** machines make up the majority of devices in the unit, with some vital signs monitors to keep track of patient conditions such as **temperature (279)**, **blood pressure (296)** and **blood oxygen (320)** levels. **Lithotripsy units (157)** may also be located here.

Kidney Complications – Jerry – Renal Unit III

Eventually, peritoneal dialysis is not cleansing Jerry's blood enough, so he is switched to hemodialysis. This means that he goes to a renal clinic three times a week, and stays there for several hours each time during the treatment process. The catheter from his peritoneal dialysis has been removed, but now he has a vascular access system in which a loop of tubing is inserted into a vein in his forearm at two points, one of which will be used to remove blood from his system and the other for returning the blood. During treatment, the blood will flow from his arm and into a ***hemodialysis machine (123)*** *so that the machine can remove impurities and excess fluids from the blood. The machine uses special filters that allow harmful material to pass through for removal while allowing the rest of the blood to circulate back into Jerry's body through the access point. The filters consist of many fine tubules that are bathed in a special fluid called a dialysate, which effectively draws wastes and excess fluid from the blood out through the walls of the tubules and into the dialysate, where it can be removed. Again, infection is a constant threat and Jerry must be very careful to keep the area around the vascular access site clean. A* ***bladder scanner (252)*** *(a small, portable, dedicated ultrasound machine that scans the bladder and calculates the volume of urine it contains) is used regularly to help evaluate remaining kidney function.*

Renal Unit Equipment Descriptions

Following are more detailed descriptions of equipment found exclusively or most commonly in this area of the hospital. Equipment that is also found in various other areas of the hospital is described in Chapter 12, p 247. Lithotripsy devices are described in the Urology section, p 156.

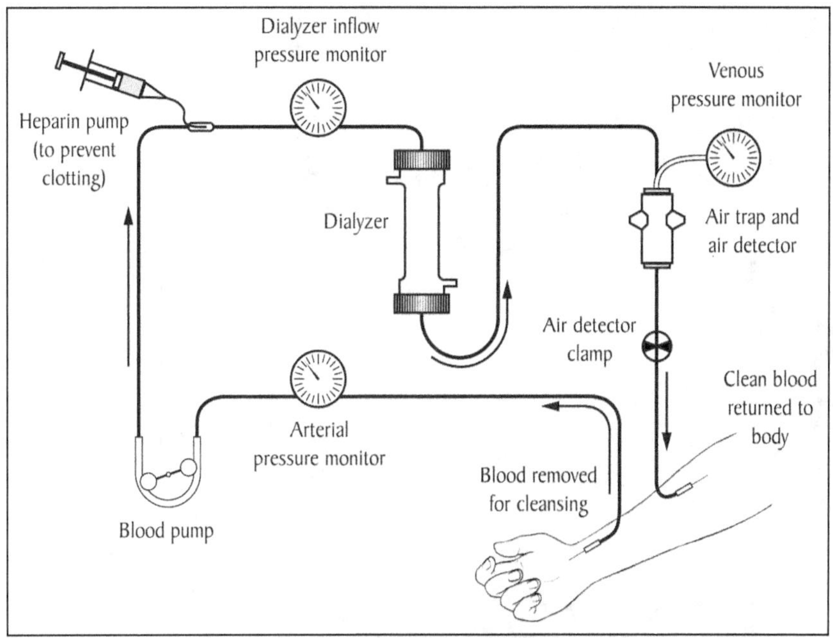

Schematic diagram of hemodialysis set–up.

Courtesy of the National Institute of Diabetes and Digestive and Kidney Diseases, National Institutes of Health.

Hemodialysis Units

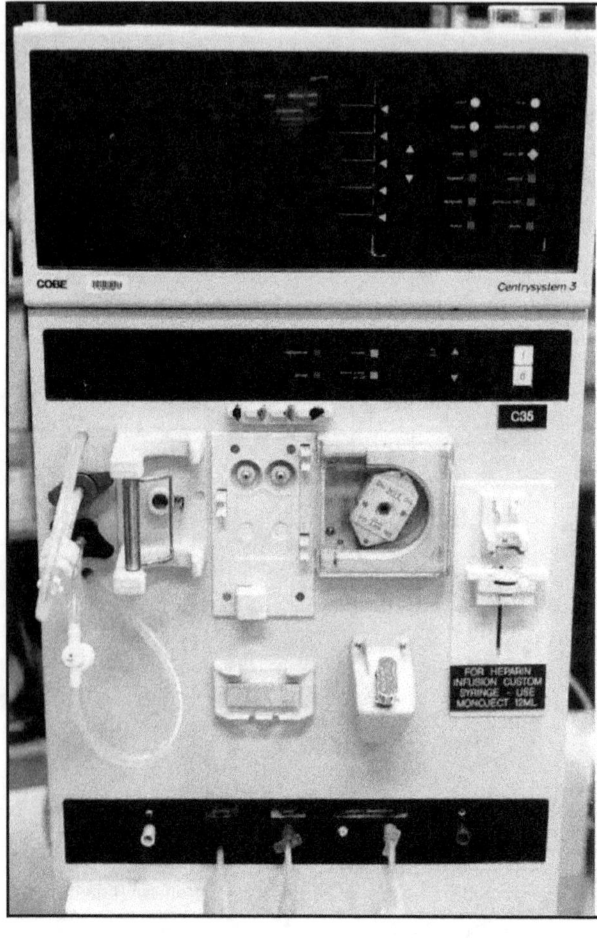

Overview □ In cases where kidney function is extremely reduced or non□existent, or where peritoneal dialysis is not appropriate, patients may have their blood purified by hemodialysis.

Function □ Blood is shunted from an artery in the patient's body and passed into a system that causes the blood to flow through a chamber where blood and a special dialysate solution are separated by a membrane film. The film allows some molecules to pass through but not others (and blocks blood cells), and the dialysate solution is formulated to encourage toxic substances and excess salts and water to move from the blood, through the membrane, and into the solution. The system adjusts the temperature of the fluids involved so that the processed blood is close to body temperature. The cleansed blood is then passed back into a vein, usually adjacent to the artery from which it was removed.

Application □ Once the arterial and venous ports have been established, the hemodialysis unit is filled with the various solutions required. Operation of the system is confirmed, and then blood flow is initiated. After the prescribed treatment time, the arterial flow is stopped and as much blood as possible is returned to the patient; then the venous line is closed.

In some patients, ports in the artery and vein can be semi-permanent so that they can be used for repeated dialysis procedures.

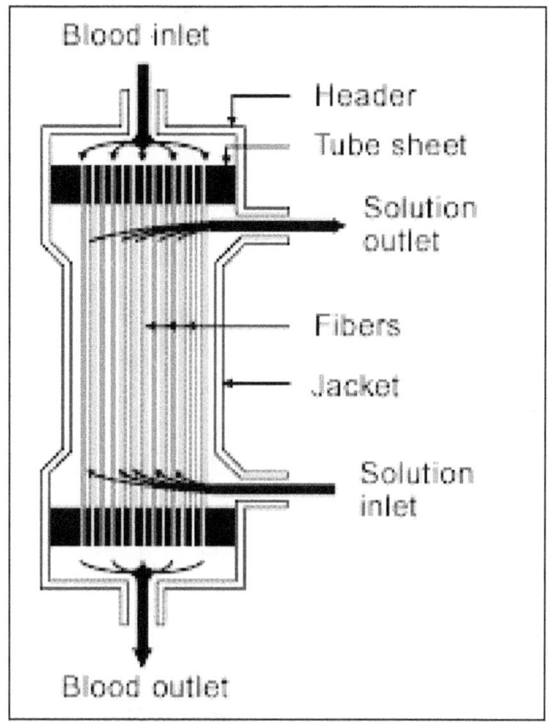

Hemodialysis filter (dialyzer).

Courtesy of the National Institute of Diabetes and Digestive and Kidney Diseases, National Institutes of Health.

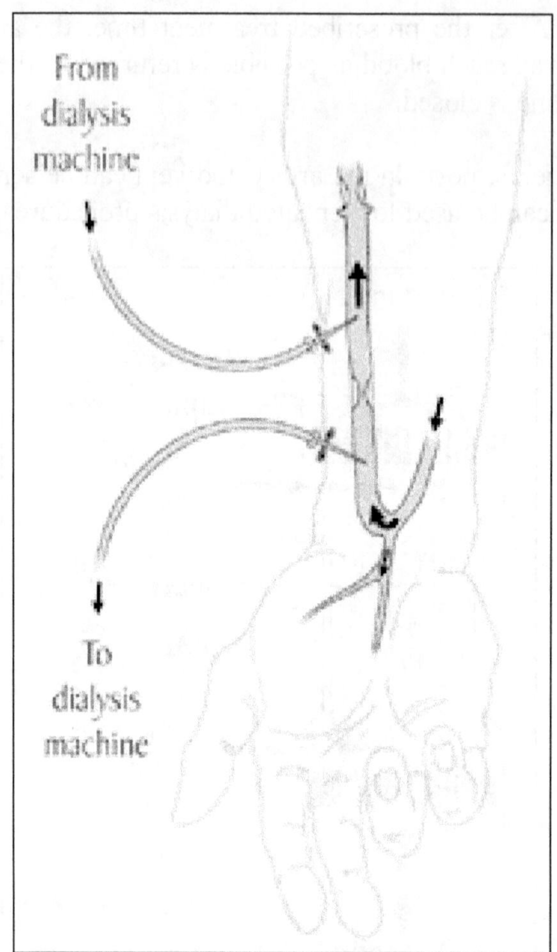

Access port for hemodialysis.

Courtesy of the National Institute of Diabetes and Digestive and Kidney Diseases, National Institutes of Health.

<u>AKA</u> □artificial kidney.

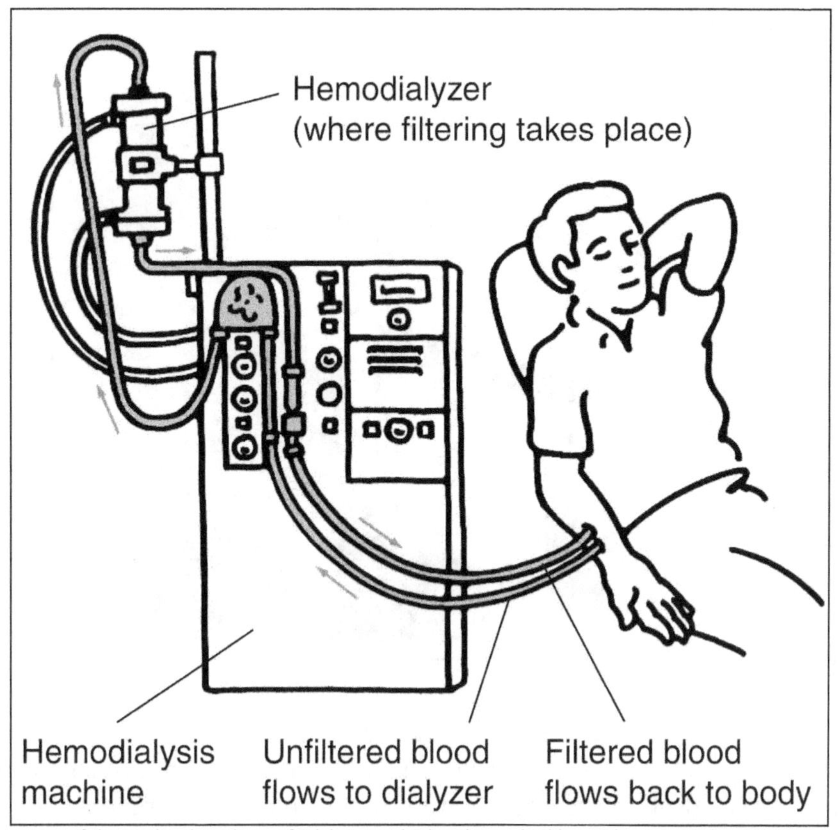

Courtesy of the National Institute of Diabetes and Digestive and Kidney Diseases, National Institutes of Health.

Related devices **peritoneal dialysis units (128)**.

Where found specialized hemodialysis units or clinics; some hemodialysis systems are small enough that they can be used by appropriately trained patients or family members in the patient's home.

Peritoneal Dialysis Units

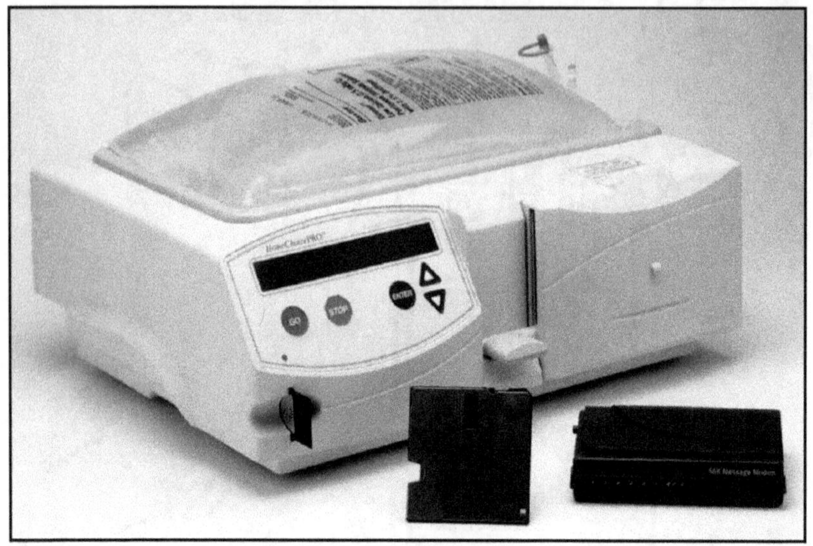

Overview □ When a patient is experiencing severely reduced kidney function, toxins and excess salts and water normally removed by the kidneys build up in the body and must be removed to prevent serious harm or death.

Function □ Peritoneal dialysis machines utilize two important principles. The first is that substances in solution tend to move from areas of higher concentration of that substance to areas of lower concentration; the second is that the inside of the abdomen (peritoneum) provides a large surface area that has an excellent blood supply. By filling part of the peritoneal space with saline solution, toxic materials in the blood will tend to move into the saline. The saline can then be drained, removing some of the toxic material as well.

Application □ A catheter is inserted into the patient's abdominal cavity; this may be semi□permanent, and closed off when not in use. Saline solution is passed through the peritoneal dialysis unit, which warms it to near body temperature and controls the flow rate. The abdomen is filled with a volume determined by body size. The unit also functions as a timer, to signal when the saline should be drained. The process is repeated several times in order to maximize toxin removal. Volumes are recorded to ensure that no significant amount of saline is left in the abdomen. This technique has a number of drawbacks, including the trauma of catheter insertion, the possibility of infection, and the fact that some toxins may not be removed effectively, while some beneficial substances may be inadvertently removed. Some systems use smaller volumes of fluid for a longer time, with fewer repetitions, while others use larger volumes for shorter times, repeated a number of times. The smaller□volume process can allow the patient to be at least partially mobile during treatment, and is thus referred to as ambulatory peritoneal dialysis. The large□volume technique requires that the patient be essentially immobile for the duration of the treatment, and is referred to as cycling peritoneal dialysis; it can be done while the patient is sleeping.

AKA □(none).

Related devices □**hemodialysis units (124)**, **fluid warmers (12)**.

Where found □ specialized outpatient clinics (note: peritoneal dialysis is often done in the patient's home or even on vacations)

Chapter 7 – Endoscopy

- <u>Function</u> □ Endoscopy units are designed for performing endoscopic examinations of patients, examining the gastro□ intestinal system, the respiratory system or joints.

  □Endoscope□ literally means □inside looking,□ and these systems are designed for just that. The general term □endoscope□ describes any device that has a tube that can be inserted into an opening in the body, either natural or surgical, for the purpose of viewing structures inside the body. This means that they must have channels both to provide lighting and to transmit visual images back out to the user. Endoscopes may also have the capacity to supply fluids such as saline solutions for irrigating sites to provide a clearer view, suction to remove the irrigation and other fluids, an air channel for insufflation, and a channel that can allow the entry of special instruments for doing various procedures inside the body.

<u>Accidents Happen – Felipe – Endoscopy I</u>

Felipe was injured in an industrial accident in which he suffered bruises and strained muscles, multiple fractures of his hand and legs as well as damage to his lungs after inhaling toxic fumes. He is now recovering from surgery to fix and set his breaks, and is about to begin a lengthy physical therapy program. He is also having breathing difficulties, and his doctor has ordered a bronchoscopy examination to check the extent of damage, in addition to x-rays of the fractures to see how they are healing. Arriving in the Endoscopy Department, Felipe is asked to remove his shirt and put on a hospital gown. An internist explains the procedure and starts in intravenous line, into which he injects a sedative drug. Felipe is soon drowsy and is positioned on his side on a gurney.

- Layout □ The unit will have one or more rooms with a procedure table, equipment cart, video monitors, recorders and printers, a computer system, storage areas for a variety of **endoscopes (135)** and endoscope washing/sterilizing equipment. Rooms may be general purpose or they may be specialized for gastro□intestinal, gynecological, respiratory or joint (arthroscopy) procedures.

- Staff □ An internist physician usually performs the actual examination, though a nurse or specialized technologist may do all the equipment set□up and patient preparation. A trained technician may help with set□up and with cleaning and organizing the endoscopes between patients.

- Equipment □ An endoscopy cart consisting of a **fiber–optic light source (142)**, a system for irrigating and suctioning the body area being examined, an **insufflator (148)**, a **video camera system (144)**, a **video recorder (146)**, a video printer, one or more **video displays (147)**, an **electrosurgery unit** for performing minor cutting and cautery, a computer system for controlling equipment, recording video and tracking patient information, a variety of **rigid and/or flexible endoscopes (135)**, and an endoscope washing/sterilizing machine.

Accidents Happen – Felipe continued

Though the drug will make it so he doesn't remember the procedure, he looks around and sees a cart with various machines on shelves and a large **video monitor (147)** *on top. The largest machine is a multi-function endoscopy unit that provides light,* **airflow (148)***, suction and irrigation. Another component is a* **camera console (144)** *that processes video signals from the bronchoscope itself. A video printer is also on the cart, and the system is connected by cables to a desktop computer. There is another video monitor mounted on the wall so that students or others can observe. On one wall are a number of bronchoscopes of various lengths and diameters. A bronchoscope must be thin enough to enter small passages in a patient's respiratory system while still allowing the patient to breathe. A technologist positions Felipe to allow best access to his trachea, and then the bronchoscope tube is passed into his mouth and down his throat. Fiber optics inside the bronchoscope tube carry bright light from the endoscopy unit to illuminate the path, and other fiber optic channels carry images from the tip of the scope to be processed and then displayed on the video monitors. The internist guides the scope carefully until she locates the opening of the trachea. Cables inside the scope are controlled by knobs on the other end to allow the tip to be turned in any direction. The tip of the scope is moved to point into Felipe's trachea, and then the scope is advanced to move down the trachea towards the lungs. Felipe gags throughout the procedure but the sedative helps him remain calm, and will also erase his memory of the procedure, making it seem as if it didn't really take place and avoiding memories of the discomfort.*

The internist makes comments throughout the procedure, noting areas of damage. The scope makes its way into the bronchial tubes that lead to the left and right lungs, and it is found that damage from the inhaled fumes apparently doesn't extend into Felipe's lungs. The doctor uses a special tool to snip a bit of tissue from some of the most badly damaged areas of Felipe's trachea, and this tissue is aspirated through the bronchoscope and collected for later laboratory examination. The scope is removed from Felipe's throat and he is wheeled into a recovery bay until the sedative wears off and he feels well enough to go home. A vital signs monitor continuously measures his blood oxygen level, pulse rate and blood pressure his temperature if staff are concerned about that.

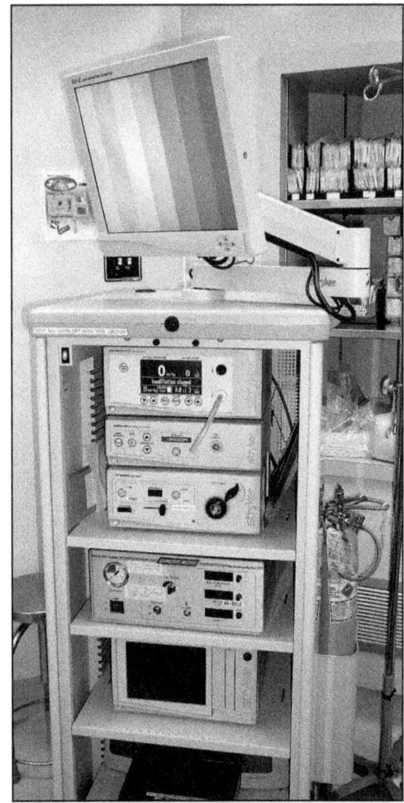

Endoscopy cart.

Endoscopy Equipment Descriptions

Following are more detailed descriptions of equipment found exclusively or most commonly in this area of the hospital. Equipment that is also found in various other areas of the hospital is described in Chapter 12, p 247.

Endoscopes

Overview □Endoscope means literally □inside viewer,□and they are used to visualize areas inside the body for diagnostic and/or treatment purposes.

Application □Varies, depending on the type, as follows:

Types of Endoscopes

Some types of endoscopes, with their target areas and insertion points, include:

- Arthroscope □joints such as knees; surgical incision
- Bronchoscope □trachea and upper bronchial passages; mouth or nose
- Colonoscope □colon; anus
- Colposcope □vagina and uterus; vagina
- Cystoscope □bladder and urinary tract; urethra
- Gastroscope □ esophagus, stomach and sometimes upper small intestine (duodenum); mouth
- Laparoscope □various abdominal organs; surgical incision
- Proctoscope □rectum and lower (sigmoid) colon; anus
- Sigmoidoscope □sigmoid colon; anus
- Thoracoscope □ organs of the thorax, including the pleura (outer covering of the lungs) and pericardium (outer covering of the heart); surgical incision

Endoscopy is less invasive and less traumatic than exploratory surgery, and while laparoscopic procedures require one or two small incisions, these are much smaller than open abdominal or thoracic surgery; recovery times are much shorter and the incidence of complications much lower.

Endoscopes are divided into rigid or flexible types, the difference being self□explanatory.

Rigid Endoscopes

Rigid endoscopes consist of a tube, usually made of stainless steel, which contains fiberoptics, a series of lenses and one or more open passages.

At the distal end of the scope, an objective lens receives light from the object and directs it into the tube. The angle at which the objective lens is set determines the viewing angle of each individual scope, from straight ahead to various angles to the side to partially in reverse.

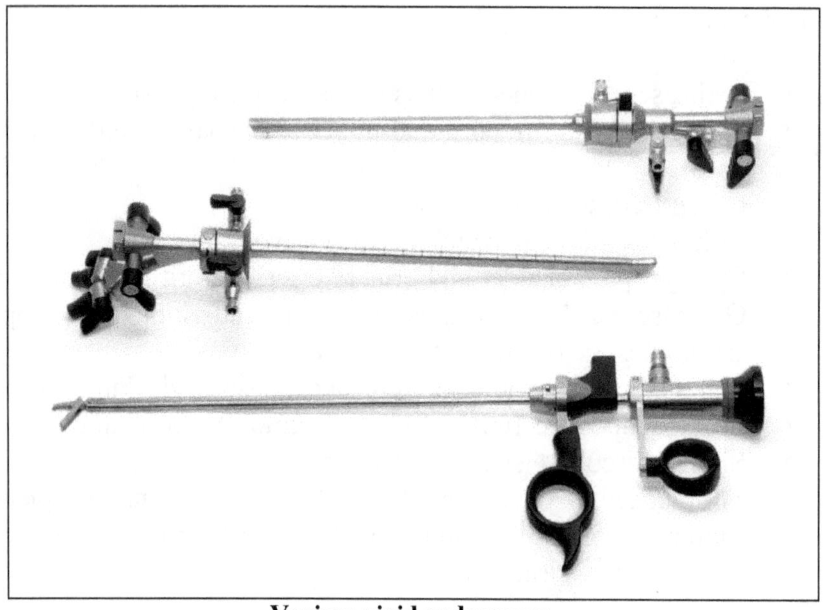

Various rigid endoscopes.
Modified from Shutterstock, Inc, www.shutterstock.com, with permission.

The other lenses, commonly referred to as the telescope, are separated by spacers. They take the light through the tube from the objective lens to the eyepiece.

Fiber optic strands are installed around the lenses to carry illumination light to the subject, and a fitting near the eyepiece allows a light cable to attach to the scope.

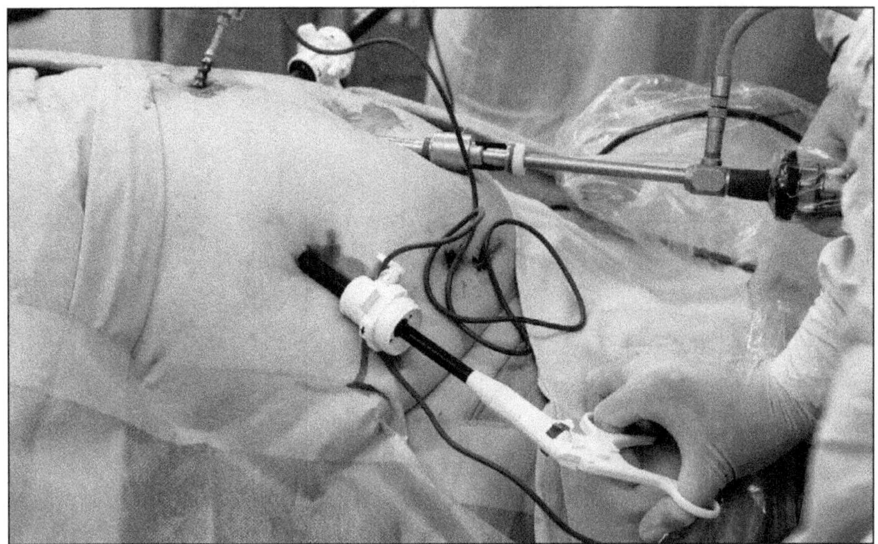

An endoscopic surgical procedure in progress – note the rigid scope on the right, the lower bipolar ESU (51) instrument, also note abdominal distension due to insufflation (147).
Modified from Shutterstock, Inc, www.shutterstock.com, with permission.

The open passages in the scope allow for irrigation and suction of the observation site to remove obscuring material such as blood. Also, pieces of tissue that have been cut or otherwise separated from structures such as tumors or polyps can be withdrawn for disposal or examination. The passages can also be used to fill the area around the object of observation with either clear fluid or air in order to allow a clearer view. Finally, the passages can allow the entry of special tools used for such purposes as excising tissue or cauterizing structures.

Flexible Endoscopes

Flexible endoscopes carry both illumination and visualization light through fiber optics, which allows the flexibility in their name. Flexibility allows the scopes to pass around corners to reach the object of observation; it also means that flexible scopes can be much longer than rigid scopes.

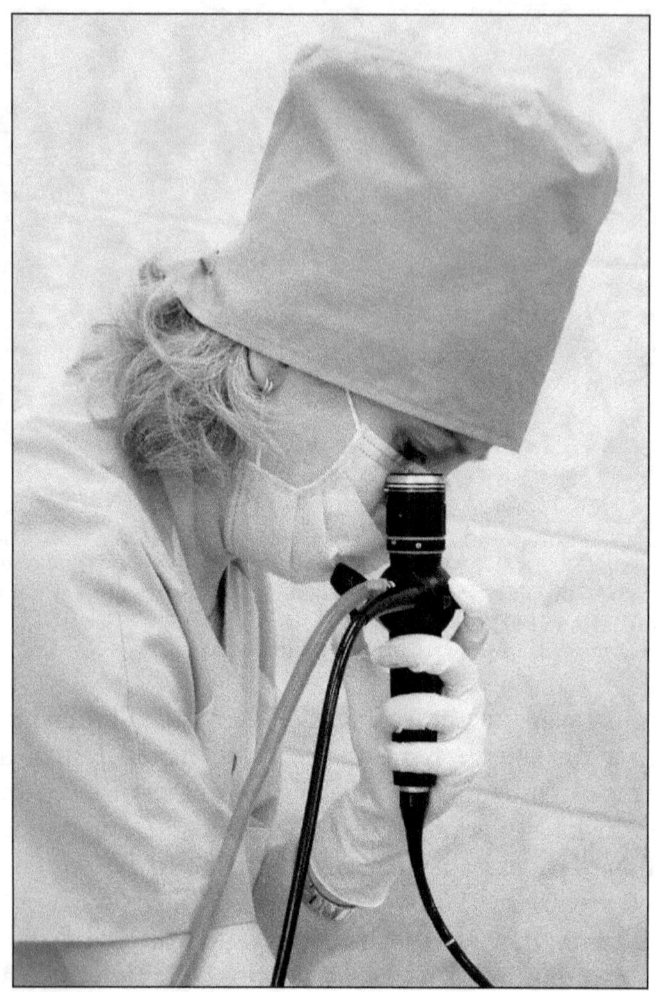

A surgeon during an endoscopic procedure, viewing directly through a flexible endoscope.
Modified from Shutterstock, Inc, www.shutterstock.com, with permission.

Flexible endoscopes generally carry markings on the outside to indicate depth of insertion. Some models have special mechanisms operated by cables that allow the operator to turn the end portion of the scope in different directions. Otherwise, flexible scope function is similar to that of rigid scopes.

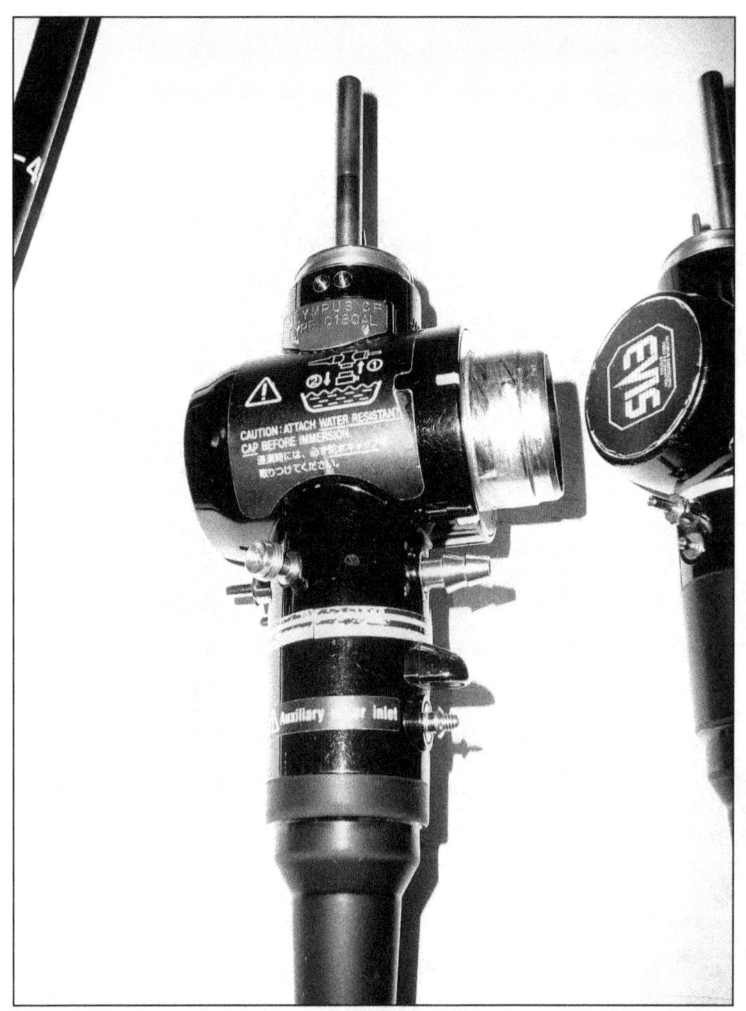

A flexible endoscope, connector end, showing the connector for a light source and ports for insufflation (148), irrigation and suction (149).

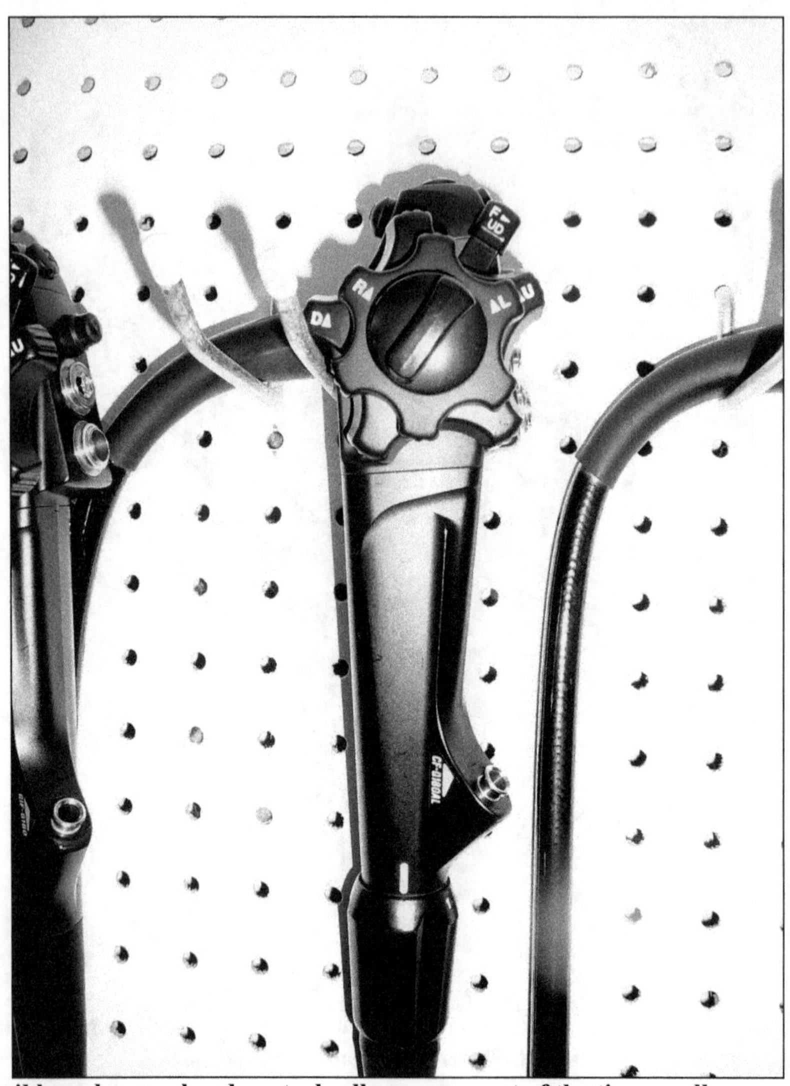

Flexible endoscope hand controls allow movement of the tip as well as adjustments to focus and light intensity.

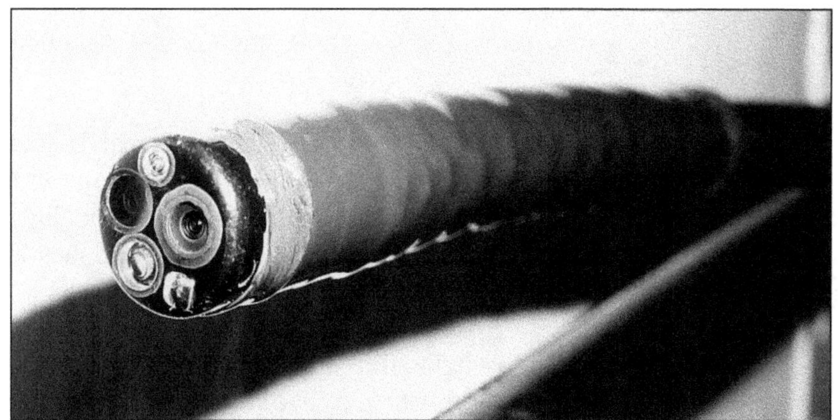
The distal end of an endoscope – note the various channels for light, viewing, irrigation, insufflation and suction.

Some flexible scopes mount directly onto the **light source (142)**, which makes video and other connections simpler and more effective. Viewing images from such scopes is done via **video monitors (147)** rather than direct eyepieces.

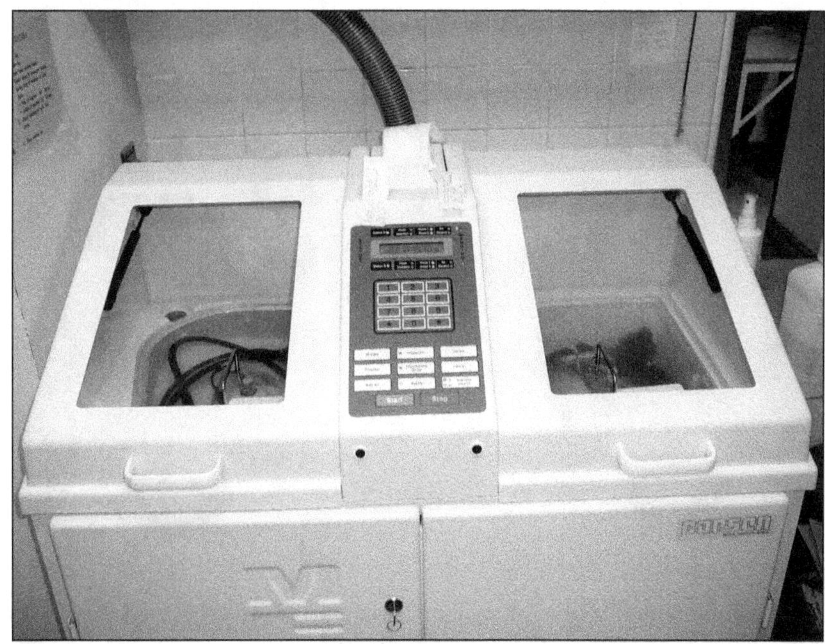
A dual–chamber flexible endoscope washer.

Light Sources

Overview Accurate recognition of normal and abnormal tissues during an endoscopic procedure requires bright illumination with light having a specific spectrum and color temperature. The light also must not impart any significant amount of heat to the tissues in the target area.

Application Most endoscopy light source use quartz halogen bulbs that run in a controlled environment to avoid overheating, with accurate power supplies, since both temperature changes and supply voltage variation can change light characteristics.

Higher intensity bulbs are fitted with heat sinks and fans to help keep them in the correct temperature range.

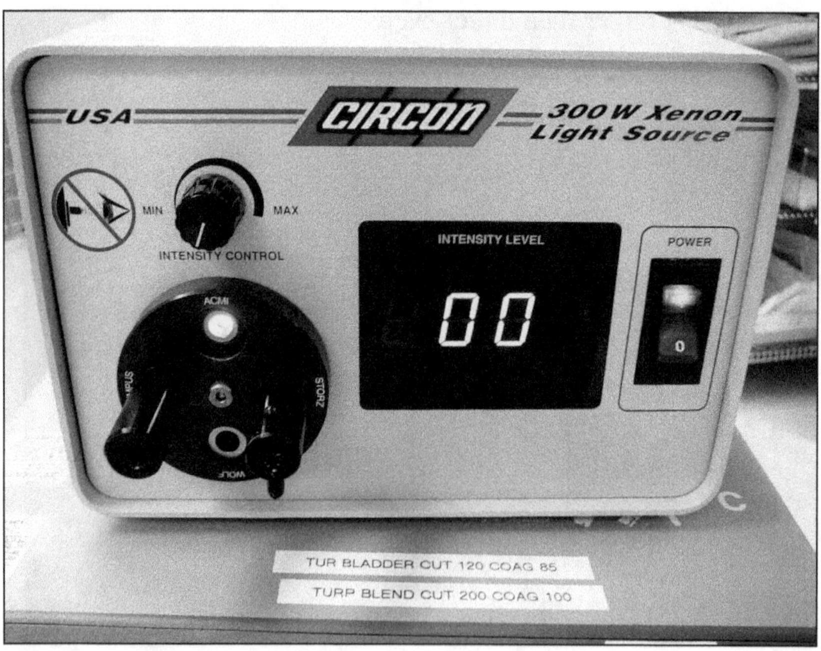

An older endoscopy light source. The connector at lower left rotates to allow connection of scopes from different manufacturers.

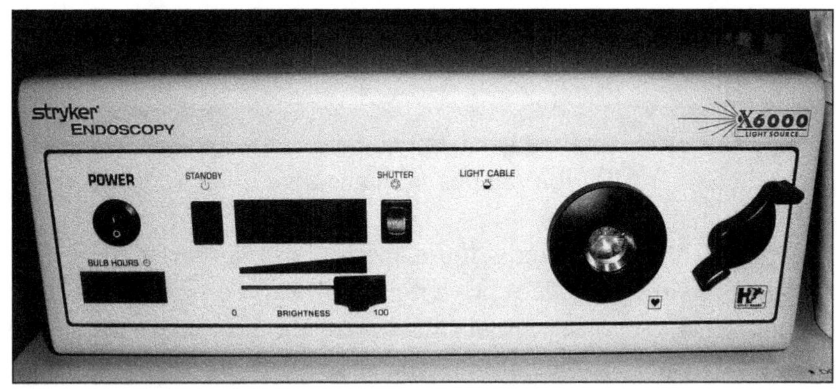

A current endoscopy light source. The connectors are now dedicated to scopes from the light source manufacturer.

In order to accommodate requirements for different light intensities, a mechanical device is used to block some portion of the light. Changing voltage to the lamp would also vary intensity, but would also affect light color temperature, which is why mechanical methods are used, allowing the lamp itself to remain in a constant state to provide consistent light quality. Simpler light sources have manual controls for intensity, while more sophisticated units can be controlled by the video portion of the system in order to maintain optimum illumination.

Light source units have a connector on the front panel to accommodate the fiberoptics for the scope; this may be a simple, single purpose plug or it may be a more complex connector that can carry optical or electronic images and control signals, as well as air, irrigation and suction.

By using fiberoptics to carry light from the source (bulb) to the viewing area, an adequate amount of light is delivered with very little heat.

Cameras

Overview — Video cameras used in endoscopy systems must be able to generate high-resolution images with accurate color reproduction.

Application — In most systems the camera is in two parts: the image sensor portion and the video-processing portion. Some systems have the image sensor on a head that attaches to the proximal part of the scope, while newer systems mount the sensors at the distal tip of the scope.

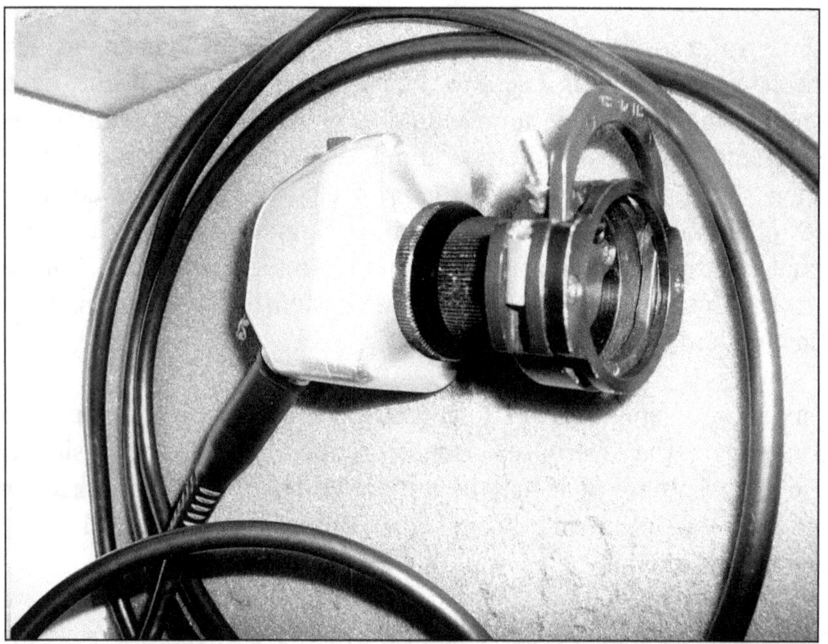

An endoscopy camera head, which clips on to the end of the scope and picks up light signals with its image sensor, converting them into electronic video signals that are then carried by cable to the camera console, where they are further processed.

Image sensors may consist of a single chip array, or three chip arrays. With the single chip arrangement, colors are differentiated electronically, while with three chip systems each chip responds to a single primary color. Single chip systems tend to be smaller and less expensive, while three chip systems tend to provide higher image quality. Both single chip and three chip cameras are available with high-definition resolution; again, higher resolution means higher costs.

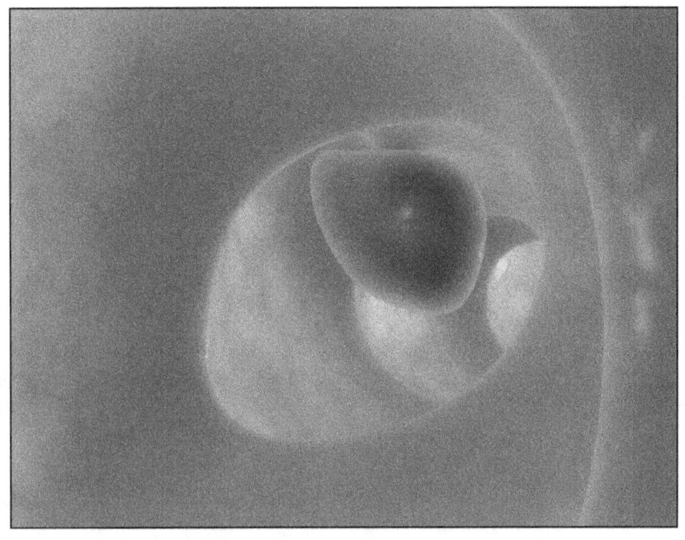

Endoscopy image showing a colon tumor.

Modified from Shutterstock, Inc, www.shutterstock.com, with permission.

In each system, video signals are taken from the sensors to a processing component, usually cabinet mounted. This part of the camera handles the video signals to adjust for light intensities and can perform such tasks as white balancing to help ensure color accuracy.

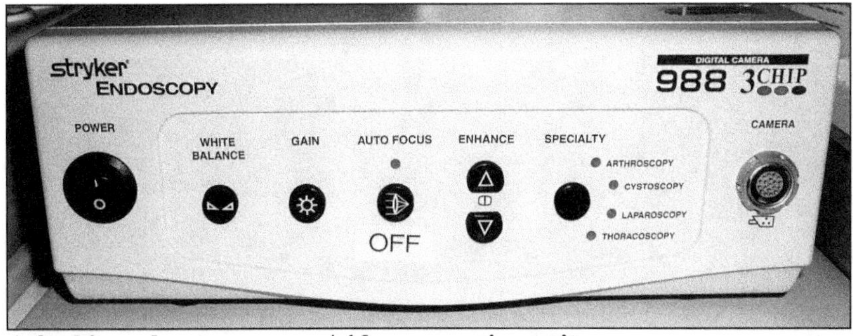

A 3–chip endoscopy camera/video processing unit.

The video processor interfaces with **light sources (142)** as well as **video image recorders (146)**, printers and **video displays (147)**.

Video Recorders/Storage

Overview □ Systems may record video as either motion or still pictures, or both, so that clinicians can later examine the images for specific details, or use them for teaching purposes. Recorded images from one test on an individual patient may be compared to those from a later test in order to see if changes in tissues or structures have taken place.

In the past, endoscopy systems recorded video on videocassette recorders, but new systems use recordable optical disks and/or hard drives, which provide much quicker access to images.

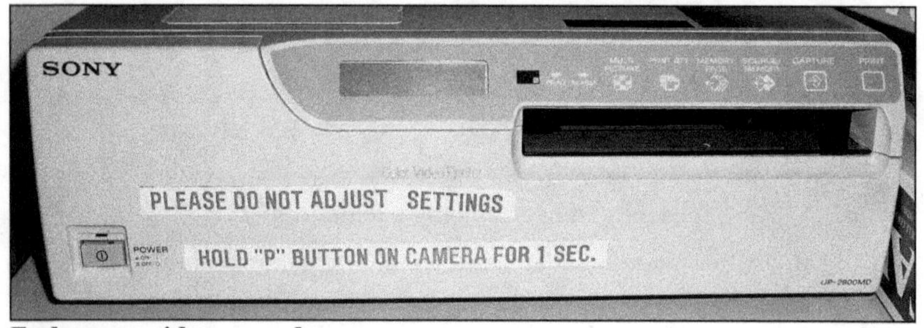

Endoscopy video recorder.

Video monitors

Overview □ As part of the system, video monitors must have equal capabilities to other links in the imaging chain in terms of resolution and color reproduction.

Application □ Both CRT and LCD monitors are used, with the size and weight advantages of LCD making them increasingly common, and universal in new installations.

Monitors are mounted to give the person performing the test a clear view, and secondary displays are often used to provide a good view to other staff or students.

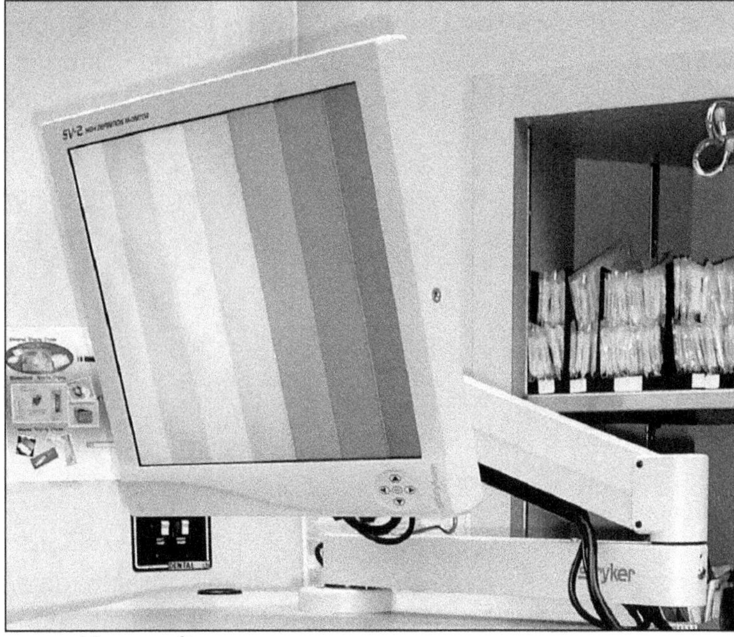

Endoscopy video monitor.

Insufflators

Overview □ Obtaining a clear view of many internal structures can be difficult when other organs or tissues get in the way; there is normally very little open space inside the body. To alleviate this problem, an inert gas such as carbon dioxide may be introduced to the target area.

Application □ Obviously such insufflatory pressures must be carefully limited to avoid damage, and so systems are equipped with regulators and over□pressure alarms. Insufflating gas usually comes from pressurized tanks since most facilities don□t have carbon dioxide wall outlets.

Room air is not used for insufflation because it isn□t absorbed by tissues as well as carbon dioxide. Excess non□intestinal gas remaining in body cavities after scope procedures can cause pain and discomfort for the patient.

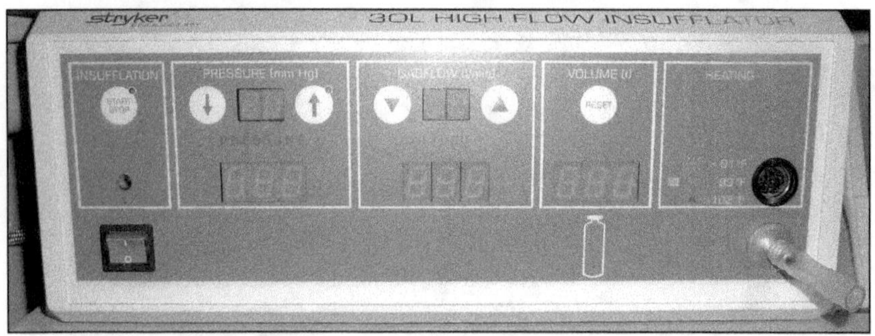

An insufflator front panel.

Insufflators typically have controls and displays (usually digital) for patient pressure, gas flow rate and total volume delivered. Since there may be some leakage of gas from the scope and also since carbon dioxide can be absorbed quite easily by internal body tissues, some level of continuous flow must be maintained after adequate insufflation is achieved. The insufflating gas may be heated by the unit to help maintain patient body temperature.

Irrigation and Suction Units

Overview □Isotonic saline is usually used for irrigation, and in some circumstances it is used to distend the viewing area to provide more clearance, when gas insufflation wouldn□t work, such as in the confined spaces of joints when performing arthroscopic procedures.

Application □ The saline is pumped in through the scope lumen using a low□pressure pump.

Removing blood, tissue particles or the debris from surgical procedures is necessary to maintain good visibility, but as with any body fluid, the evacuated material must be handled using appropriate precautions. A low□suction vacuum pump or line suction is used via the scope lumen.

Tools

Overview A wide range of procedures can be accomplished with endoscopy, using an equally wide range of tools.

Function For some laparoscopic or thoracoscopic procedures that might require bulkier or multiple tools, a separate tube may be inserted in to a second small incision.

A common goal of endoscopy, in addition to simple observation, is the removal of small samples of suspect tissue in order to examine the sample in detail to help diagnose or eliminate conditions such as cancer. Special, fine grasping and cutting tools allow such biopsies to be performed quickly and accurately.

Larger amounts of tissue can be excised and removed as well, for example in the removal of tumors or polyps. Since the suction lumen of an endoscope is limited in size, such tissue must be reduced to relatively small pieces before suction is applied. Gall bladder removal is commonly performed in this manner, a procedure called a laparoscopic cholecystectomy.

Electrosurgery (see p. 51) can be performed laparoscopically, using long, thin electrode probes that are well insulated except for the tips. These tips can be snares or pincers, and can be used for such things as polyp ligation or fallopian tube sealing. The inner conductor must be insulated from the outer sleeve. A flat electrode may be used to cauterize highly vascularized tissue that is causing blood loss, such as in the liver or uterus.

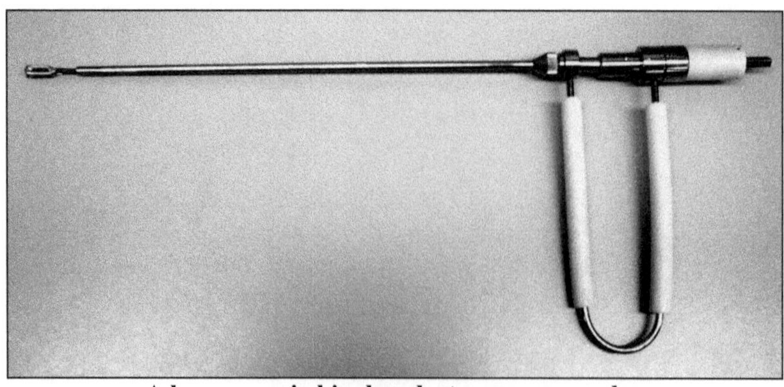

A laparoscopic bipolar electrosurgery probe.

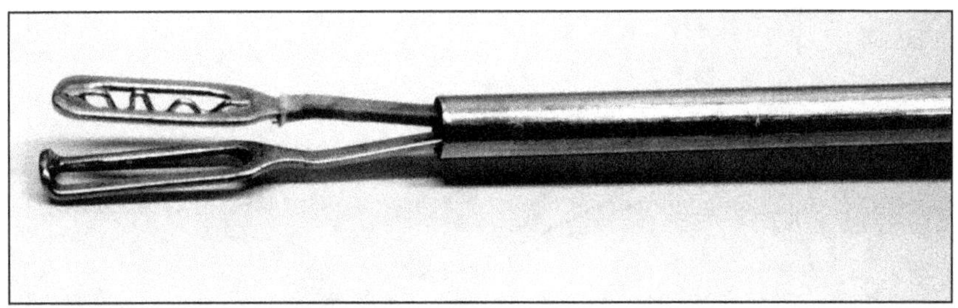

The tip of a bipolar ESU probe.

In arthroscopy, harder material such as cartilage or bone may need to be removed, in which case rotating grinding tools can be used through the scope.

Application Examples of various endoscopic procedures:

Arthroscopy of the knee This surgery may be done under local or general anesthesia. Several small incisions are made into the knee joint and arthroscopic instruments are inserted. The joint area is **insufflated (148)** to allow for viewing and working. The remaining process is determined by the condition of the knee joint. Cartilage damage due to arthritis can be alleviated by removal of some of the cartilage; detached portions are washed and suctioned out, while damaged portions may be cut away and then washed and suctioned. Some researchers are working on methods of transplanting cartilage into the joint, which involves removing some of the old tissue and replacing it with cartilage either taken from another part of the body or grown from the patient's cells in a lab culture. Rough bone surfaces can be smoothed out, improving mechanical function and reducing pain. Cartilage damage due to injury is treated in much the same manner as that due to arthritis, though the structural changes are different. Ligament damage can be repaired by realigning ligaments, rejoining and strengthening torn ligaments, or grafting new sections of ligament into the damaged area. Patellar misalignment can be corrected by adjusting and repairing the ligaments that normally hold it in the correct position.

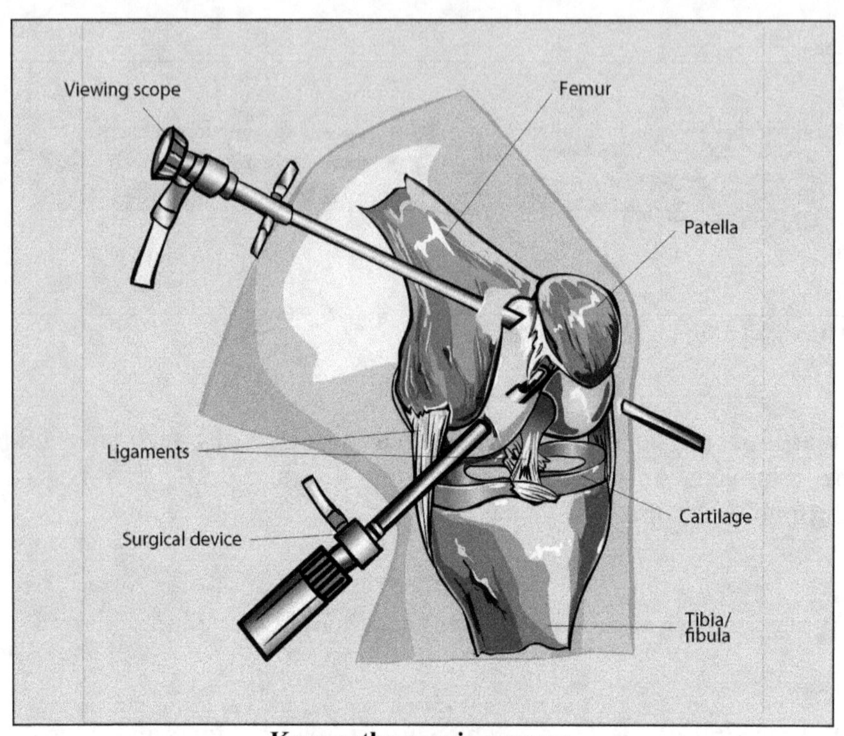

Knee arthroscopic surgery.
Modified from Shutterstock, Inc, www.shutterstock.com, with permission.

Bronchoscopy (Gastroscopy) The flexible bronchoscope (gastroscope) is inserted through the mouth, down the trachea (esophagus) and into the bronchial tubes (stomach). The scope has facilities for providing **illumination (142)** and acquiring **visual images (144)**, as well as **irrigation and suction (149)** plus channels for specific surgical procedures. Images are recorded for later examination and diagnosis. Tissue samples may be excised and aspirated for examination, and small lesion such as polyps may be removed. The scope is then withdrawn.

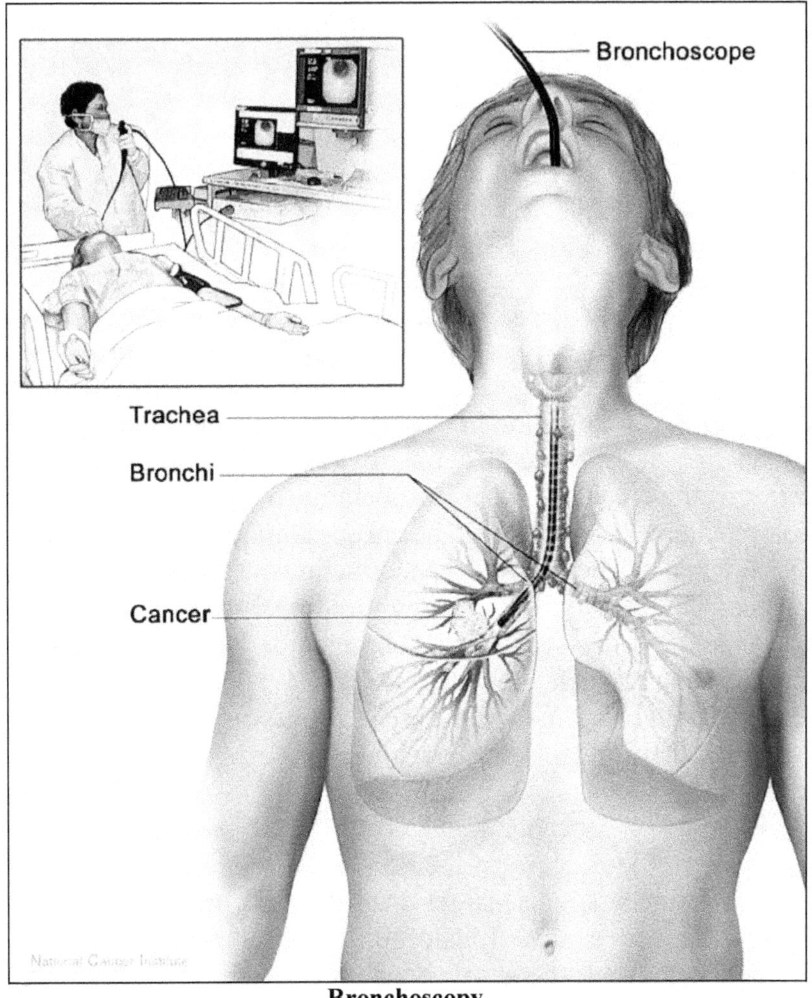

Bronchoscopy.

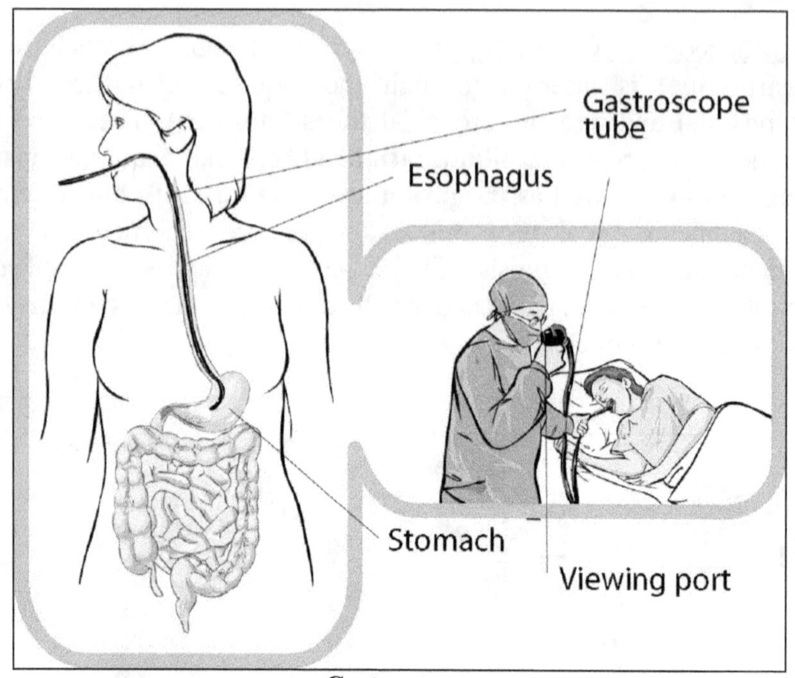

Gastroscopy.

Modified from Shutterstock, Inc, www.shutterstock.com, with permission.

<u>Colonoscopy</u> The colonoscope is lubricated and inserted slowly through the anus. Video images provide a continuous view of the interior of the colon, allowing the operator to guide the instrument to areas of interest. Images may be taken continuously or still photos may be taken of specific sites and structures. Tissue samples can be obtained with the use of the cutting tool on the scope; these can then be aspirated up the scope and collected for later lab examination. Some structures such as polyps or small tumors can be excised during colonoscopy. When sufficient images and/or tissue samples have been obtained, the scope is withdrawn.

<u>Colposcopy</u> A speculum may be inserted into the vagina and opened to provide access to the cervix. A series of tapered cervical dilation instruments, each larger than the last, are pressed into the cervix to slowly expand (dilate) the cervical opening. When the opening is sufficient, the hysteroscope is inserted. The uterus may be **insufflated (148)** with carbon dioxide to provide better visual access. The scope provides illumination and an optical channel that allows the physician to observe the inside of the uterus. There is also a lumen inside the scope that permits the insertion of devices to take

tissue samples or remove small lesions such as polyps or fibroid tumors. When the examination is complete, the scope is removed.

Cystoscopy □ The cystoscope, a thin tube that may be rigid or flexible, is lubricated and inserted into the urethral opening. Fluid is pumped in through the tip of the scope to increase visibility, and light for video viewing is carried in both directions by fiber□optic channels in the scope. Another channel in the scope can be used to remove tissue samples or small stones. Video images are recorded for diagnostic purposes. When the desired images and samples have been obtained, the scope is removed.

AKA □scopes

Related devices □**anesthetic machines (47)**

Where found □endoscopy clinics, operating rooms

Chapter 8 – Urology

- Function □ The urology unit may be stand□alone or it may be part of the surgical department. It provides treatments for patients with conditions related to their urinary system (other than kidney failure, which is handled in the renal unit.) Procedures such as prostate resections, bladder cyst removal, **lithotripsy (157)** for kidney stones, vasectomies and incontinence treatments are provided here.

- Layout □ Urology ORs are similar to general□purpose ORs, with the addition of special facilities for delivering and flushing fluids during procedures. ESWL equipment, due to its size, may be located in an adjacent room or even in an entirely different area.

- Staff □ Same as a typical OR. Urology specialist MDs are called urologists.

- Equipment □ Typical OR equipment (**anesthetic machines (47)**, **ESUs (51)**) plus special devices for lithotripsy such as **ESWL and laser lithotriptors (157)**. A **C–arm x–ray machine (212)** is usually available to help in monitoring procedures.

Urology Equipment Descriptions

Following are more detailed descriptions of equipment found exclusively or most commonly in this area of the hospital. Equipment that is also found in various other areas of the hospital is described in Chapter 12, p 247.

Lithotriptors

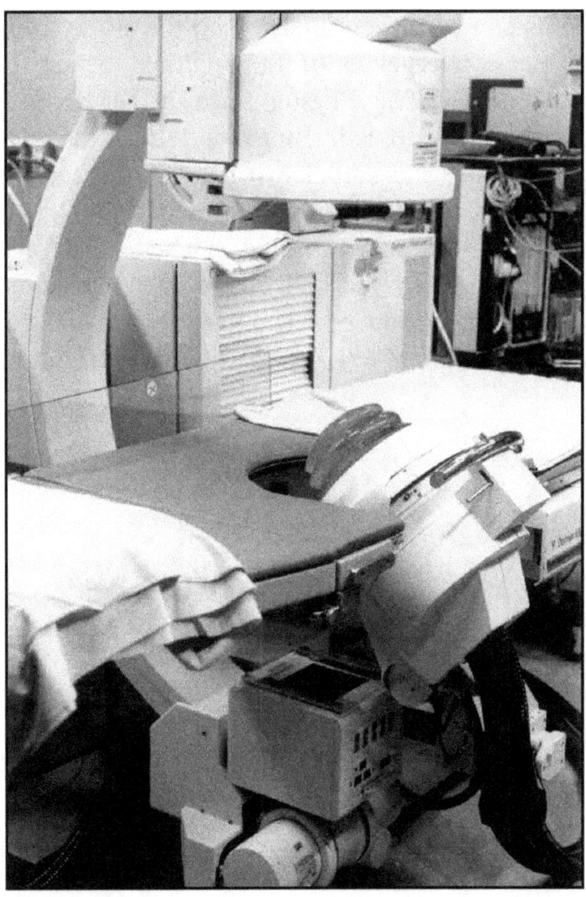

Overview □ Kidney and gallstones (calculi) can be extremely painful, and often dangerous to the patient. Surgical removal is possible, but, like any surgery, carries a degree of risk, as well as an extended recovery time. If these stones can be broken up into small□enough fragments, they can be passed with minimal discomfort, thus avoiding the drawbacks of surgery.

Function □Lithotriptors (literally, stone breakers) use high□powered, high□frequency sound waves to shatter stones. Because the stones are much harder and more brittle than the surrounding tissues, the sound pulses affect them much more. When pulses are of sufficient magnitude and duration, they cause the stones to gradually break apart. To avoid soft tissue damage as much as possible, treatment times are generally extended.

There are two general types of lithotriptors: direct contact and focused.

Direct contact units consist of a special tip on a catheter. Circuitry passes a high-voltage pulse through the tip, causing a micro-burst of vaporized water. This burst in turn generates a sound shock wave, which begins to break the stone apart.

Focused systems utilize a number of sources that produce narrow sound beams. These beams can be closely focused on the stone from outside the body, and the convergence of the multiple beams is sufficient to break up the stone(s). These systems are further divided into two types, immersion and coupled. Immersion units have a bathtub in which the patient sits, and sound waves are produced by transducers in the water. The water transmits the sound waves well, and they are transferred into the patient's body, where they are focussed on the stone. Coupled units (pictured) use a rubber bladder in which the sound waves are produced. The bladder is pressed against the patient, with a coupling gel between to aid in sound transmission.

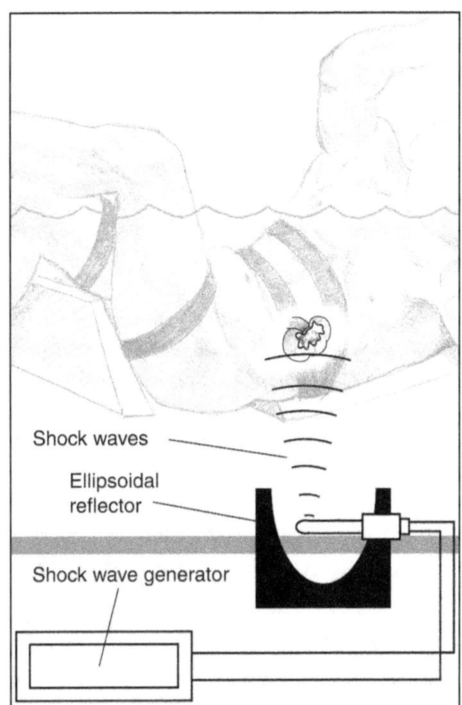

ESWL diagram. The shock waves would actually be curved in the opposite direction so they would focus on the stone.

Courtesy of the National Institute of Diabetes and Digestive and Kidney Diseases, National Institutes of Health.

Kidney Complications □Jerry □Lithotripsy

In the past, Jerry would have been condemned to suffer extreme pain while eventually passing the kidney stones out of his kidneys, down the ureters to his bladder and finally though his urethra to the outside. If the stones would not pass, various complications would quite possibly have lead to death. Somewhat more recently, a small basket may have been threaded into his kidneys and the stones captured and pulled out, a procedure at least as painful as passing the stones but at least in a situation where painkillers could be administered. Surgery to cut the stones out of the kidneys was also an option if they would not pass.

Kidney Complications – Jerry – Lithotripsy

Fortunately, such methods are no longer used in modern hospitals. Some perform a procedure called extracorporeal shock-wave lithotripsy, or ESWL (literally, breaking stones from outside the body using sound), in which extremely intense bursts of sound waves are focussed on the stones by a ***lithotripsy system (157)****. Depending on the system design, the patient is either be immersed in a water bath, allowing the water to help conduct the sound pulses, or they have a water-filled rubber bladder pressed against their back, which again carries the sound pulses into the body. The pulses are repeated once a second or so for an hour or more, gradually breaking the stones into smaller pieces, with the process being monitored with an* ***x-ray C-arm unit (212)****. When the attending physician feels that the stones are broken down sufficiently, the procedure ends. Over the next few days, the patient can then pass the smaller particles more easily, though still not without some pain. Due to the long exposure to high intensity sound waves, kidney tissue may be bruised, resulting in some blood being passed in the urine.*

Jerry will have his stones broken up by a newer technique in which a very thin optical fiber is threaded in a small tube up through his urinary tract until the tip comes in contact with the stones in his kidney. High-powered laser light pulses from a urological laser system are then passed through the optical fiber, gradually vaporizing the stone. This has advantages over the ESWL method, being faster and less likely to damage kidney tissue, producing no stone particles that have to be passed (all the stone is vaporized) and using much less bulky apparatus. The targeting and progress of the procedure is again monitored by fluoroscopy. The procedure is done under general anesthesia *(see page* Anesthesia*364)* *in an operating room and takes about an hour, after which Jerry is observed for a few hours in the recovery area and then allowed to go home.*

A newer technique uses a very thin optical fiber threaded in a small tube up through the urinary tract until the tip comes in contact with the stones in the kidney. High□powered laser light pulses from a urological laser system are then passed through the optical fiber, gradually vaporizing the stone. This has advantages over the ESWL method, being faster and less likely to damage kidney tissue, producing no stone particles that have to be passed (all the stone is vaporized) and using much less bulky apparatus. The targeting and progress of the procedure is again monitored by fluoroscopy. The procedure is done under general anesthesia (see p. 364) in an operating room

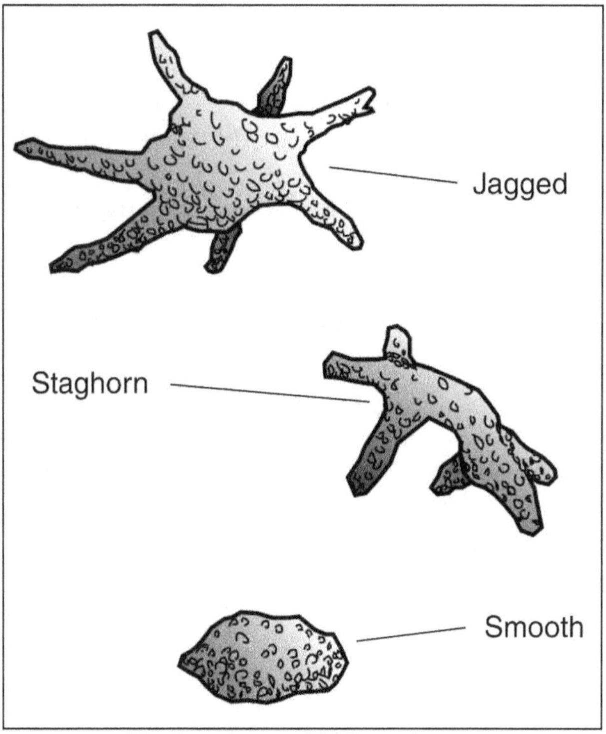

Various types of kidney stones.

Courtesy of the National Institute of Diabetes and Digestive and Kidney Diseases, National Institutes of Health.

Application □Direct contact lithotriptors require that the patient be sedated; a catheter is then introduced via the urethra, bladder, and ureter (for kidney stones) or through a small abdominal incision (for gallstones). The tip is positioned with the aid of a fluoroscope or an

ultrasound machine (217). Pulses are initiated when the tip is in position, and continue, with regular monitoring to ensure correct position, until the stone is sufficiently reduced. This system requires a semi-invasive procedure, and some stones are inaccessible to the catheter.

Focused beam lithotriptors are non-invasive, but tend to take longer to produce the same results as direct contact units. This means that the patient must remain essentially immobile for the duration of treatment, which can be an hour or more. The patient is either immersed in a special water-filled tub, which houses the sound generators, or placed firmly on a rubber bladder (using a special gel to help couple the sound waves between the bladder and the patient's body). Sedation is required, partly to help the patient remain motionless and partly because the effects of the treatment on soft tissue adjacent to the stone can cause discomfort. The stone must be visualized and triangulated with a fluoroscope system; this location information is used by a computer system and the operators to keep the beams focused on the stone.

In all cases, patients are **monitored (314)** to watch for possible adverse reactions to the treatment.

Some time (from hours to several days) after the treatment, stone fragments are passed by the patient. If treatment was ideal, the particles are small enough that little discomfort is experienced. Since kidney tissue is relatively delicate and highly vascularized, some bleeding into the urinary tract is likely to occur after treatment; this may also occur when stones are located in the ureter or bladder.

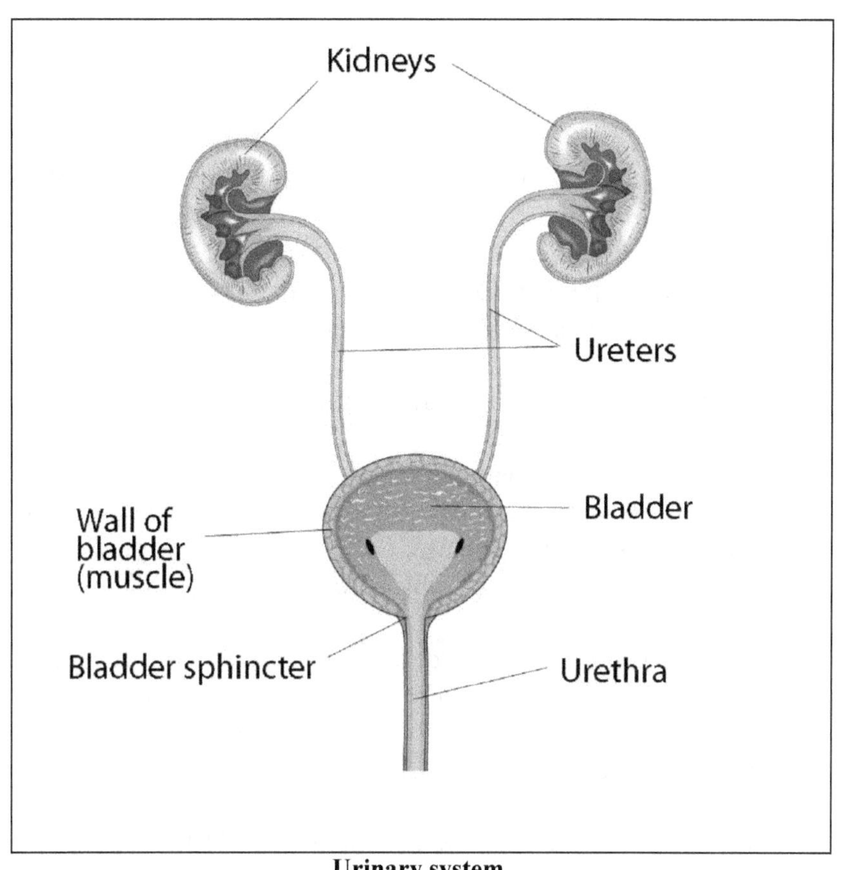

Urinary system.

Modified from Shutterstock, Inc, www.shutterstock.com, with permission.

AKA stone breakers.

Related devices fluoroscopes, **ultrasound machines (217)**, **physiological monitors (314)**.

Where found special treatment units, special x-ray rooms, operating rooms.

Chapter 9 – Cardio–Respiratory

- Function □ Cardio□Respiratory departments provide specialized diagnostic testing of the heart and circulatory system and the respiratory system. Tests may include ambulatory ECG monitoring, cardiac stress testing, 12 lead ECG tests, plethysmography, spirometry, respiration testing and detailed pulse oximetry testing.

- Layout □ Cardio□Respiratory functions may be combined into one unit or they may be divided into cardiology and respiratory units, with larger facilities possibly having sub□sections of each. A sleep studies lab may be included as part of the department. 12 lead ECG tests may be performed in the department or on patient wards using a portable machine.

- Staff □ while tests are ordered, supervised and interpreted by cardiologists and internists, cardiology technologists and respiratory therapists perform most patient preparation and testing procedures.

- Equipment □ **12 lead ECG machines (270)**, **cardiac stress test systems (184)**, **ambulatory ECG monitors (166)** (sometimes called Holter monitors), **plethysmograph systems (173)**, **spirometers (180)**, **respiration test systems (180)**, **pulse oximeters (320)**. A **defibrillator/monitor (259)** will be either in the department or easily accessible since many patients will be susceptible to heart attacks.

Cardio□Respiratory Equipment Descriptions

Following are more detailed descriptions of equipment found exclusively or most commonly in this area of the hospital. Equipment that is also found in various other areas of the hospital is described in Chapter 12, p 247.

Devices typically found in these areas, in addition to the equipment listed in this section, include: **defibrillators (259)**, **ECG machines (270)**, **manual (325)** or **non–invasive blood pressure units (296)**, **pulse oximeters (320)**, **stethoscopes (327)**, **aspirators (250)**, and **ventilators (334)**.

Ambulatory ECG Recorders

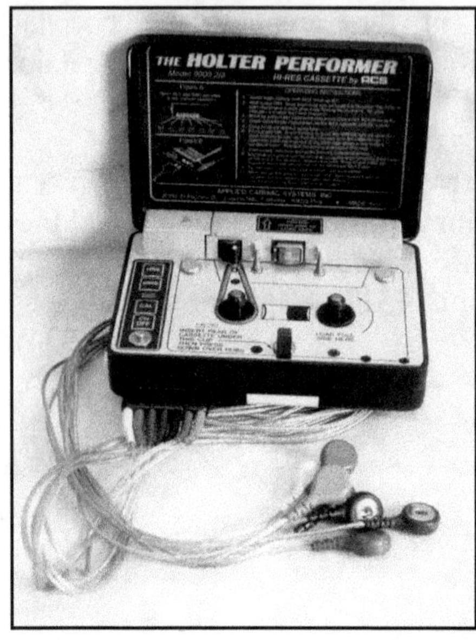

Overview □ It can be important to track the ECG signals of patients for an extended period of time, as they go about their daily activities.

Function □ Ambulatory ECG recorders perform mobile ECG measurement, by putting the input and processing circuitry for ECG signals into a small, battery powered package, along with a means of recording the signal. In the past, this was done with magnetic tape (often a standard cassette, geared down to run for 24 hours), but newer units use electronic memory modules which have the advantage of needing no moving parts or mechanical alignment, thus, being lighter, more durable, and requiring less maintenance. Picking up the ECG signals from the patient involves the same type of skin electrode and lead wires as other **ECG monitors (314)** and **recorders (270)**, but since there is no need for display or print□out of the signal in the device itself, the large and high□power□consumption monitor/recorder can be eliminated. Also, since the signal is not analyzed on the machine and there are no alarms or other parameters to be considered, the electronic circuitry can be relatively simple.

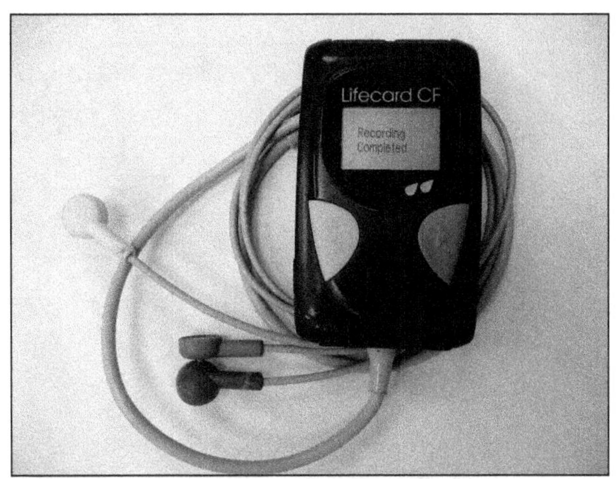

A digital solid–state ambulatory ECG recorder.

These units have a clock that records a coordinating signal along with the ECG, and there is normally a button that the patient can use to mark times of exertion, chest pains, meal times, or other circumstances as requested by their physician.

<u>Application</u> □ Electrodes are placed on the patient□s skin in prescribed locations, and the device is connected and started. To ensure the proper functioning of the device at the start of recording, there is usually a port that connects to the circuitry after amplification and processing, allowing the operator to check that everything is working at least to that point. The unit is worn in a comfortable pouch that allows access to the □mark□ button while protecting it from the elements. The patient is asked to keep a diary of activities and symptoms, to complement the □marks□ made by pressing the button. Since timing is an important factor in these recordings, the units have an internal clock which must be checked and set, if necessary, before recording starts.

After the recording period (usually about 24 hours), the signal is read by an analysis machine that can display the whole track on a video screen or print it out on a recorder.

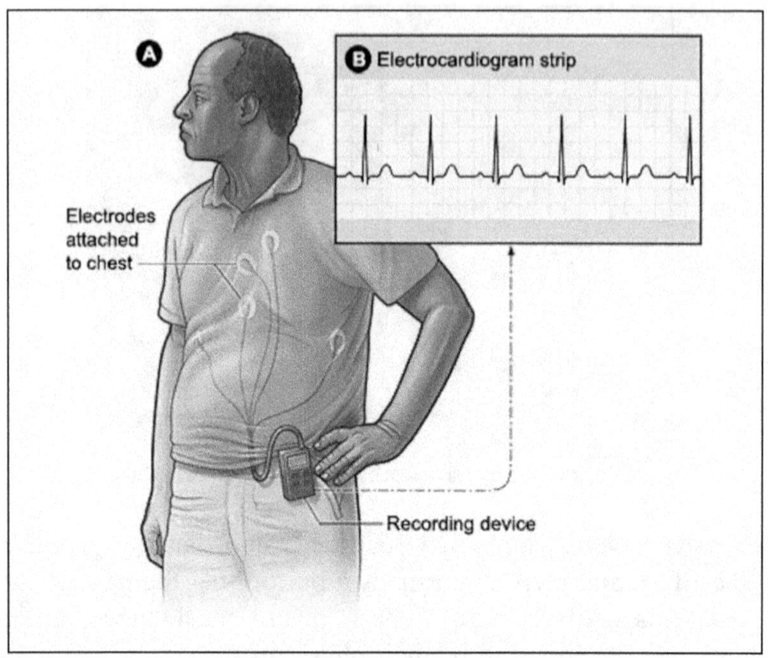

“Holter” or ambulatory ECG monitoring set–up.
Courtesy of the National Institute of Diabetes and Digestive and Kidney Diseases, National Institutes of Health.

Clinically□significant sections of the trace can be magnified and viewed or printed in more detail, and the analyzer can perform various measurements and analyses, such as average, minimum, and maximum heart rates, frequency of abnormal beats, and others. The signals can be correlated to the diary and the mark signals to help in understanding the condition of the patient□s cardiac system.

<u>AKA</u> □ AECG machines, long□term ECG recorders, Holter recorders (after one of the first manufacturers of this type of device).

<u>Related devices</u> □ **ECG monitors (314)**, **ECG recorders (270)**, **cardiac stress test systems (184)**.

<u>Where found</u> □ Cardiology department, laboratory outpatient department.

Cardiac Catheterization Systems

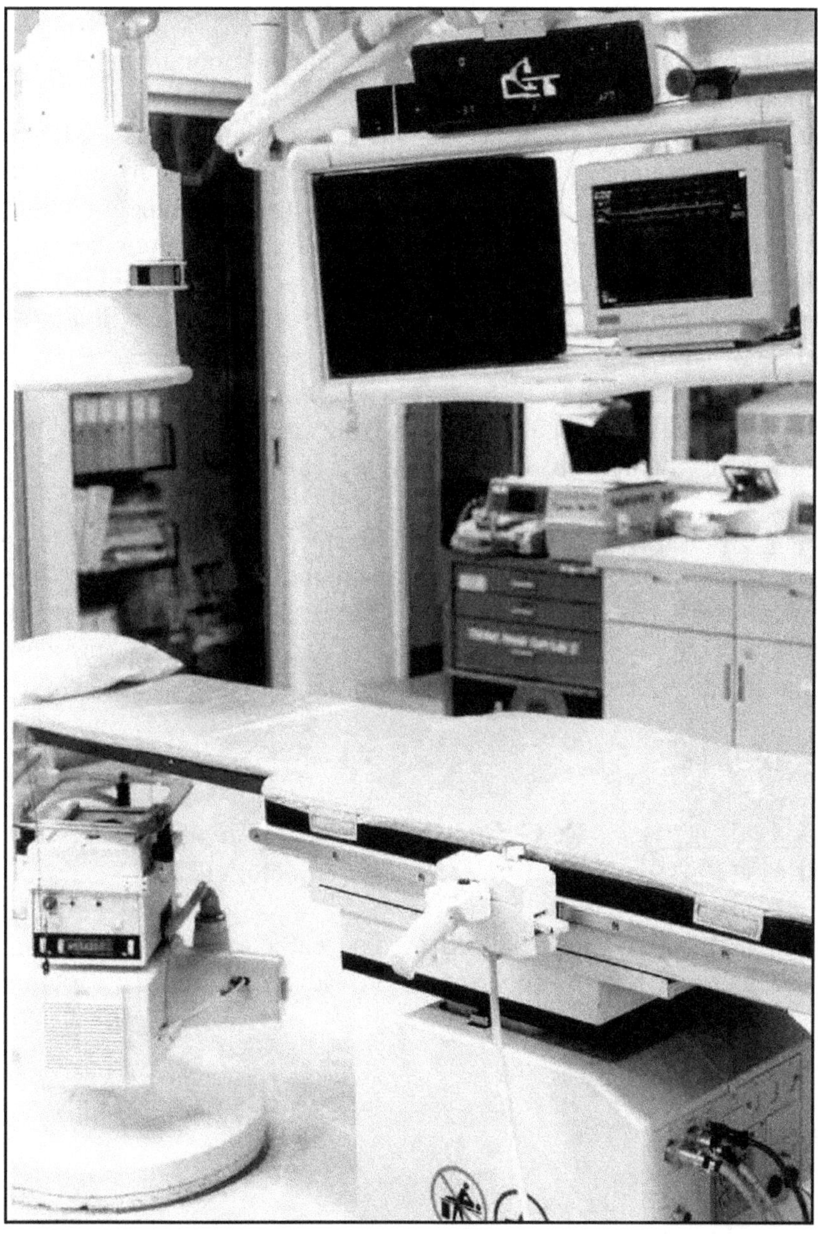

Overview □The diagnosis of certain heart conditions can be aided by visualizing the coronary arteries.

Function □ Cardiac catheterization (□cath□) systems allow this visualization by injecting contrast medium (radiopaque dye) into the target arteries, then taking x□rays as the dye moves through the vessels.
The system is made up of several components. A monitoring system measures, displays, and records pressure values from the catheter, along with the patient□s ECG signal. **X–ray apparatus (241)** is required to visualize the progression of the catheter and the movement of the injected dye (recorded on video tape or other storage medium for later analysis). There is specific equipment for handling the catheter itself. Finally, a **dye injector (222)** delivers the contrast medium. Since it is a critical procedure, a **defibrillator (259)** is normally kept on hand as well.

The injector must be capable of delivering precise quantities of dye very quickly, which means that high pressures are involved.

Application □Operators insert a catheter into the heart (usually from a point in the patient□s groin), through the aortic valve and into the coronary artery, and then inject a radiopaque dye; the catheter is then withdrawn. X□ray images are taken and ECG and pressure measurements are made throughout the procedure.

AKA □cath lab.

Related devices □ **ECG monitors (314)**, **invasive pressure monitors (294)**, **defibrillators (259)**, **dye injectors (222)**.

Equipment location □ specialized cardiac catheterization lab, which may be in a cardiology department, in radiology, or in a separate unit.

Cardiac Output Systems

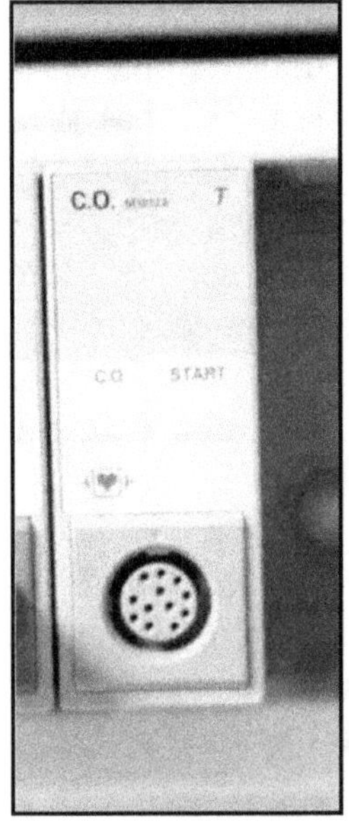

Overview □ One of the ways of determining a patient□s state of cardiac health is to measure the amount of blood pumped by each cycle of the heart. This value is the cardiac output, and though it cannot be measured directly, techniques have been developed to determine this value very accurately.

Function □ There are two basic methods of measuring cardiac output. One uses colored dye; the other uses cold saline solution. Both rely on the same principle.

In each case, a double□walled catheter is inserted into the patient□s venous system and guided to the vena cava, through the heart, and into the pulmonary artery. An injectate opening is located a precise distance from the end of the catheter, in the right atrium of the heart; on the end of the catheter, in the pulmonary artery, is a sensor.
In the dye dilution method, a specific amount of dye is injected through the catheter into the right atrium at a specific rate. As blood flows through the vessel, it mixes with the dye, diluting it. When the diluted mixture passes the tip of the catheter, a special optical sensor measures the concentration of dye. This measurement is done for a period of time, and the results are entered into a computer. A graph is obtained of dye concentration versus time, and by performing calculations on the measurements, an accurate measure of blood flow over time can be determined; this value is the cardiac output.

The cold saline method is similar, except the saline substitutes for the dye, and a temperature sensor is used in place of the optical sensor. Saline is less likely to produce side effects in the patient than dye, and the temperature sensors tend to be more stable than the optical probes.

Either method can be performed by a stand□alone device, or by a module that is part of a **physiological monitoring system (314)**. Stand□alone units need a display for prompting injection times, etc., and showing results; they also usually have a built□in recorder.

Modules can use the display and recorder of the monitor system for these functions.

Application — The special catheter is inserted into the patient's venous system, often via the subclavian vein in the neck. It is then advanced until it reaches the correct location, determined by observing pressure measurements taken from the catheter tip. At a precise time, the injection is started. Temperature or dye concentration measurements are taken throughout the procedure. The process may be repeated, though too much dye or cold saline can cause difficulties. When satisfactory results have been obtained, the catheter is withdrawn.

Because most cardiac output measurements are performed on patients with heart problems, and because the procedure can cause side effects such as cardiac arrhythmias, staff must be well trained and alert, and emergency equipment such as **defibrillators (259)** must be immediately available.

AKA — (none).

Related devices — **physiological monitors (314)**, **electronic probe thermometers (279)**.

Equipment location — intensive/cardiac care units, cardiology labs.

Doppler Blood Flow Detectors

Overview □Tissue health throughout the body depends on adequate blood circulation. Circulation can be impaired by various disease conditions or by trauma including surgery. If impaired circulation can be detected before damage occurs, preventive measures can be taken.

Application □ Blood behaves like an ideal fluid in some ways, but not in others, mainly because it contains particles in the form of red blood cells. (White blood cells and others make up an insignificant portion of blood from a hydrodynamic point of view).

Particles moving in flowing blood can provide a target for ultrasound signals, in that the frequency of ultrasound waves reflected back from them is subject to the Doppler effect (see p. 93). This Doppler frequency shift can be detected and analyzed in such a way as to provide information about blood flow, with a non□invasive technique.

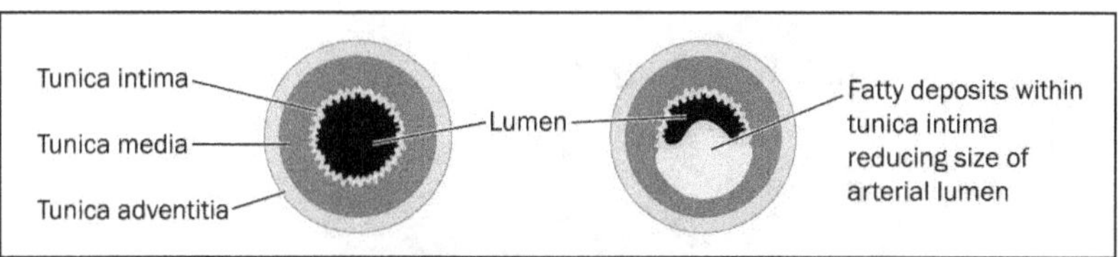

Blood vessels showing narrowing which can cause changes in blood velocities that can be detected with Doppler technology.
Modified from Shutterstock, Inc, www.shutterstock.com, with permission.

Ultrasound waves can be beamed into various parts of the body and positioned in such a way that they intersect with blood moving in a target vessel. Some of the ultrasound energy is reflected by the red blood cells, the frequency is altered according to the Doppler effect, and a transducer picks up the reflected waves. By filtering out non□ Doppler shifted signals and analyzing the degree of shift, a measure of the blood flow in the target vessel can be derived.
Such Doppler blood flow detectors range from relatively simple hand□held devices that provide feedback about blood flow via sound from a speaker or headset. Moving blood produces a rushing sound, which varies with the pulsatile flow. This provides a quick means of determining if there is circulation in various parts of the body,

usually the limbs. These devices are very similar to ultrasound **fetal heart detectors (93).**

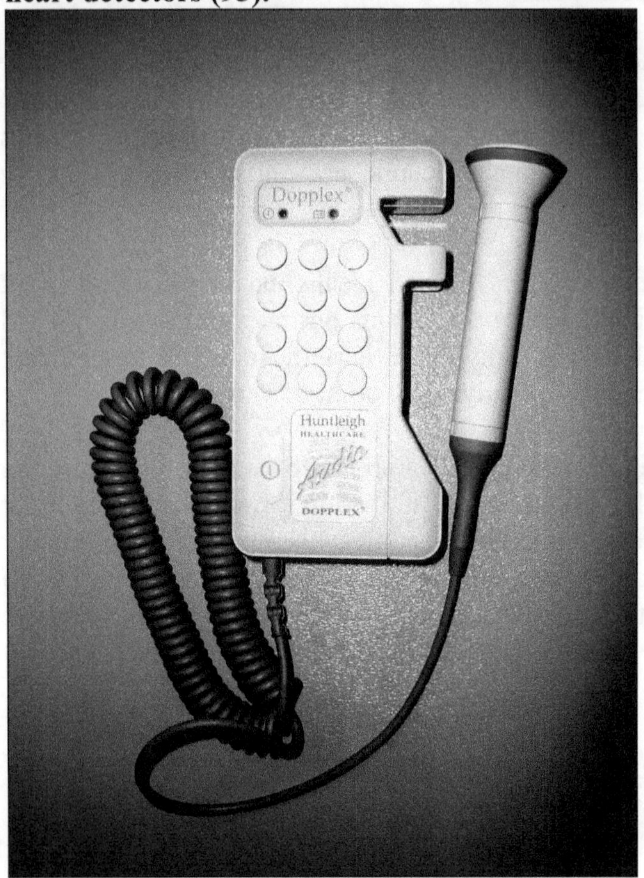

A simple Doppler blood flow detector.

Computerized blood flow systems (plethysmographs) utilize the same principle as the simpler systems, but can provide quantitative and graphical data about blood flow that can be analyzed and stored, along with information about which blood vessels were being targeted, patient parameters, transducers in use, and more.

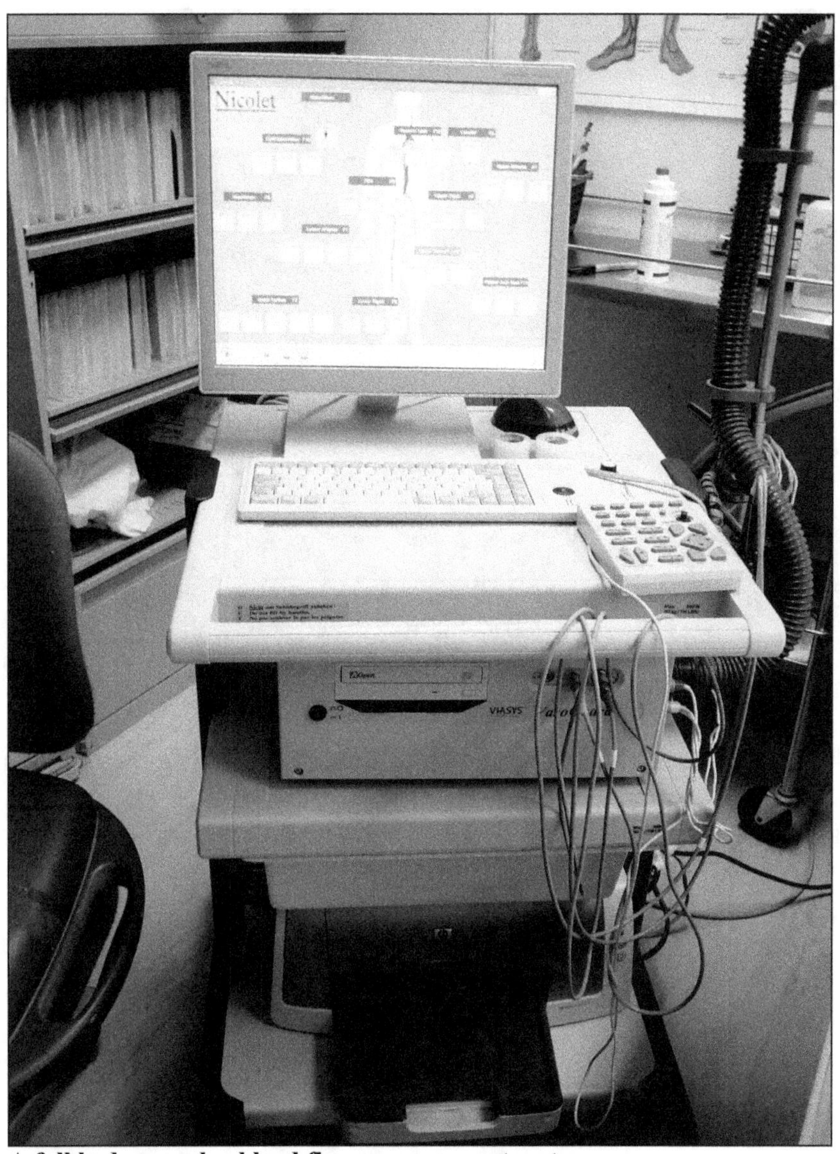

A full body vascular blood flow measurement system.

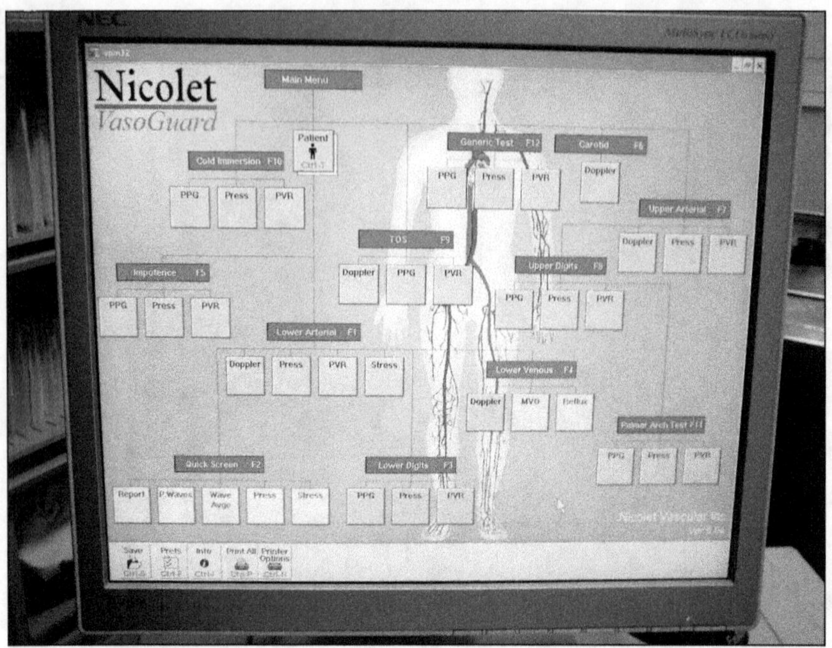

Vascular blood flow system screen shot. Flow values will appear in the boxes related to specific blood vessels.

Ultrasound transducers consist of piezoelectric crystals mounted on a probe. When stimulated with an electrical signal, the crystals emit ultrasound waves. The crystals can be arranged in such a way that the beams from the different crystals intersect at a specific depth, or they may use a frequency that penetrates to a specific depth range.

Different transducers may be available for blood flow analyzers, since lower frequencies penetrate more deeply than higher frequencies.

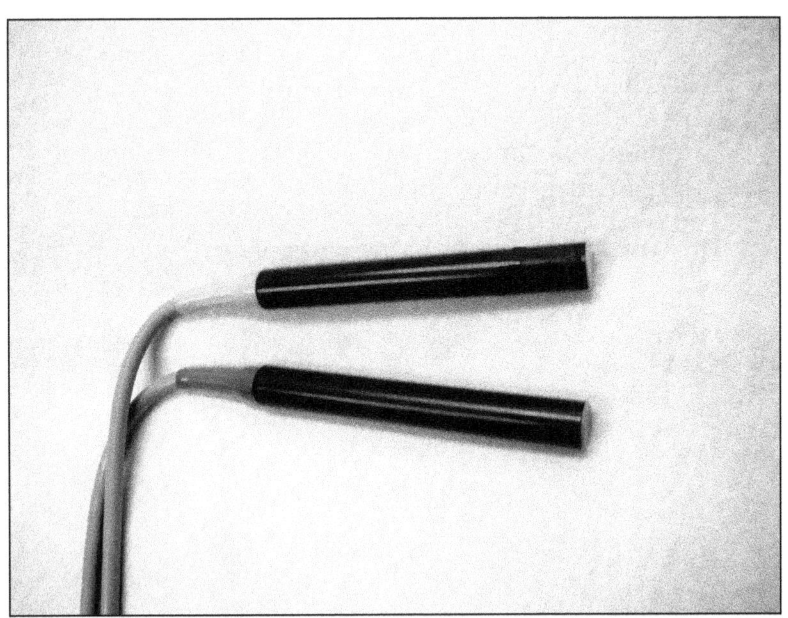

Two vascular blood flow probes.

As with all ultrasound technology, a gel is used to provide better coupling between the probe and the patient, improving wave transmission in both directions and reducing noise.

AKA □vascular lab, pleth.

Related devices □**fetal heart detectors (93), diagnostic ultrasound machines (217)**.

Where found □Cardio□respiratory departments.

Pacemaker Programmers

Overview **Implantable pacemakers (25)** have to be able to be programmed to suit patient requirements.

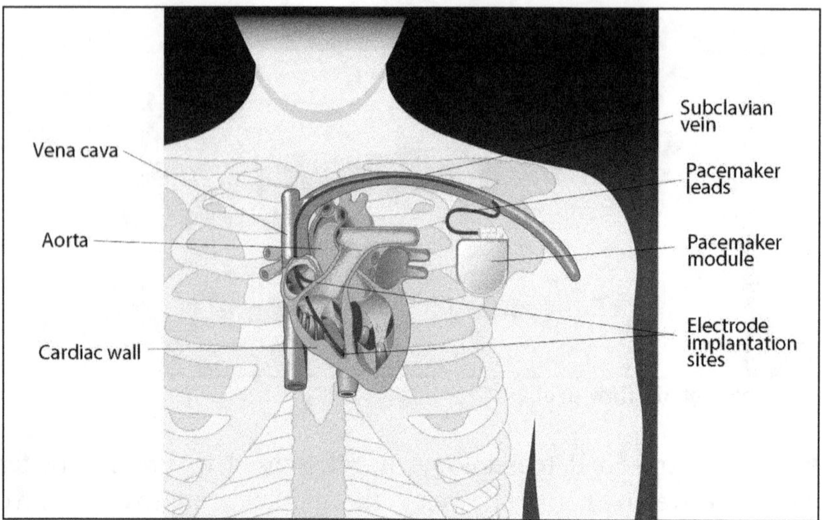

Pacemaker implantation diagram.
Modified from Shutterstock, Inc, www.shutterstock.com, with permission.

Application Programmers use an antenna placed over the pacemaker site to communicate with the device, and a terminal allows users to see current programming parameters and enter new ones.

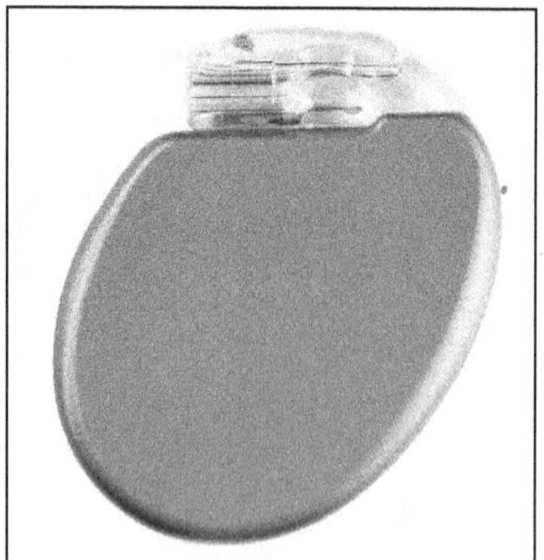

An implantable pacemaker module.
Modified from Inmagine Corp, www.123rf.com, with permission.

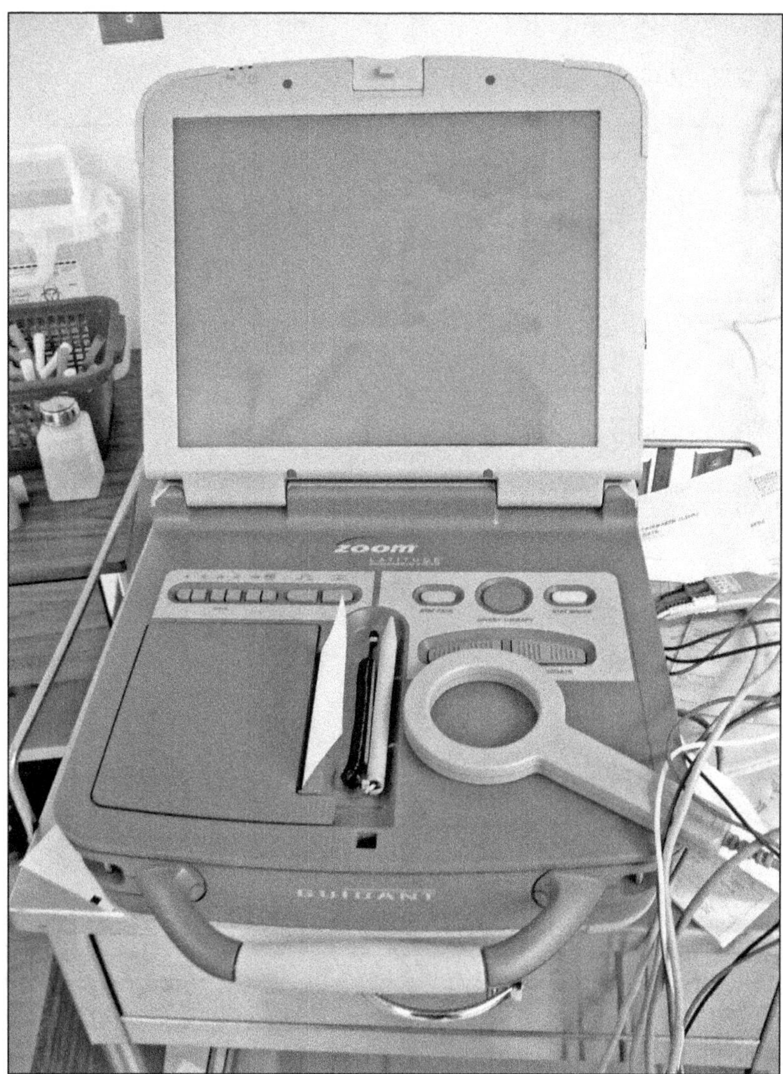

A pacemaker programmer. The "lollipop" shaped section is the electromagnetic wand that carries programming signals to the pacemaker.

AKA □none.

Related devices □**Implantable pacemakers (25)**.

Where found □ Operating rooms, cardio□respiratory departments.

Spirometers/ Pulmonary Function Analyzers

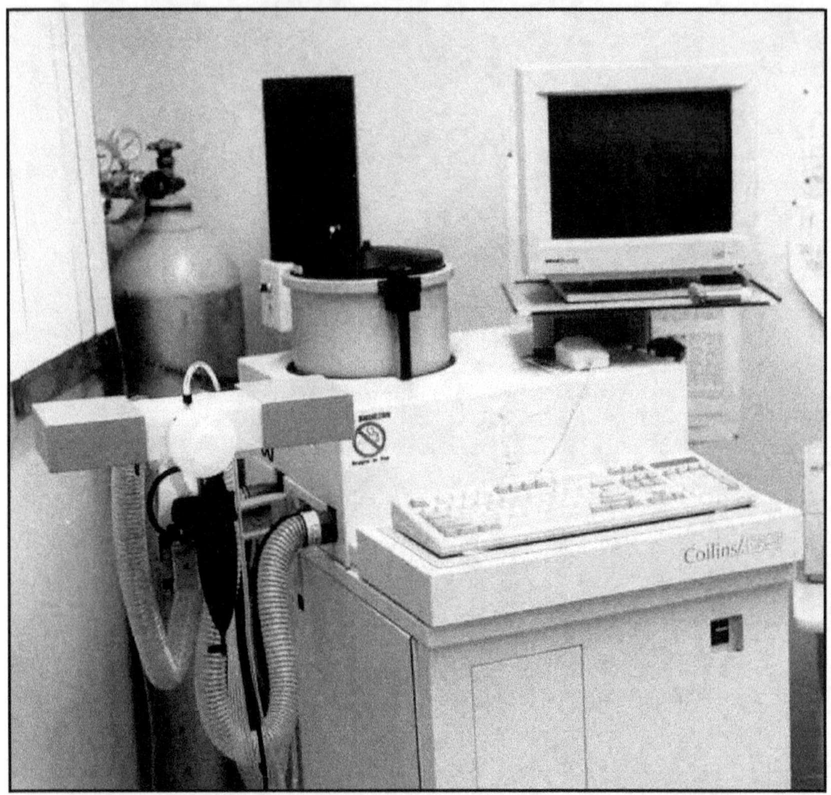

Overview □ Measuring lung function is critical in determining the state of health of many patients, especially those with respiratory disorders. Various parameters can be measured, including those of normal breathing and the extremes of inspiration and expiration.

Function □ Both the volume and the rate of airflow during breathing can be measured by a spirometer; both can be graphed against each other to produce a roughly circular chart, beginning and ending at the same point, or volume can be graphed against time to give a linear chart. Measurements are usually repeated a few times for each level of breathing (normal and maximal effort). The shape of the charts, including minimums and maximums, as well as any irregularities, can tell the caregiver a great deal about the health of the patient□s lungs. In addition, tests performed both before and after medications can give a good indication as to the effectiveness of the medication. Long□term tracking of test results provides a means of following disease and/or recovery progress.

The simplest spirometers are strictly mechanical, with the patient breathing into a bellows that has a chart pen attached, which in turn marks rotating or moving graph paper, producing a linear chart of volume vs. time. More advanced versions use some kind of electronic sensor to measure flow; once the flow rate and cross□ sectional area of the breathing tube are known, volumes can be calculated. These data can then be used to produce the circular graphs mentioned previously, either on a graph paper or on a video monitor. Electronic circuitry can perform all relevant measurements and give a print□out of the results, as well as allowing pre□and post□ medication tests to be compared directly, on a graph and/or as numerical values.

Spirometers may also form part of a system that can monitor such parameters as expired **CO2 levels (254)**, **body temperature (279)**, **ECG (314)**, **blood oxygen saturation (320)** (SpO2), and others.
The prime considerations of spirometer design are that they be accurate and repeatable, and that they provide an absolute minimum of obstruction to the patient□s breathing.

Application □A fresh mouthpiece is inserted into the breathing tube of the unit, and the patient places it in the mouth. Normal breathing is done for several cycles, and then the operator asks the patient to take in as much air as possible, hold it for a second, and then exhale that breath as thoroughly as possible, as rapidly as possible. The operator examines the results, and may ask the patient to repeat the procedure, sometimes giving specific instructions to help obtain a better result.

If pre□ and post□medication studies are being done, the patient is given medication and the test repeated, sometimes at a few pre□ determined times after medication administration.

Galling Gall Stones – Elizabeth – Cardio-Respiratory

Elizabeth has been home from the hospital for a few weeks and is recovering well from the surgery, but her COPD (Chronic Obstructive Pulmonary Disease) is causing difficulties, so when she is feeling well enough, her Doctor schedules her for some tests in the Cardio-Respiratory Department of the hospital. She is first checked with a simple spirometer, and when that confirms that her breathing is compromised, she is connected to a ***pulmonary function analyzer (190)****. She is seated on an exercise bicycle and a mouthpiece is fitted along with a gentle clamp that closes her nose so that she could only breathe through her mouth and the mouthpiece. The mouthpiece is connected by light plastic tubing to a machine that looks something like a portable dishwasher, except with a clear top-mounted cylinder, a computer keyboard and a video screen. The technologist running the tests has Elizabeth breathe normally for a few breaths, then asks her to take the deepest breath possible and then exhale as much air as possible. This is repeated a few times until the tech feels the results are the best they would get. Elizabeth is then asked to start pedaling the bicycle while continuing to breathe through the mouthpiece. She notices that a bellows inside the cylinder rises and falls with her breathing, and that the computer screen shows a lot of numbers as well as roughly circular graphs. The technologist explains that the numbers and graphs are measures of how much volume of air she is inhaling and exhaling and the flow rates of air during her breaths. These results would later be compared to "normal" values and would help determine the extent of her COPD, and thus aid in her future treatment.*

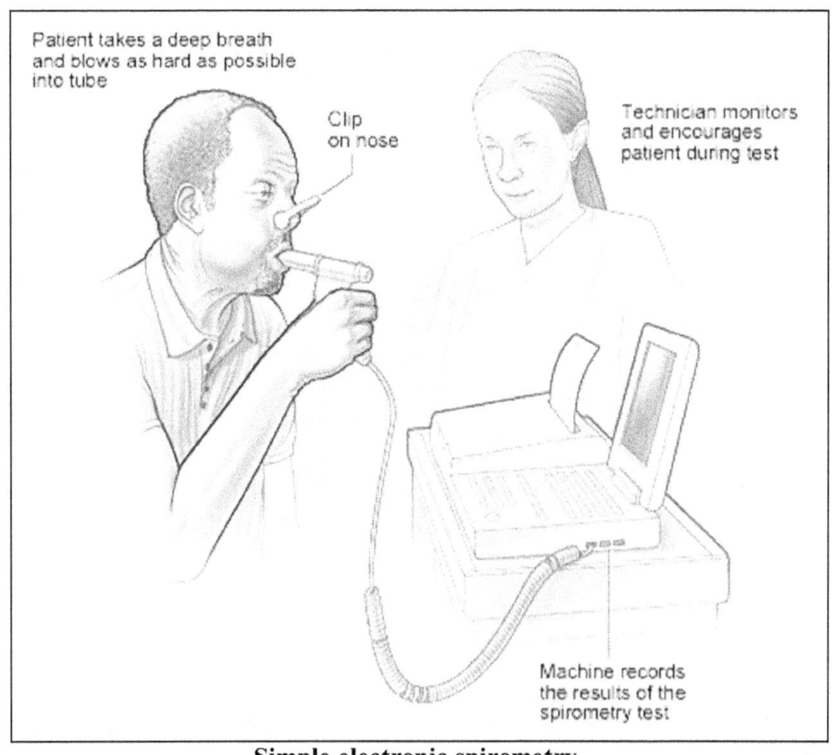

Simple electronic spirometry.
Courtesy of the National Institute of Diabetes and Digestive and Kidney Diseases, National Institutes of Health.

Avoiding disease transmission is, of course, an important consideration, and all spirometers have disposable mouthpieces, which are changed after each patient. In addition, parts exposed to patients are sterilized at regular intervals.

<u>AKA</u> □spirometers, pulmonary function testers or machines or analyzers.

<u>Related devices</u> □**stress test systems (184)**, **pulse oximeters (320)**, **capnographs (254)**.

<u>Where found</u> □ respiratory clinics, some doctor□s offices, laboratories (usually in smaller hospitals), mobile respiratory testing facilities.

Stress Test Systems

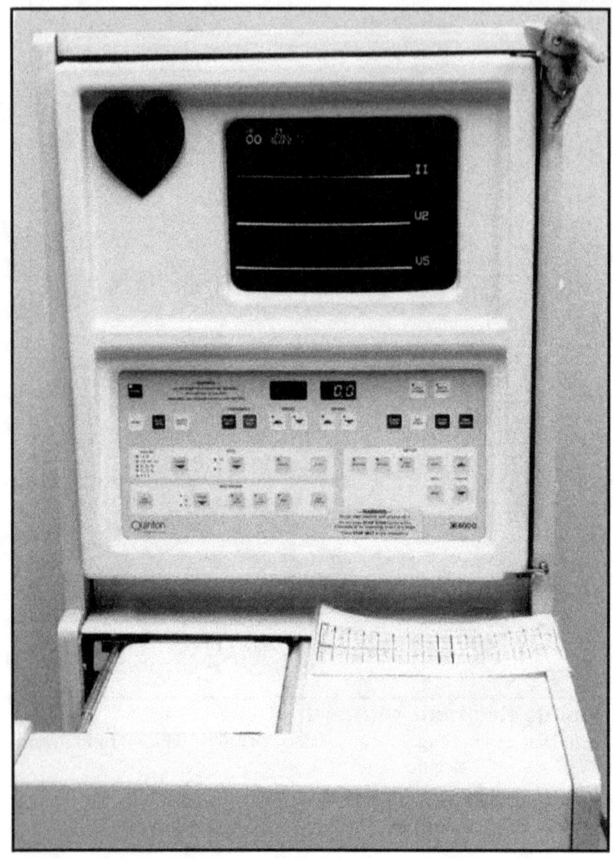

Overview □ The ECG of a patient is usually measured with the patient in bed. In diagnosing many cardiac however, the physician needs to see how the heart reacts to exercise.

Function □ Stress test systems allow the opportunity of testing ECG during exercise. They consist of a mechanism for exercise in a fixed location, such as a treadmill, and a component that combines control circuitry for the exercise device with physiological monitoring. The monitor looks at the patient□s ECG waveforms, usually on multiple leads, and displays the signals on a screen and on a chart recorder. Some systems may also monitor other parameters such, as oxygen saturation (**SpO2, pulse oximetry (320)**) or respiration.

The system controls the level of exercise according to a pre□programmed pattern. For example, by varying speed and/or slope of the belt of a treadmill, exercise levels can be changed. The exercise levels can also be controlled directly by the operator; however, the preset programs are usually used. These are developed by cardiologists who have determined the optimum exercise patterns for various patients and conditions, in order to maximize the chance of obtaining clinically useful results while minimizing risk to the patient. The operator can stop the exercise program at any time if it appears that the patient is becoming over-stressed, and systems have safety mechanisms to stop if the patient moves off the equipment during exercise.

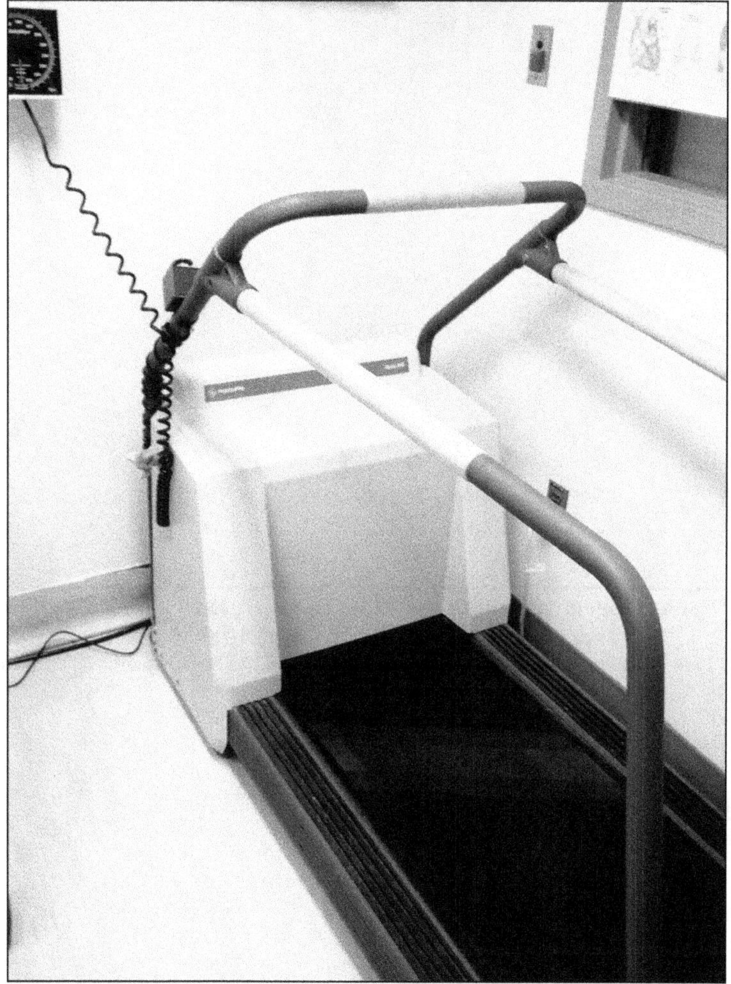

Stress test exercise treadmill.

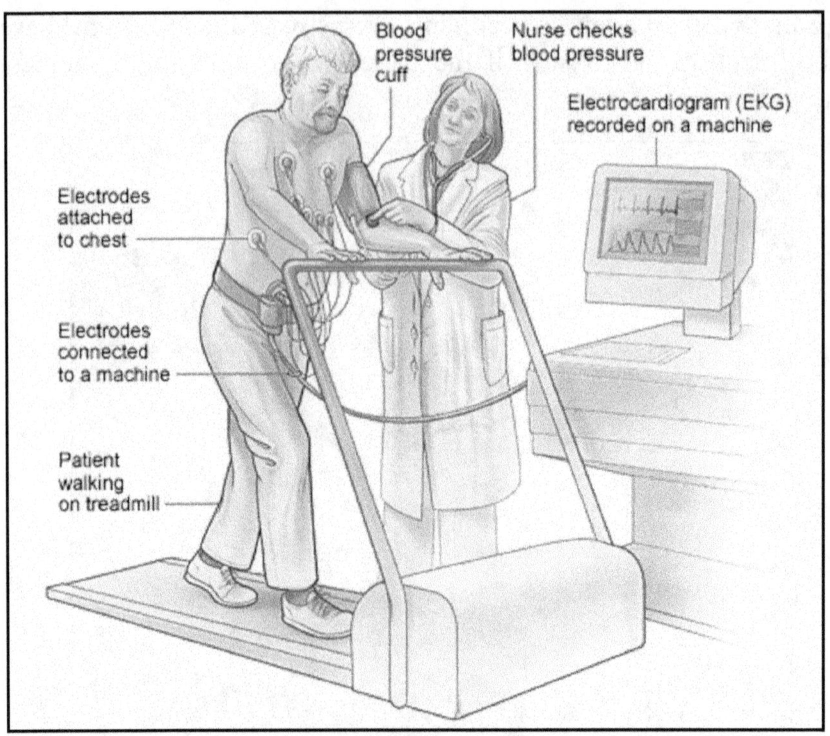

Stress test arrangement. There would be an emergency shut–off button on the treadmill front handle, and usually side rails..

Courtesy of the National Institute of Diabetes and Digestive and Kidney Diseases, National Institutes of Health.

Heart Attack! – John – Cardio-Respiratory

John is taken down to the Cardio-Respiratory Department, where a number of tests are performed including a cardiac stress test. In this test, John has a number of ECG electrodes attached to his chest and arms. These electrodes are connected to a ***stress test system (184)*** *via a long cable. John then steps onto an exercise treadmill and the technologist running the test explains how the test works. John will have his resting ECG taken by the machine, and then the test will start and be run automatically by the system, with the main unit controlling the treadmill. The treadmill will start at a slow speed, and then it will increase in both speed and slope according to a predetermined pattern called a protocol. This particular test will use the Bruce Protocol, which has seven stages of three minutes each. The system records several channels of John's ECG signals and displays information about the ECG and the test functions on a video screen. The system also has a large-format chart recorder that will printout results at the end of the test, including ECG waveforms, test parameters and notations about any abnormalities. The test results will later be analyzed by John's cardiologist. The test can be cancelled at any time by the operator if John is feeling distressed, and there is also a large, red emergency stop button that John can press himself if he feels the need to stop the test.*

ECG signals are picked up from the patient□s skin just as with normal **ECG monitors (314)**, but with certain modifications. Because the electrodes will be applied for a short time, but must be able to withstand (sometimes vigorous) patient movement and possible perspiration, they are designed somewhat differently than those used for longer□term monitoring. Suction cup electrodes may be used, with rubber bulbs to create suction and silver cups to make contact with the patient□s skin. A conductive cream is usually used with this type of electrode. A harness of some sort may be used to keep the electrode lead wires and cables in place, and, of course, the cable must be quite long to allow adequate patient movement.

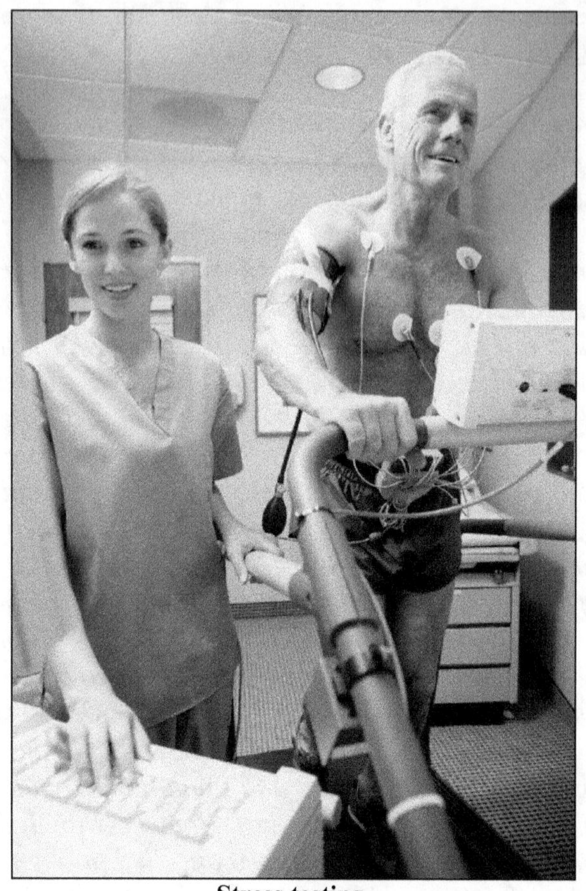

Stress testing.
Modified from Shutterstock, Inc, www.shutterstock.com, with permission.

<u>Application</u> □ After skin preparation, electrodes are applied to the patient□s skin. They may be held more securely in place with a harness or vest. The patient moves onto the exercise machine, and the operator initiates the procedure. While the operator (and sometimes the monitoring system) watches for signs of problems, the control system runs through the pre□set exercise program, which usually includes a slower □warm up□ phase, a longer, high□intensity phase, and a □cool down□ phase.

Recordings may be made continuously during the exercise program, or for shorter periods, either at pre□selected times or when the operator decides something should be examined more closely.

Since many of the patients undergoing this type of testing have cardiac problems, a **defibrillator (259)** is normally kept nearby during procedures.

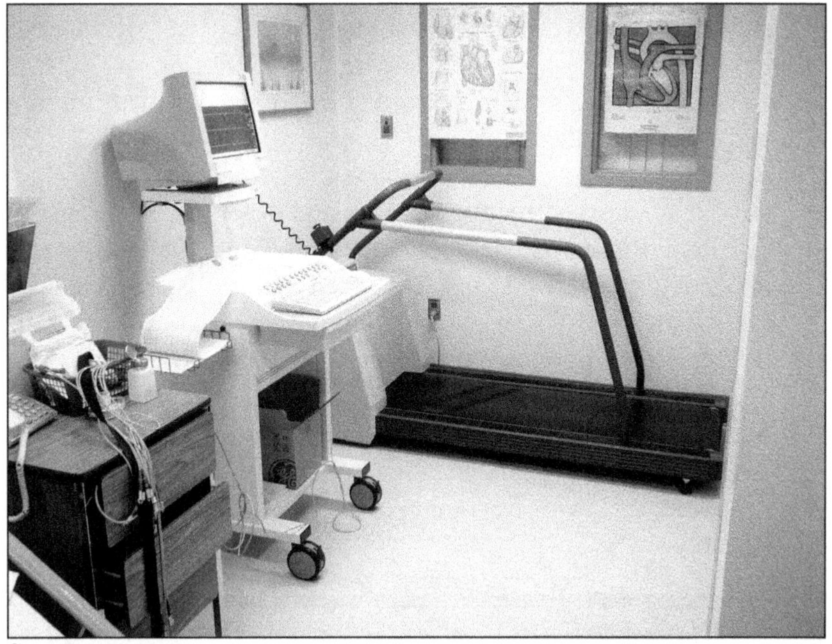

Stress test system.

<u>AKA</u> exercise systems, treadmills.

<u>Related devices</u> **ECG monitors (314)**, **ECG machines (270)**, **pulse oximeters (320)**, **spirometers (180)**, **defibrillators (259)**.

<u>Where found</u> cardiology, outpatient, physiotherapy, or respiratory therapy departments; laboratories.

Chapter 10 – Physical Therapy

- Function □ Patients who have had surgery or who have suffered serious illness or injury often have significantly reduced mobility, strength and range of motion, as well as pain and stiffness of muscles and/or joints. Physical therapy aims to reduce these

- Layout □Various treatment tables and other large devices are distributed in a (usually) spacious area, sometimes separated into cubicles with curtains. An open area is usually included for patients to walk or move under observation. Hydrotherapy pools are usually in a separate room.

- Staff □Physiotherapists and assistants.

- Equipment □ A wide range of devices is used in physical therapy.

Accidents Happen – Felipe – Physical Therapy

Felipe hobbles his way into the Physical Therapy Department and is greeted by one of the staff physiotherapists (sometimes called physical therapists). He has been coming to the unit for a couple of weeks and knows the routine. He gets comfortable on a table while an aide brings hot packs from ***a hot pack heater (198)*** *and places them on the leg that had suffered the most damage. After warming up his muscles and doing some stretching and strengthening exercises, Felipe gets on his back and places his foot in the stirrup of a* ***continuous passive motion (CPM) machine (193)****. This unit simply moves his leg back and forth, bending his knee to a degree set by the physio. Felipe is still having trouble moving the leg much on his own, so the machine provides movement for him.*

Accidents Happen – Felipe continued

After some time on the CPM machine, one of the physiotherapists has Felipe lie on a treatment bed while she uses a ***laser therapy unit (196)*** *on his forearm to produce deep heating and increase blood circulation to aid in healing as well as providing a measure of pain relief. She then has Felipe sit up and she applies a set of four suction cup electrodes to the damaged muscles in his back. These electrodes are connected to an* ***interferential therapy unit (194)*** *that sends electrical pulses through the electrodes as well as developing alternating suction pressures in the cups that produce a massage-like effect. The electrical signals cross each other and cause muscle contractions and increased circulation deep in the tissue as well as providing pain relief. After half an hour on this unit, a small* ***TENS (203)*** *(Transcutaneous Electrical Nerve Stimulator) pack is connected to electrodes on his shoulder, where it delivers similar electrical signals to a smaller area, but with the same kinds of effects as the interferential unit, though mainly pain relief. After this, Felipe is still feeling some discomfort in his injured hand, so he is take to a* ***wax bath (210)*** *and instructed to dip his hand repeatedly into the hot, melted wax, building up layers of warm wax that produce deep heating. The bath uses special wax that melts at a lower temperature than candle wax so it is pleasantly hot without burning. When the wax has cooled Felipe peels it away from his hand. The physio has noticed that Felipe has eczema on his arms so she suggests a session in the* ***UV therapy booth (205)****. Felipe strips to the waist and stands inside a cylindrical chamber that is lined with long, bluish fluorescent light bulbs, something like a vertical tanning booth. He is provided with protective goggles for his eyes and then the door is closed and a timer set, turning the UV lights on. After a pre-set time a buzzer sounds and the lights go off. Felipe exits the booth, gets dressed and says goodbye to the staff until his next visit.*

Physical Therapy Equipment Descriptions

Following are more detailed descriptions of equipment found exclusively or most commonly in this area of the hospital. Equipment that is also found in various other areas of the hospital is described in Chapter 12, p 247.

Continuous Passive Motion (CPM) Systems

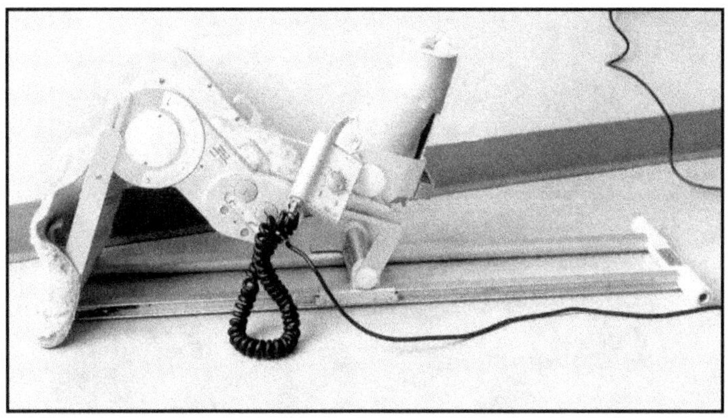

Overview □Patients are often unable to move their limbs enough for adequate rehabilitation. A mechanism that performs repetitive motion of the limb automatically is useful in promoting recovery.

Function □ A continuous passive motion machine consists of a comfortable frame into which the patient□s limb can be inserted and effectively immobilized, with mechanical hinges corresponding to the joints involved. A motor and gear or belt assembly then moves the frame back and forth on a track, flexing and extending the limb. The degree of motion is adjustable to suit each patient, as is the rate of operation. Systems often include a timer to signal the end of the selected treatment time.

Application □ The patient is moved to a comfortable position that allows the range of motion developed by the continuous passive motion device. The target limb is placed in the frame, which is lined with a soft material such as sheepskin, and strapped in place. The frame has to be on a stable surface, though not necessarily smooth or horizontal. After determining the most effective range of motion and rate of action and setting the controls, the operator starts the machine, which can then function for a pre□determined time.

AKA □CPM units or machines.

Related devices □**TENS (203), sequential compression (201).**

Where found □ physiotherapy departments or clinics, patient bedsides where physiotherapy is administered.

Interferential Therapy Units

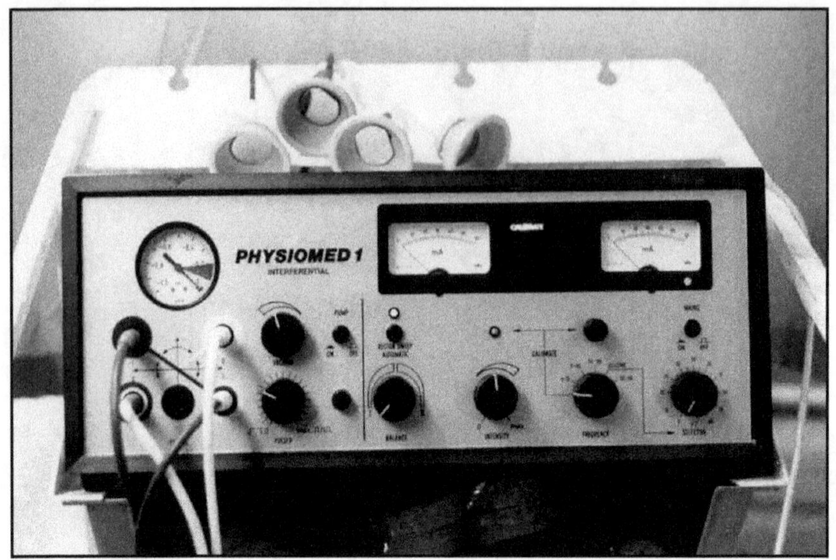

Overview □ Pain reduction is a goal in the treatment of many medical conditions. Pain may not respond well to pain□killing medications, and even when it does, the medications used may have undesirable side effects, especially at high doses. Non□chemical means of alleviating pain can be very valuable.

Reduction of swelling (edema) in disease or surgical sites is also important to promote healing.

Function □In a manner similar to that of **trans–cutaneous electrical nerve stimulator (203)** (TENS) units, interferential therapy units apply electrical signals to specific areas of the patient□s body. These signals can reduce pain by either disrupting the normal pain nerve transmissions in the body, preventing them from reaching the brain to cause a sensation of pain, or by causing the body to produce endorphins, which are natural painkillers. The exact mechanism of operation is under debate.

Interferential therapy units use two pairs of electrodes, and pass signals in various patterns between the pairs so that an interference pattern of high and low intensity levels is produced in the tissues between and around the electrodes. This pattern apparently helps to reduce pain as well as reducing edema.

Some interferential units incorporate an alternating vacuum system, in which large suction cups fit over the electrodes. Vacuum is applied alternately to the suction cups, producing a massaging action. Units with this option are considerably larger than those without, since a vacuum pump and switching apparatus are required.

Application □ Electrodes (and suction cups, if used) are applied to the patient□s skin in a criss□cross arrangement over the target area. Power levels, rates, and patterns are set, as well as treatment time. An audible and/or visual alarm indicates the end of treatment, at which time the signals and vacuum are switched off.

AKA □(none).

Related devices □ **trans–cutaneous electrical nerve stimulator units (203)**, **sequential compression units (201)**.

Where found □physical therapy departments and clinics.

Laser Therapy Units

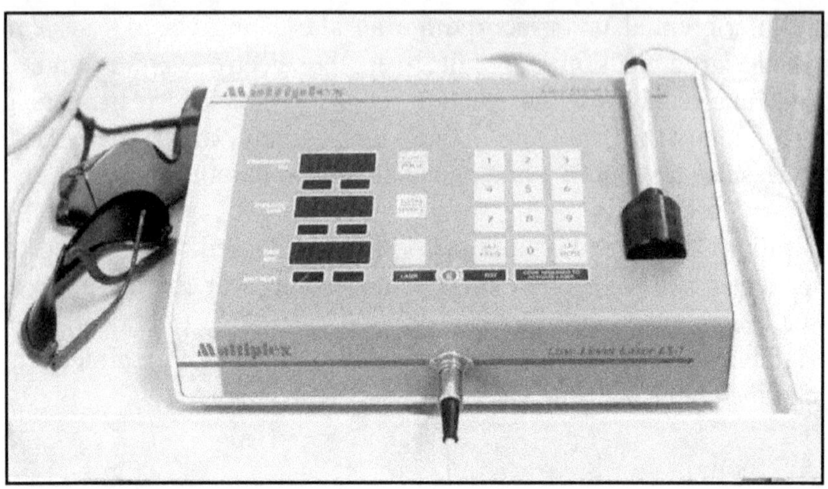

Overview □Reduction of pain and increased healing are two important goals in physiotherapy.

Function □ Laser therapy units utilize a relatively low□power red and/or infrared laser beam to stimulate the skin. This stimulation can produce increased blood flow to the area, thus aiding healing. It has also been found to aid in reducing inflammation, as well as increasing electrolyte activity in target tissues, both of which can be beneficial to healing.

Laser therapy can also act in a similar manner to **TENS units (203)** or acupuncture by either blocking nerve signal transmission or stimulating endorphin (natural pain killer) production.

Units have controls for beam intensity, frequency, and treatment time.

Application □ The patient is placed in a comfortable position with the target area exposed, and the operator sets treatment power, frequency, and duration. The laser beam is directed over the target region for the length of the procedure, possibly without further operator involvement.

Even though the laser beam used in these units is of relatively low power, it can still cause damage to eyes. The eyes of both patient and operator must be protected by goggles at all times and the laser beam must never be directed at eyes.

AKA (none).

Related devices **TENS (203), hot pack heaters (198), wax baths (210), ultrasound therapy (208), surgical lasers (70).**

Where found physiotherapy departments.

Moist Heat Units

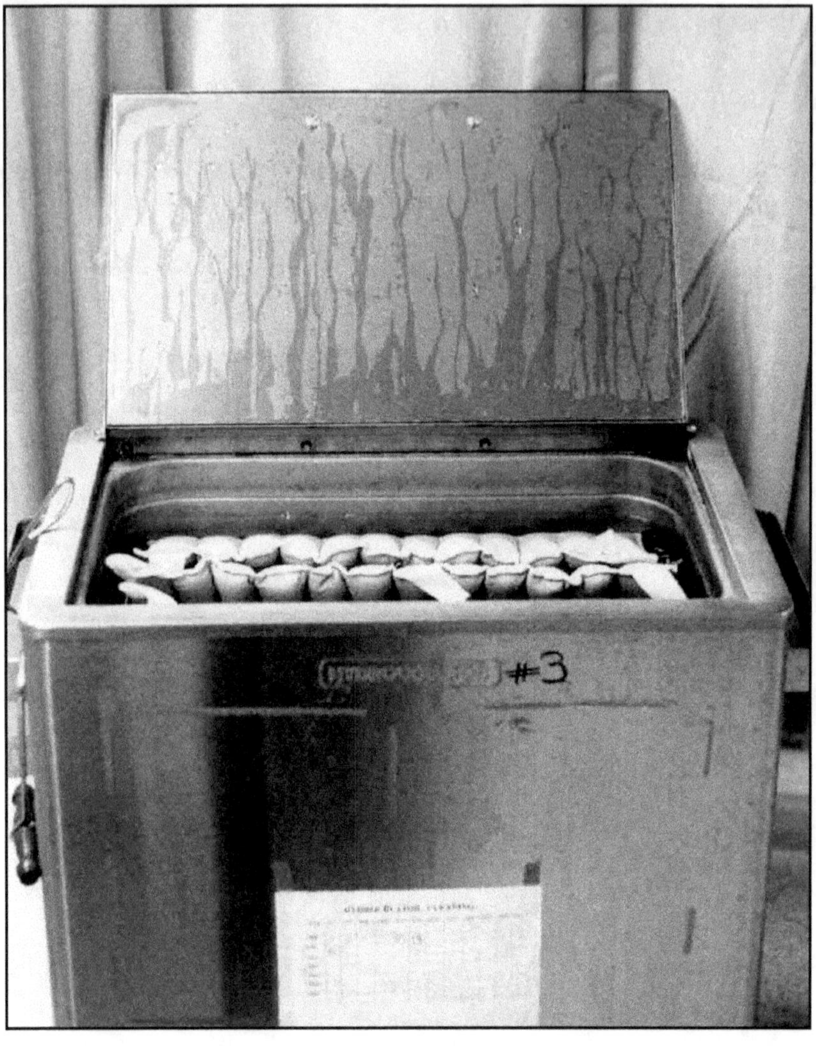

Overview □ The application of heat can relieve some of the pain associated with tissue inflammation caused by injury or diseases such as arthritis. It can also promote healing by increasing blood flow to that area.

Function □ Moist heat units are simply water heaters that store hot packs, which are cloth□covered bags that hold heated water and can be moulded to the shape of the body part to which they are being applied. A thermostat maintains a constant, therapeutic water temperature in the water tank.

Application □Hot packs are placed against the skin of the patient to provide maximum heating of the target tissue. Towels or other insulating materials may be placed over the hot packs to help retain heat. After a pre□determined treatment time, the packs are either replaced or removed.

To avoid the possibility of contamination, water in the heater unit must be changed on a regular basis and tested for organism growth.

AKA □ hydrocollators (after the model name of an early version), hot pack heaters.

Related devices □**wax baths (210)**, **ultrasound therapy (208)**.

Where found □physiotherapy departments and clinics.

Percussors

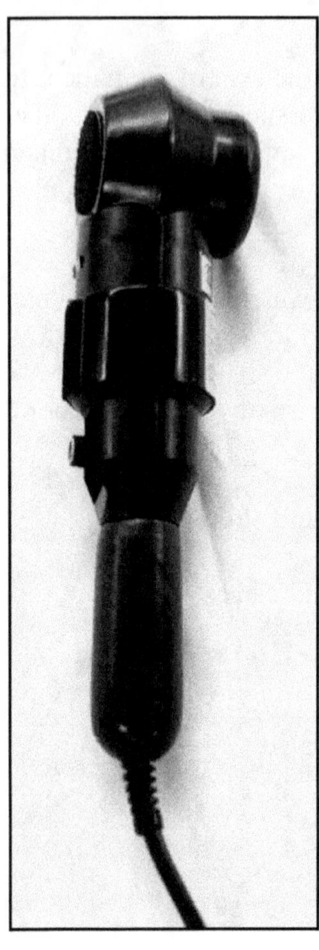

Overview □ Various medical conditions (such as cystic fibrosis) can result in an excessive build□up of mucus in the patient□s lungs. It is vital that these build□ ups be removed on a regular basis, otherwise pulmonary function will be seriously impaired.

Function □ Percussors are simple mechanical vibrators that send low frequency, relatively high power shock waves (□thumps□) into the patient□s body. The shock waves help to loosen the mucus so that it can be drained or expelled from the lungs.

Application □ The patient is positioned head□down on a tilted table or frame and the percussor is applied to their chest and slowly moved around. The patient may need to be turned to various angles in order for treatment to be most effective.

AKA □(none).

Related devices □(none).

Where found □ physiotherapy departments or clinics, patient wards, patient□s homes.

Sequential Compression Devices (SCD)

Overview □ Fluids may collect in the limbs, particularly the legs, of patients with compromised circulation. This fluid build□up can lead to serious complications.

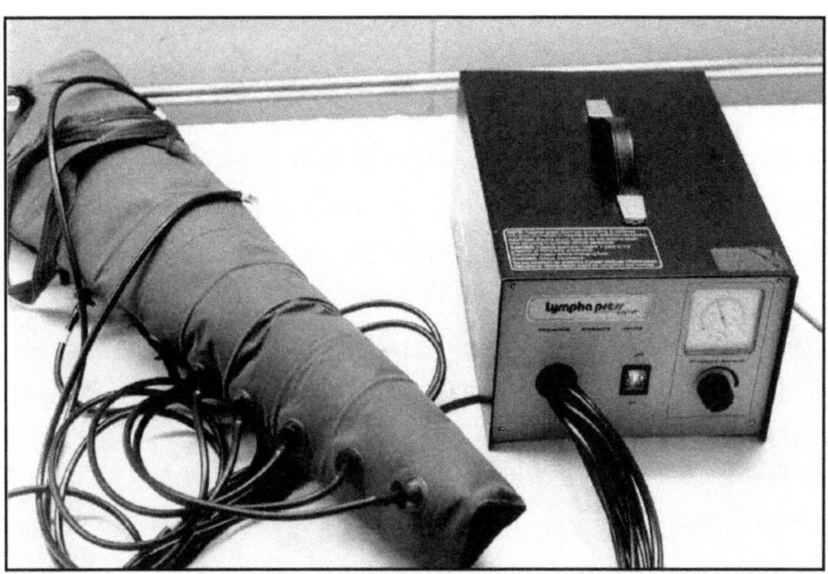

Function □ A sequential compression unit consists of a sleeve that fits over the patient□s limb. A series of air bladders in the sleeve can be inflated one after the other, from the distal part of the limb inwards, thus squeezing the limb with a peristaltic wave, pushing fluids toward the body. Some systems allow two such sleeves to be used at once, so that both legs can be treated simultaneously. An air pump feeds a controller unit, which directs air to the various bladders in proper sequence. Pressure and rate are adjustable, and a timer signals the end of treatment.

Application □ Different sleeves are available for different limb sizes. Once the appropriate sleeve has been selected, it is pulled over the target limb and connected to the air hoses coming from the controller. After selecting pressure, rate, and treatment time, the pump and timer are started. Treatment is passive on the part of the patient.

AKA □ (none).

Related devices **continuous passive motion machines (193)**.

Where found physiotherapy departments or clinics, patient bedsides.

Transcutaneous Electrical Nerve Stimulators (TENS)

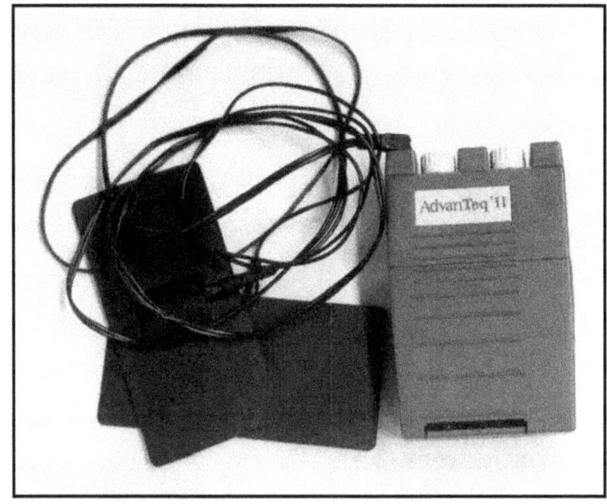

Overview □ Pain reduction is a goal in the treatment of many medical conditions. Pain may not respond well to pain□killing medications, and even when it does, the medications used may have undesirable side effects, especially at high doses. Non□chemical means of alleviating pain can be very valuable.

Function □ By applying controlled electrical signals to the skin at specific locations, a transcutaneous electrical nerve stimulator unit can produce significant pain relief. The exact mechanism of this relief is under debate, but it is thought that either the transcutaneous electrical nerve stimulator signals disrupt the normal pain nerve transmissions in the body, preventing them from reaching the brain and causing a sensation of pain, or that the electrical stimulation causes the body to produce endorphins, which are natural pain killers.

The unit producing the signals is generally quite small, and consists of a set of controls for signal amplitude, frequency, and shape, as well as visual indicators of treatment activity and connectors for electrode wires. The electrode wires carry the signals to electrodes (usually made of conductive rubber), which have been placed on the patient□s skin.

Application □ The operator may do some testing to determine the optimum placement of electrodes, by applying signals and checking for reactions from the patient. Sometimes electrodes are applied according to precise diagrams that specify locations for various sources of pain. In either case, the electrodes are affixed to the skin, treatment parameters are set, and the stimulation signals are turned on. Both the parameters and the electrode location may be adjusted during the course of the treatment, depending on patient response.

Since the electrical signals may interfere with pacemaker function, the use of transcutaneous electrical nerve stimulator with such patients is not advisable.

Pain relief may be an ongoing process, in which case patients often learn to use the transcutaneous electrical nerve stimulator unit on their own.

AKA □nerve stimulators, TENS units.

Related devices □**interferential therapy units (194), laser therapy units (196), muscle/nerve stimulators (63)**.

Where found □ physiotherapy departments or clinics, doctor□s offices, patient□s homes.

Ultraviolet Therapy Units

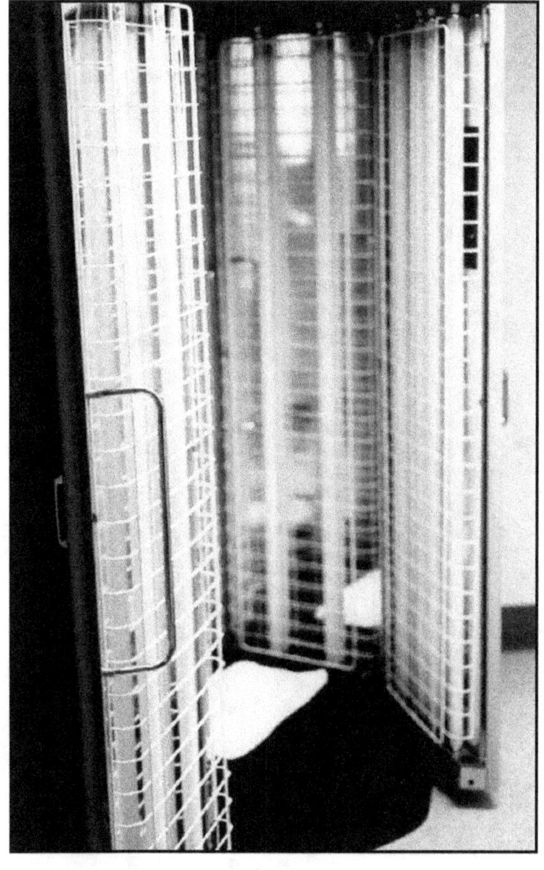

Overview □Exposing the skin to ultraviolet (UV) light can aid in the treatment of some skin conditions. Particular wavelengths of UV have been found to give the maximum benefit with minimal harmful effects. The timing of exposure is critical, as a balance must be reached between effective treatment and skin damage.

Function □ UV therapy units are similar to commercial tanning booths, except that the special fluorescent UV lamps are designed to emit light most beneficial to medical conditions rather than to provide maximum tanning effect. Also, safety concerns are more carefully addressed, with timer circuits to prevent overexposure.

Fluorescent tubes in the units are parallel to each other and are arranged in a circle, so that 360□degree, head□to□foot exposure is possible.

Because UV light output can vary with the age of the fluorescent tubes, operators must periodically check for light levels using a calibrated UV light meter, located a prescribed distance from the bulbs.

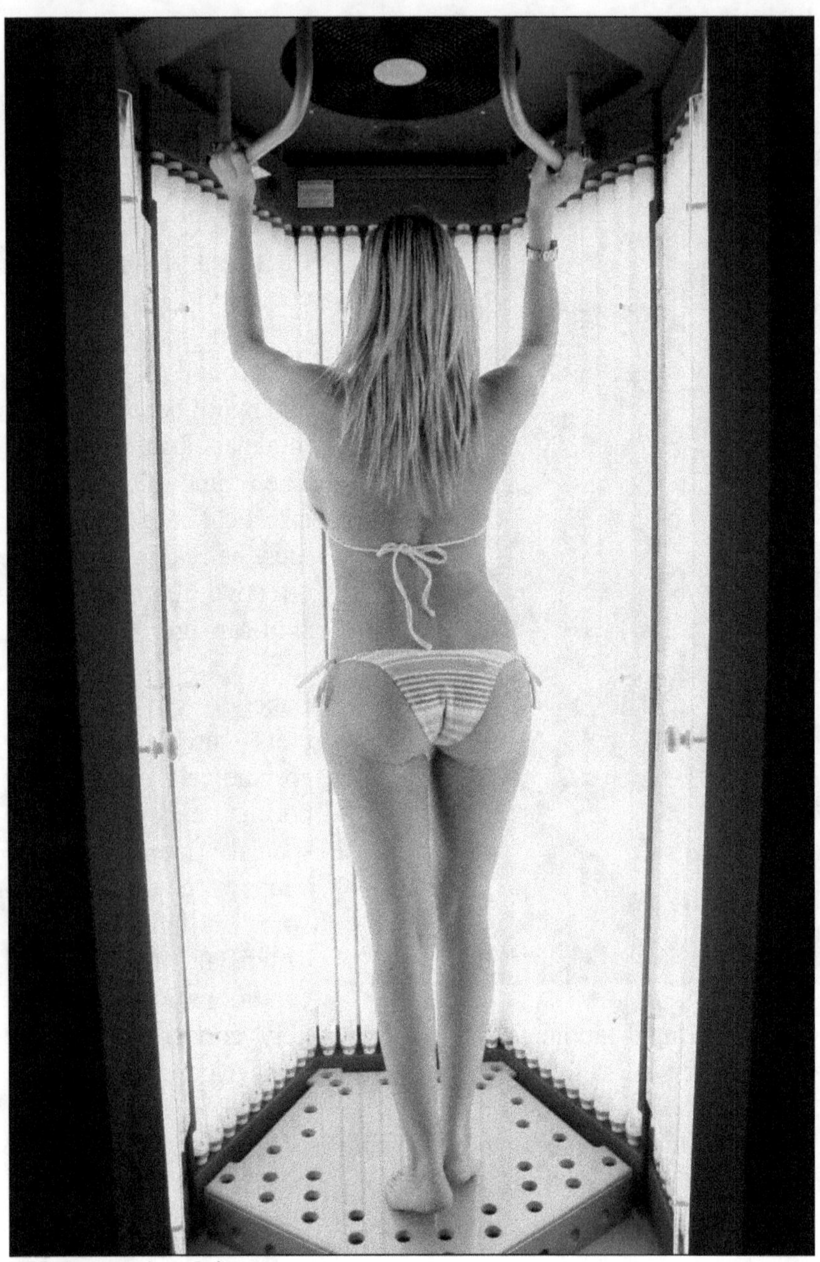

UV therapy booth in use.
Modified from Inmagine Corp, www.123rf.com, with permission.

Application The patient removes as much clothing as is required to provide adequate exposure, applies eye protection (as inadvertent UV exposure can be damaging to the retina), and then stands or lies in the treatment booth. The operator sets exposure time and turns on the lamps; at the end of the treatment period, the timer turns the lamps off and initiates an audible signal.

AKA □UV booth, tanning booth.

Related devices □**bilirubin therapy systems (87)**.

Where found □ physiotherapy departments, special skin treatment units.

Ultrasound Therapy Units

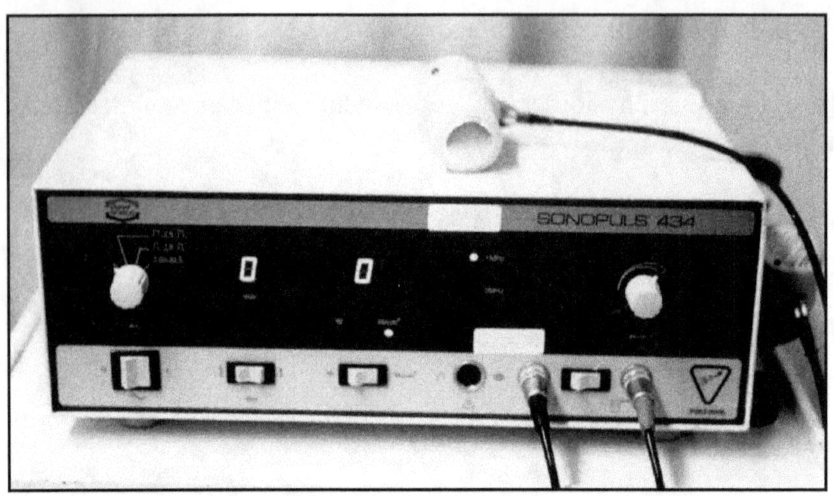

Overview – The application of heat can relieve some of the pain associated with tissue inflammation caused by injury or diseases such as arthritis. It can also promote healing by increasing blood flow to that area.

Function – High-frequency sound waves can cause localized heating in tissue. Ultrasound therapy units utilize this fact to provide such heating for therapeutic purposes. An electronic circuit develops high frequency signals that are applied to a crystal, which in turn emits sound waves. By applying the crystal face (mounted in the head of a handle) to the patient's skin, the underlying tissue is heated. To ensure maximum transfer of sound energy from the crystal to the patient, a sound-conducting gel is placed between the two.

Devices often come with two or more treatment heads, each with different frequencies of operation. The different frequencies produce heating at different depths.

A means of controlling power output and a timer circuit complete the basic design of these devices. Some units have a visual indicator of contact quality, and possibly a means of reducing or cutting off power when coupling is inadequate.

Application □Ultrasound gel is applied to the face of the treatment head, which is then placed on the patient□s skin before power is turned on. Either the operator or the patient moves the head to various positions to attain maximum heating benefit to the target area.

Power levels must be selected carefully to prevent burns, and care must be taken not to use the unit on areas with closely underlying bones for the same reason. Further, since an improperly coupled or open ultrasound head can get extremely hot (if the unit is not equipped with a contact quality safety monitor), power must never be applied unless the head is in proper contact with the patient.

AKA □US therapy, ultrasound.

Related devices □**wax baths (210)**, **hot pack heaters (198)**.

Where found □physiotherapy departments or clinics.

Wax Baths

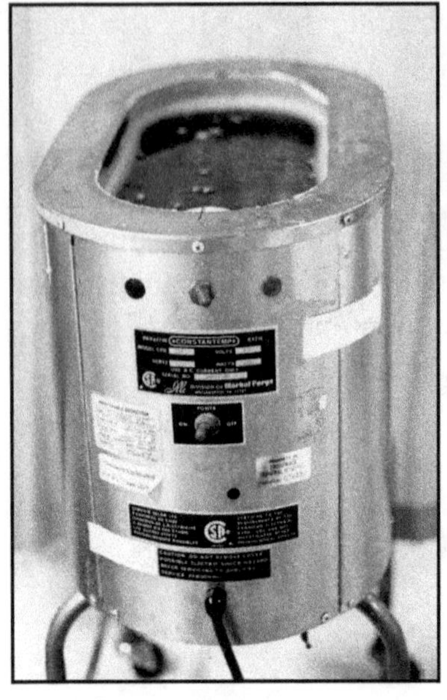

Overview □ The application of heat can relieve some of the pain associated with tissue inflammation caused by injury or diseases such as arthritis. It can also promote healing by increasing blood flow to that area.

Function □ A wax bath consists of a tub of paraffin wax that is kept just above its melting point by a thermostat and heater. The wax is formulated to have a relatively low melting point, so that it is liquid at non□scalding temperatures. A lid retains heat when the unit is not in use, and it is on a stand that places it at an accessible height.

Application □ A patient□s body part, such as a hand or an elbow, is dipped in the liquid wax and then removed, so that the wax coating solidifies. Repeated dipping produces many layers of wax, which retains heat for a considerable time. This heat is effective at penetrating into the tissue and effecting relief from inflammation.

Temperature of the wax bath must be monitored at all times to guard against overheating, even though most units have a double□ thermostat control system.

AKA □paraffin bath.

Related devices □ **ultrasound therapy (208)**, **hot pack heaters (198)**.

Where found □physiotherapy departments or clinics.

Chapter 11 – Diagnostic Imaging

Diagnostic Imaging Equipment Descriptions

Following are more detailed descriptions of equipment found exclusively or most commonly in this area of the hospital. Equipment that is also found in various other areas of the hospital is described in Chapter 12, p 247.

Devices sometimes found in diagnostic imaging departments, in addition to the equipment listed in this section, include: **aspirators (250)**, **intravenous pumps (289)**, and **stethoscopes (327)**.

C□arm Units

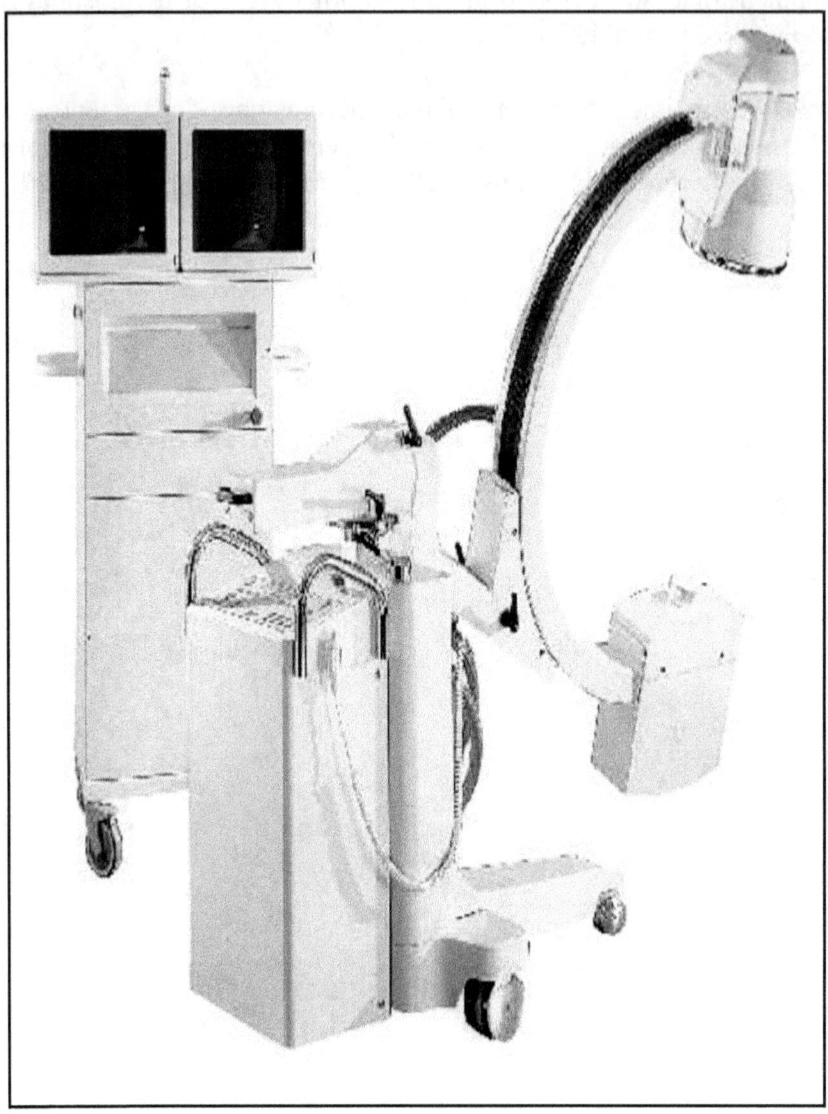

Overview □ It is often necessary to obtain x□rays of patients from various angles without having to move them from their current position. This requires an x□ray machine that can be positioned so that its source is over the patient and its receiver is under the patient, and the whole assembly can be rotated to obtain the angled exposures needed. Some units are mobile, for use in situations where the patient cannot be moved to the x□ray department.

Function □ Units were designed so that they could be moved, and then placed at the patient□s location, with arm extensions that reach both over and under the patient. Since these extensions were in the shape of a □C□ the devices were called C□Arm units. The upper extension houses the x□ray source and associated mechanisms, while the lower extension contains a chamber for film cassettes. The base of the unit allows for vertical positioning as well as rotation of the arm and extensions so that exposures at various angles can be obtained. In mobile C□Arm units, the base is wheeled and has batteries to power not only the x□ray and positioning mechanisms, but also to propel the whole unit, as they are very heavy.

Application □ The patient is prepared as much as possible and shielded if necessary. The C□Arm is brought into place and adjusted much like a room X□Ray unit, for position and exposure power and time. The operator (and any other personnel in the area) moves to a safe location, and exposures are made. The unit is then moved clear, and film cassettes taken for developing.

AKA □(none).

Related devices □**room X–ray units (241)**.

Where found □ diagnostic imaging departments, any area of the hospital where patients might be immobile but still require x□rays.

Computerized Tomography (CT) Scanners

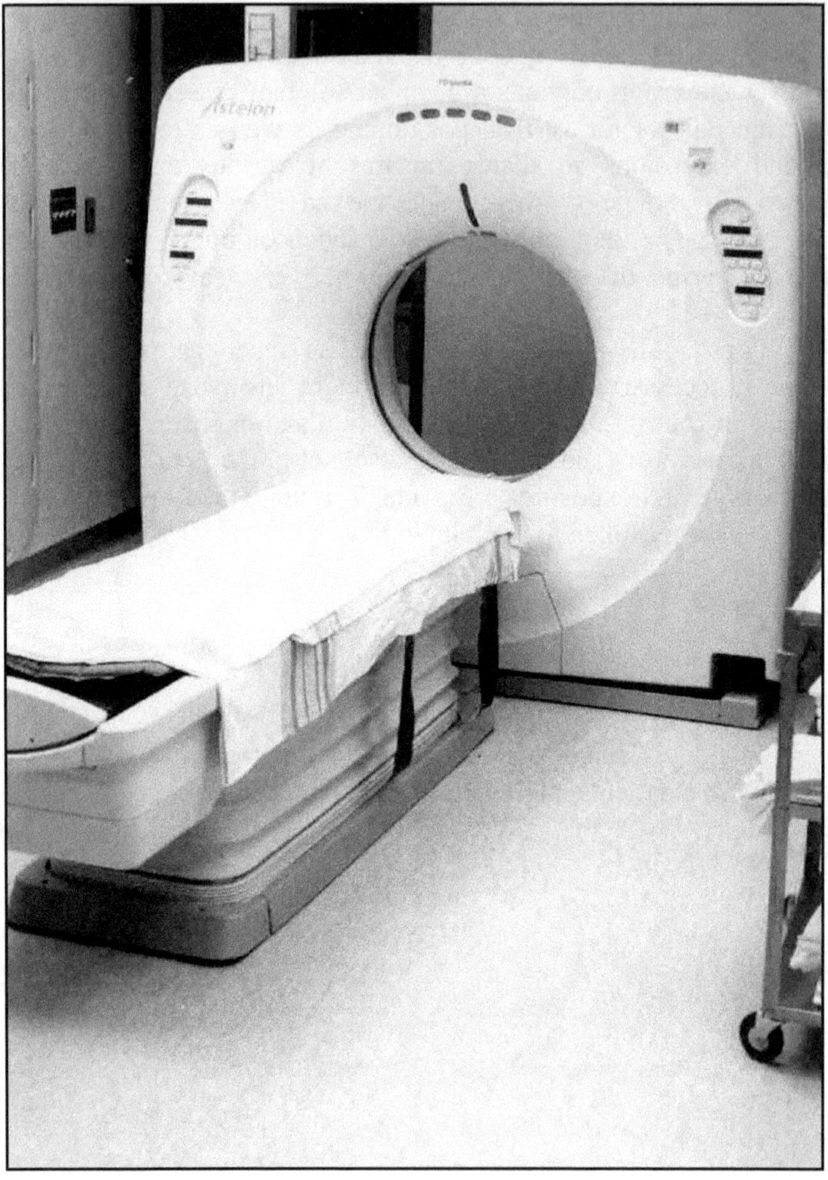

Overview □ Conventional x□rays produce a "shadow" image of the tissues through which the x□rays pass. Many disease conditions or abnormalities can be visualized better when a "slice" view is available, so that structures are not obscured by tissues above or below, as may be the case with regular x□ray images.

Function □ CT (Computerized Tomography) scanners pass a series of narrow beam x□rays through the target area of the body in a circular pattern, and then combine the information from each exposure with computers to develop a "slice" image. With enough individual exposures and accurate computer analysis, very detailed images can be produced. Because the system uses narrow beams and a combination of many sub□images, each total image exposure can be relatively low, and the total radiation dose is acceptable. Newer devices use more sensitive x□ray receptors and faster computers to reduce the total radiation exposure and both the time required to acquire an image and the time to process the image and have it available for viewing. Images may be presented as an x□ray□like transparency, a printed picture, or on a video display; they can be stored as computer files for later retrieval and analysis. By taking a series of CT images, each adjacent to the next, a three□dimensional representation of structures can be developed.

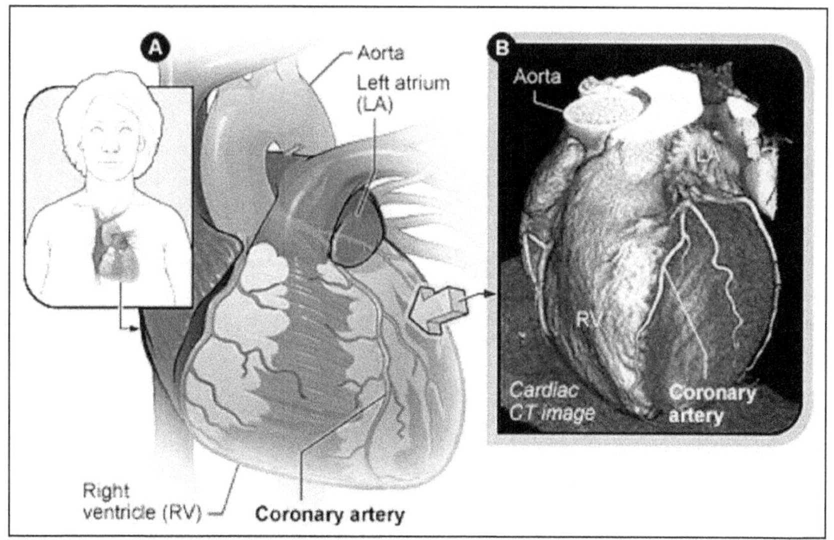

CT of the heart, with reference diagram.

Courtesy of the National Institute of Diabetes and Digestive and Kidney Diseases, National Institutes of Health.

Application □ Patients are moved by a powered table surface into the scanning chamber, where exposures are made. Because exposure times can be somewhat prolonged, the patient must remain as still as possible; newer systems have reduced exposure times, but this is still a factor. The range of "slices" that can be obtained is limited by the size of the scanning ring and the shape of the human body. Most systems have a ring not much larger than a human torso. Patients may find the enclosed interior of the unit to be claustrophobic, something the operators need to discuss beforehand and be aware of during the procedure.

AKA □CAT scanner, computerized axial tomography scanner.

Related devices □**room x–ray systems (241), MRI scanners (229), PET scanners (237)**.

Where found □dedicated rooms in diagnostic imaging departments; some regions may have mobile units housed in a semi□trailer.

Diagnostic Ultrasound Machines

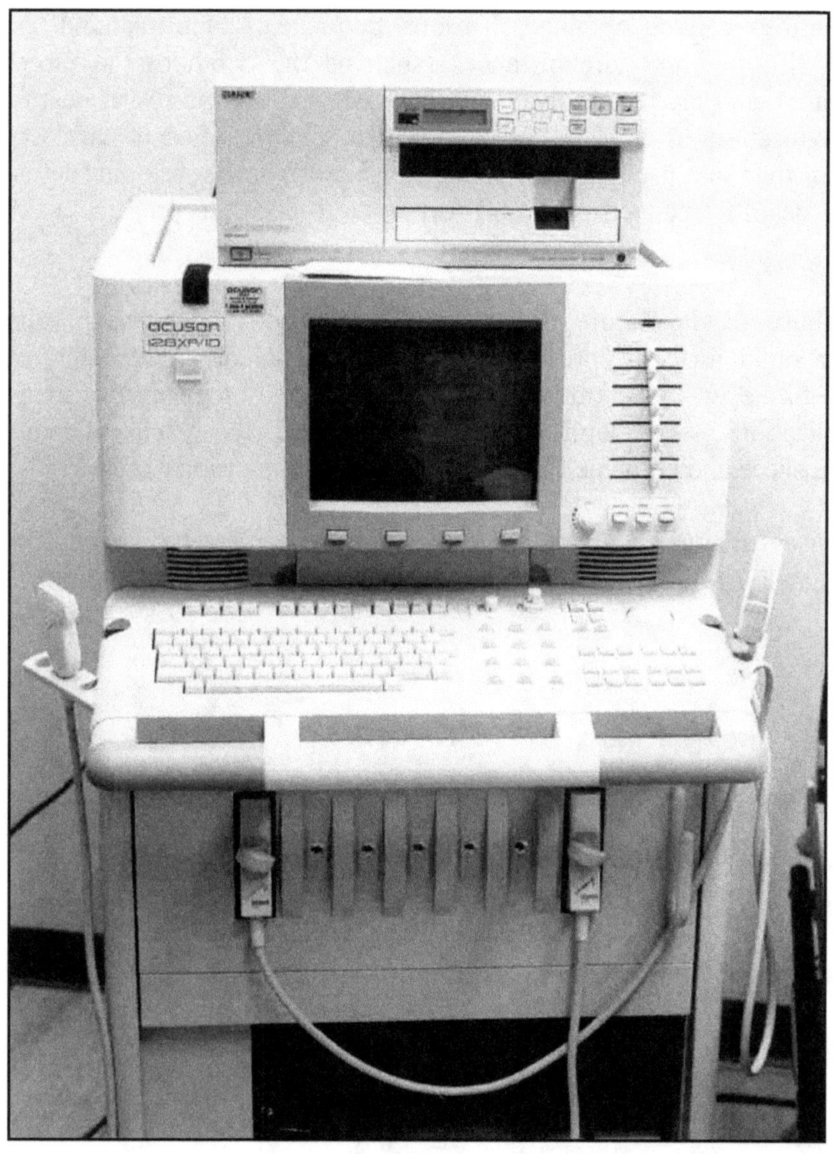

Overview □ Certain tissues cannot be visualized well with x□rays, and some situations (such as pregnancy) require that x□rays be avoided if at all possible, but visualization of internal structures is still needed.

Function □ Diagnostic ultrasound machines produce beams of ultrasonic sound waves, which can be directed into the patient□s body. The sound waves are reflected by tissues of different densities, and by the boundary layers between different tissues. By picking up and processing the reflected signals, an image of the internal structures can be obtained. Various frequencies of ultrasound are used for different circumstances (such as the depth of the target organs), and probes are available that give wider or narrower beams. Visualization of a heart valve, for example, requires a narrower beam than one used for visualizing most or all of a developing fetus. The beam is scanned back and forth electronically to produce a full image.

Because of the nature of the wave generation and pick-up, raw ultrasound images represent a two-dimensional or "slice" view of the tissue in question. While this may be sufficient for many applications, more sophisticated units can take the results of many such slices and combine them to give a three-dimensional view.

Devices may be general-purpose, or they may be specifically designed for particular applications, such as cardiology or maternity.

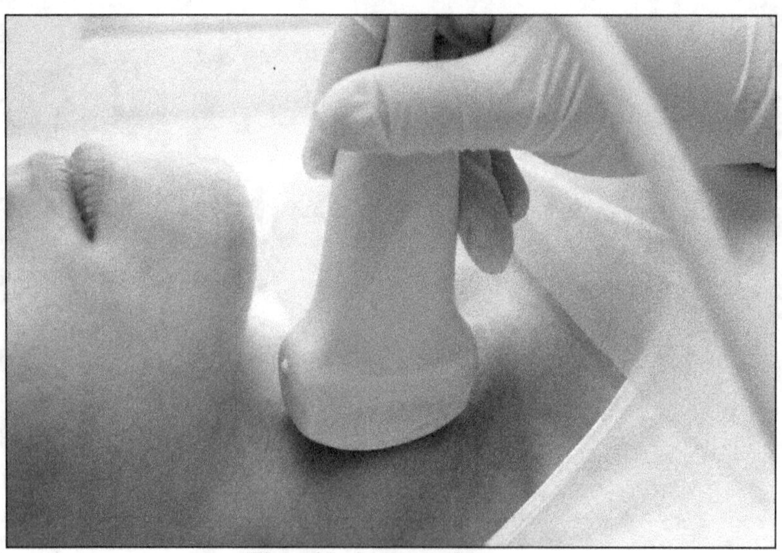

Thyroid ultrasound exam.

Modified from Shutterstock, Inc, www.shutterstock.com, with permission.

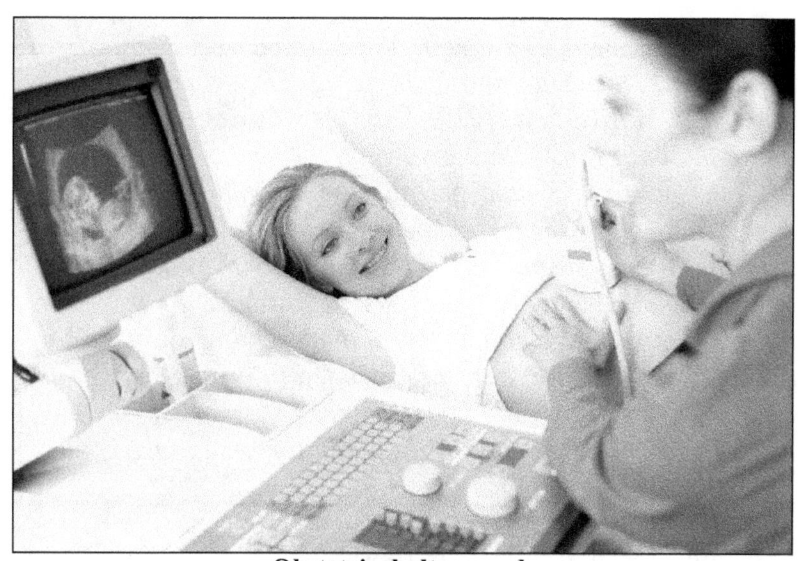

Obstetrical ultrasound.
Modified from Shutterstock, Inc, www.shutterstock.com, with permission.

Angie visits the Diagnostic Imaging Department for an ***obstetrical ultrasound (217)****, and is looking forward to seeing the image of the baby form on the screen. Her belly is slathered with ultrasound gel and the technologist places a large probe against her abdomen. The baby is too big now to show up entirely in one scan, but the machine adds images together and does a 3-D analysis to produce a very clear image. She asks the technologist to avoid giving away the sex of the baby so certain areas are avoided in the scanning. She wishes her husband could have come with her to see this, but the tech burns a DVD copy of the exam for her to take home.*

Application The patient is positioned as required, and the ultrasound probe is applied to the skin. Because sound waves are partially blocked when they encounter a boundary such as between the probe surface and the skin, especially if there are any air gaps, a special gel that helps to couple the sound waves more efficiently is used. This also helps lubricate the skin to make positioning the probe easier. Particularly for fetal imaging, because images are taken from a variety of angles, large quantities of coupling gel are required. If the operators are nice, they keep the gel in a heated chamber so that it is warm when applied.

Galling Gall Stones – Elizabeth – Diagnostic Imaging

Elizabeth has experienced severe abdominal pain and her Doctor ordered an ***abdominal ultrasound (217)****. On the examining table, her abdomen is liberally covered with ultrasound gel and a technologist places a large probe on the area. Images that mean little to Elizabeth are fascinating to the tech, and she calls a Radiologist in to go over results. When she gets up from the bed, her breathing is wheezy and she winces when she puts weight on her left leg. A few days later, her Doctor calls to tell her that she has gallstones and that she needs surgery soon.*

Some systems use a probe that can be inserted into the patient□s esophagus, which allows it to come closer to the heart for better images of heart details.

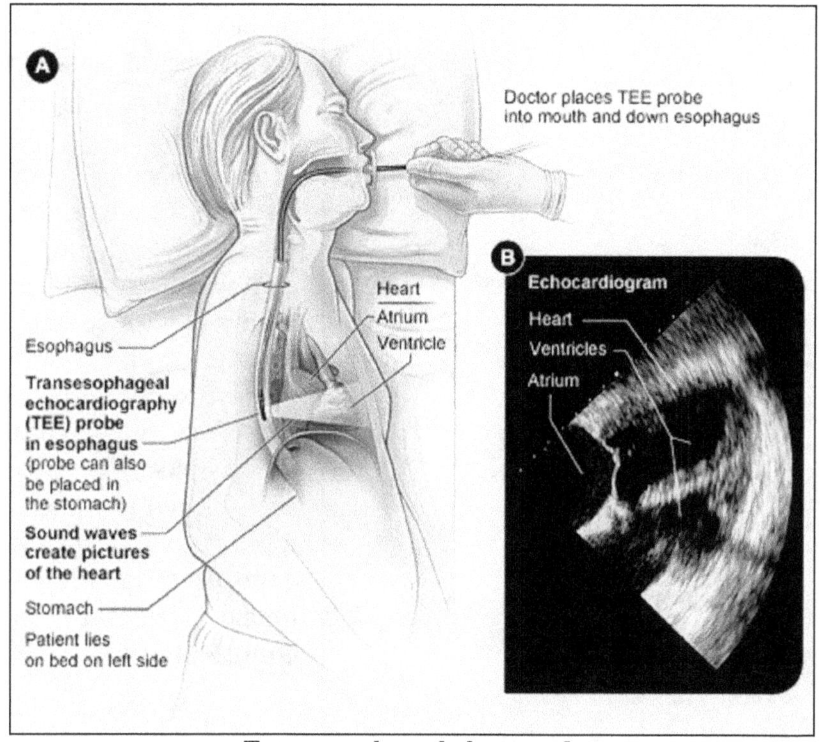

Trans–esophageal ultrasound.

Courtesy of the National Institute of Diabetes and Digestive and Kidney Diseases, National Institutes of Health.

AKA □US machines.

Related devices □**room x–ray units (241)**, **doppler units (93)**, **fetal monitors (95)**, **plethysmograph systems (173), bladder scanners (252)**.

Where found □special sections of diagnostic imaging departments, dedicated ultrasound departments; some devices are mobile and can be taken to the patient□s bedside.

Dye Injectors

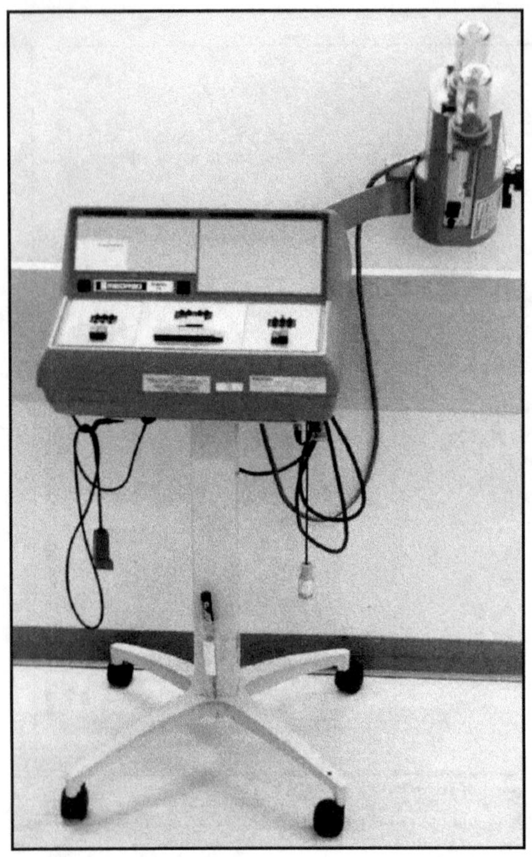

Overview □ Some soft□tissue body structures, such as blood vessels, the urinary or digestive systems, and cerebrospinal fluid channels, can be better visualized on x□rays if a dye which is opaque to x□rays is injected into the structure in question before x□ray exposures are taken. In the case of the circulatory system, such injections must be rapid and precisely controlled in order to obtain useful and consistent results.

Function □Dye injectors consist of a syringe to hold the dye material and a mechanism to activate the syringe and inject the dye into the patient. Because high pressures are involved, the syringe and associated components must be designed to withstand these pressures. Also, since excessive length of tubing between the syringe and the patient will reduce the effectiveness of the injection, the syringe must be mounted on an articulating arm, which can position the components very close to the injection site.

Kidney Complications – Jerry – Diagnostic Imaging

Jerry has been suffering from abdominal pains for a few weeks before finally visiting his doctor, who makes a preliminary diagnosis of kidney stones, also known as renal calculi. The doctor orders blood and urine tests as well as an abdominal ultrasound to confirm the diagnosis, and a renal pyelogram for further clarification should his suspicions prove correct.

After visiting the lab, Jerry goes to Diagnostic Imaging, where he will have the ultrasound examination. The ***ultrasound machine (217)*** *is basically the same as that used for obstetric exams, and the technologist spreads coupling gel on Jerry's back as he lies on his stomach on the examination table. The tech places an ultrasound probe against the skin, with the gel helping to carry the ultrasound waves in and out of Jerry's body more effectively. The probe sends very high frequency sound waves into his abdomen, where they are reflected by surfaces that have a change in density. The probe picks up the reflected waves and the machine processes and analyzes them to produce a 3-D image of the target tissues, in this case Jerry's left and right kidneys. The images are displayed on a video screen as they are captured, and after processing. Jerry has a degree in Biology and has been with his wife for numerous obstetrical ultrasounds, so he is able to recognize his kidneys and see the shapes of several stones inside the organs. The images are recorded and made available on the hospital* ***PACS (232)*** *system, where both a renal specialist and Jerry's family doctor can view them. The tech cleans the gel from Jerry's skin and he proceeds to the next test.*

<u>Kidney Complications – Jerry continued</u>

*Still in Diagnostic Imaging, Jerry checks in at the special procedures desk where he is instructed to empty his bladder and then go to change into a hospital gown. Once positioned on an **x-ray table (241)**, a special solution containing iodine is **injected (222)** intravenously. The iodine compound shows up on x-rays and collects in his kidneys and then his bladder; x-ray exposures are taken at intervals as this is happening. This gives a clearer outline of the kidney stones, showing their size and shape.*

Injection mechanisms must operate smoothly and have adequate power and control to deliver precision doses. The unit has controls to adjust volume and rate of injection, and a remote activating switch.

<u>Application</u> □ An intravenous line is established at the required injection site, and the injector is loaded with dye and positioned close to the site and connected to the line. When the patient has been positioned for x□ray exposures, the operator moves to a shielded location and begins the injection. X□ray exposures are taken before, during, and after the injection, until the necessary information has been obtained.

<u>AKA</u> □angiography or angio injectors.

<u>Related devices</u> □**room x–ray equipment (241)**.

<u>Where found</u> □diagnostic imaging departments.

Mammography Units

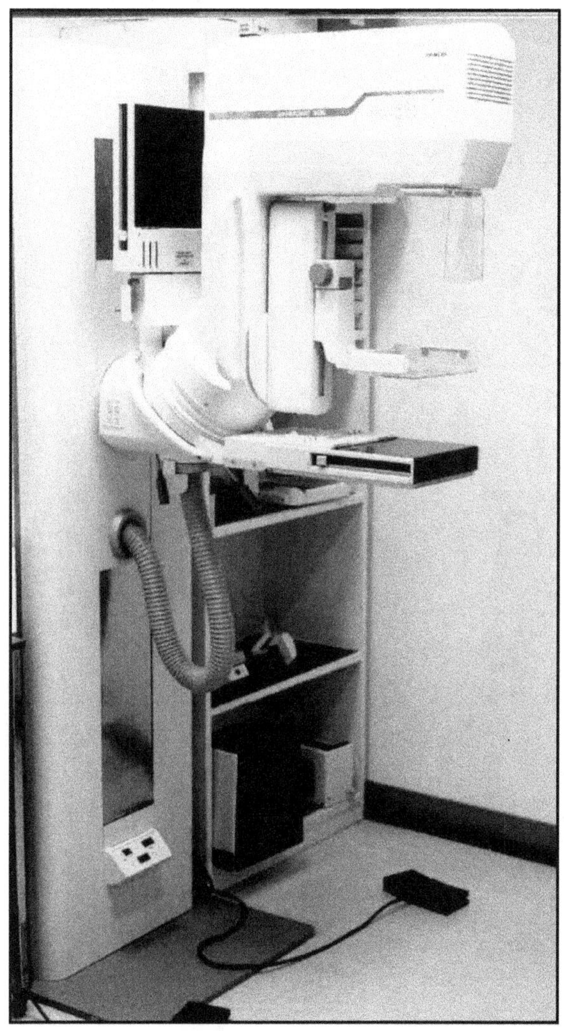

Overview □ Early detection of breast cancer is critical in reducing harm from the disease, including mortality. X□ray imaging is one means of aiding such detection. Since cancer tissue is relatively close in x□ray density to normal breast tissue (as compared to bone, for example), and because tissue nodes that may be clinically significant are often small, means that can increase the effectiveness of imaging must be adopted. A reduction in the thickness of over□ and under□lying tissue surrounding possible tumors is an important factor.

Function □ Mammography units are similar to normal x□ray units, with x□ray characteristics optimized for breast tissue. They have attachments that compress the breast, horizontally and vertically, in turn. With the breast compressed, thus having a much thinner profile, x□ray film exposures are taken. If lumps have been detected by other means, these areas may be examined more closely.

Application □ The operator sets power and exposure times for the procedure, and then adjusts the x□ray head to the patient. The patient, with the assistance of the operator, places one breast on a clear plastic plate. A motorized mechanism then lowers a second plastic plate onto the opposite surface of the breast until the tissue is adequately compressed. The operator then moves to the control area (shielded by lead glass and walls) and makes the exposure. The breast is then compressed along the other axis and exposures taken again.

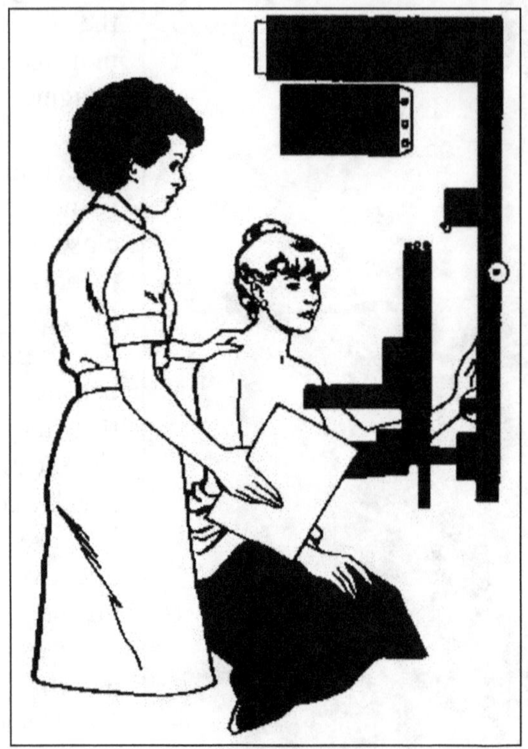

Mammography exam.
Public domain image.

Mammograms for the Masses – Sundeep – Diagnostic Imaging I

Sundeep, 72, comes in to the Diagnostic Imaging Department accompanied by her son. They check in at the reception desk to say they are here for a mammogram appointment for Sundeep. They are directed to the mammography waiting area and she is instructed to remove her clothes down to the waist. Sundeep is in the early stages of Alzheimer's and her son has to reassure her that everything is OK, and remind her of the instructions. Once she is ready in a hospital gown, a technologist leads her into the mammography room, where she explains the procedure in both English and Punjabi. The gown is removed and Sundeep is positioned in front of the ***mammography machine (225)****, which is then adjusted for height. The technologist positions Sundeep's right breast on the lower compression plate and then lowers the clear Plexiglas ® upper compression plate to squeeze the breast. This procedure is somewhat painful and the tech reassures Sundeep that it will be done soon, but is necessary to reduce tissue thickness for better images and also to help separate any structures (including possible tumors) so they will show up better in the x-rays. This also allows for lower doses of x-rays to be used. The tech asks Sundeep to stay still and hold her breath and then she moves behind a shield and triggers the x-ray exposure. The process is repeated with the left breast and then the compression mechanism is rotated 90 degrees, which allows lateral breast compression for another set of images. Since this is a digital system, no film is involved and the images are available almost instantly on the hospital* ***PACS (232)*** *system.*

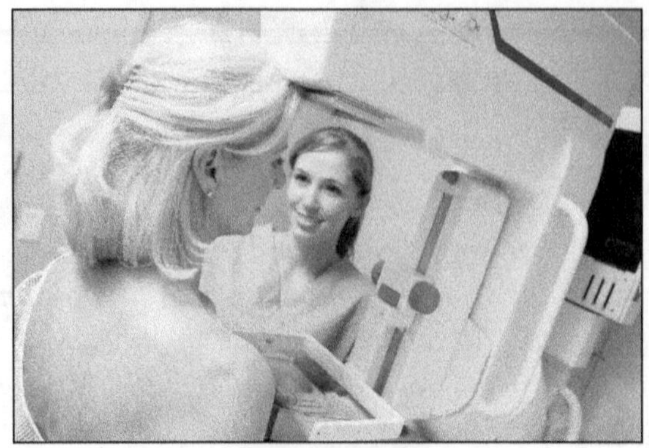

Mammography.
Modified from Shutterstock, Inc, www.shutterstock.com, with permission.

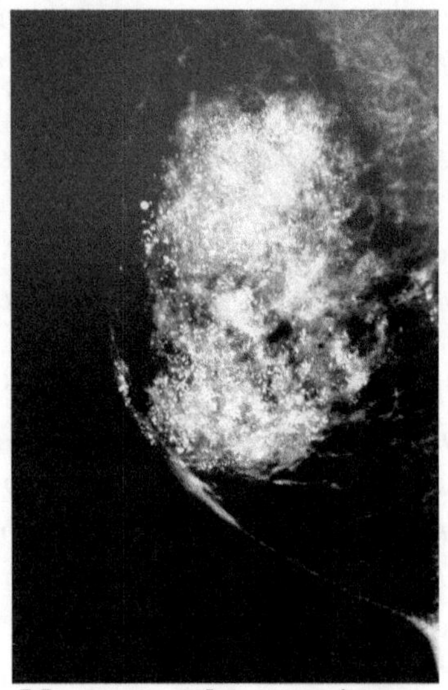

Mammography x–ray image.
Modified from Inmagine Corp, www.123rf.com, with permission

Patients are shielded appropriately to reduce x□ray exposure to non□ target areas of the body.

As the compression required for good images is significant, this procedure can be quite uncomfortable for the patient.

AKA □Mammo unit.

Related devices □**room x–ray units (241)**.

Where found □ diagnostic imaging departments, special mammography units (including mobile ones).

Magnetic Resonance Imaging (MRI) Scanners

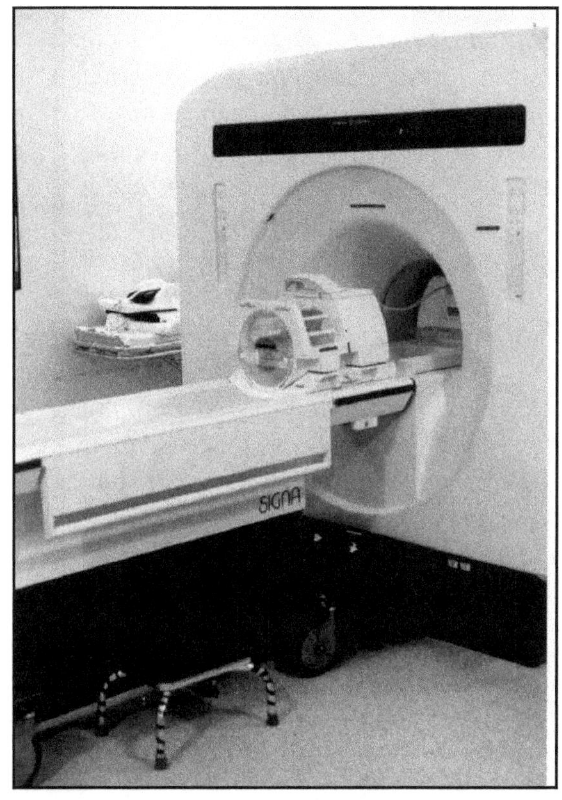

Overview □ Since the human body is composed largely of water, a means of imaging the distribution of water in the body provides a picture of various structures giving a different kind of information than that provided by x□rays or other scanning technologies.

Function □ Water molecules consist of two atoms of hydrogen and one of oxygen. When they are within a powerful magnetic field, radio waves of a precise frequency can interact with the hydrogen atoms and cause them to resonate and emit their own radio signals. These signals can then be detected and analyzed, and an image of hydrogen (and thus water) distribution within the body can be obtained. With sufficiently advanced detection and analysis, very detailed images of body tissues can be obtained. These images can then be displayed on a video monitor and stored and/or printed out for later examination.

Application □ Since extremely powerful magnetic fields are used in MRI procedures, all magnetically active metallic objects must be removed from the patient. This means that patients with stainless steel implants or pacemakers may be excluded from such studies. The operation of pacemakers is also affected directly by magnetic fields, so that further restricts MRI use with these patients. Dental fillings and crowns are not usually affected.

***Accidents Happen – Felipe – Diagnostic Imaging* I**

Some of Felipe's knee pain seems to be resulting from damage to soft tissue, that is, other than bone, so an MRI was ordered. The MRI machine is in the same area as the X-ray room so Felipe is able to have both procedures done consecutively. The operator has him remove any metal objects such as jewelry, and he is positioned on a hard, narrow table. The table is on a track that can move into the large, donut-shaped imaging chamber. The operator positions the table so that the first images will be from just above Felipe's knee, advises Felipe to remain still, and the process is started. There is a loud humming and banging sound from the machine, which continues until the scan is complete. This noise is produced by the equipment generating very intense magnetic fields and radio waves, which interact with molecules in Felipe's tissues, causing them to emit their own radio wave signals which are detected by the equipment, processed and analyzed to produce a 3-dimensional image of his knee, clearly showing the muscle, tendon and cartilage structures as well as bones.

The patient is positioned on an examination table, which can be moved around to facilitate imaging of different areas. The operator moves to a shielded location, and the magnetic field is initiated. To obtain the images desired, patient position is adjusted by the table, under both operator and program control.

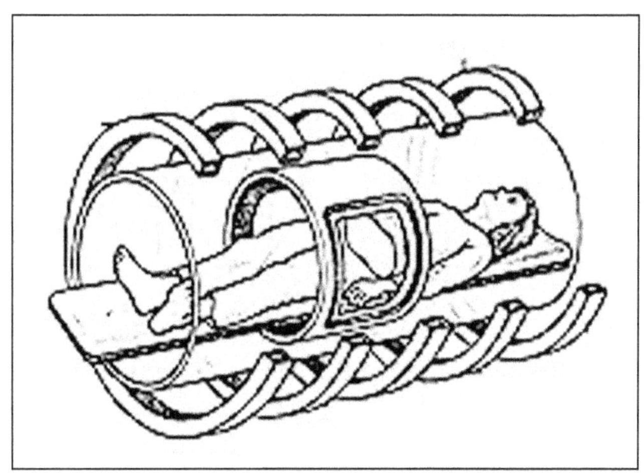

MRI cross section showing magnetic rings.
Public domain image.

Typically, two to six images are taken during a procedure, and since each image takes a few minutes for positioning and exposure, the whole procedure may take 15 to 45 minutes. This time may be longer for especially detailed or complex studies. Patients must remain still during the actual imaging, but can shift to a limited degree between exposures. Patients may find the enclosed interior of the unit to be claustrophobic, something the operators need to discuss beforehand and be aware of during the procedure.

A contrast medium may be injected into the patient for some studies, in order to improve image quality

AKA MRI scan, magnetic resonance imaging.

Related devices **room x–ray equipment (241)**, **diagnostic ultrasound unit (217)**, **PET scanner (237)**, **CT scanner (214)**.

Where found diagnostic imaging departments, special clinics, mobile MRI units.

Picture Archiving and Communication System (PACS)

Overview □ With the advent of digital image techniques, powerful and relatively inexpensive computers and high□speed data networks, it became possible to handle diagnostic images in a coordinated manner. Images could be stored, distributed and presented in a consistent format, allowing various medical personnel to have access to high□quality images from many different locations.

Such systems came to be called picture archiving and communication systems, or PACS.

Application □ Any digital image can be handled with a PACS system, including x□rays, and CT, MRI, PET and ultrasound scans, as well as endoscopy or microsurgery images.

Specialists can evaluate images from a distant location where such expertise may not be available, without the delays and inconvenience of having to ship hard□copy images from place to place. Various people can look at the same image simultaneously for collaborative or educational purposes.

Digital storage is much more compact and less expensive than the huge archives used in keeping traditional film images.

A PACS network consists of a central server connected to various client workstations though a local and/or wide area network. Several PACS systems can be connected together, and the Internet can also be used as a communications channel.

Because diagnostic images are large and of high resolution, system data rates must be high enough to allow image transfers in reasonable time periods.

Workstations must be capable of displaying images at diagnostic□ quality levels and be able to handle them quickly. Two video displays are usually included to allow comparison of images.

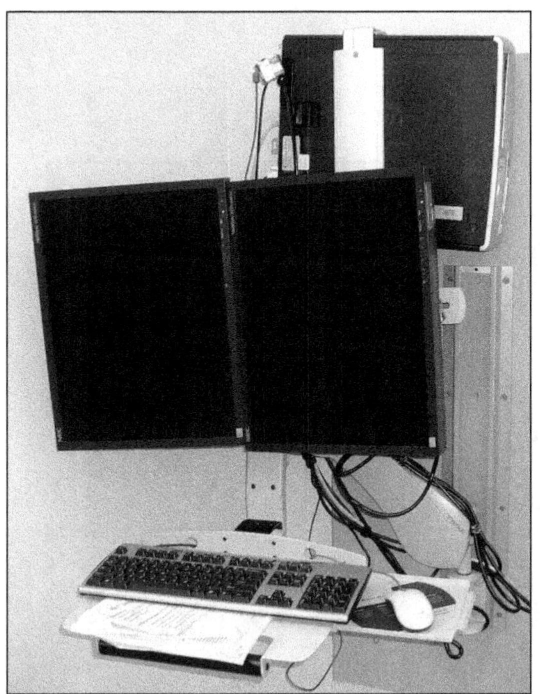
PACS terminal with dual displays, keyboard and mouse.

The central server stores images in a database and handles requests for access to existing images or storage of new images. Functions such as database maintenance such as data backup and system upkeep are performed as with any other database.

Since images can come from many sources, there must be a very effective means of naming and organizing them.

AKA □ Digital image handling systems, various other terms. PACS is almost universal.

Related devices □**All diagnostic imaging equipment (210)**.

Where found □Servers are usually located in the IT area, terminals can be located anywhere in the hospital where access to images might be required.

Radiation Therapy Systems

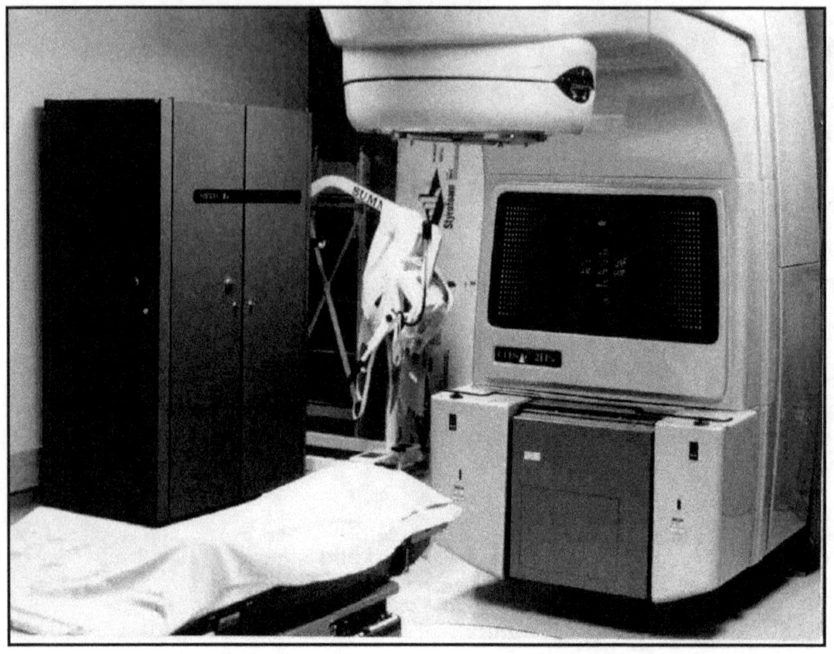

Overview □ Some types of cancer cells can be killed by exposure to radiation; they tend to be more sensitive to radiation than normal cells because their rapid reproduction rate is disrupted by the radiation.

Function □ By focusing the radiation from one or more sources on the area in which cancer cells are likely to be present, a radiation therapy unit allows the selective removal of cancer cells, while leaving most of the surrounding tissues relatively undamaged. A block of radioactive material (produced in high□technology nuclear facilities) is enclosed in a lead container, which has a window that can be opened to allow radiation to escape in a narrow beam.

Application □ The patient is positioned so that the radiation beams can reach the target area with minimal penetration of healthy tissue. Because treatment times are quite long, the patient must also be made as comfortable as possible while remaining motionless. When the patient has been positioned and non□target areas shielded, an operator remotely opens a window in the container holding the radioactive source, allowing the target area to be exposed to radiation. During the course of a treatment session, the angle of the radiation may be changed so that healthy tissue above and below the tumor site is irradiated less than the tumor.

Mammograms for the Masses – Sundeep – Diagnostic Imaging II

Based on the results of the mammogram, Sundeep's doctor orders a biopsy, which shows that one node identified in the mammogram is cancerous. Because of its location and other characteristics, a relatively simple lumpectomy is performed, to be followed by radiation therapy. Sundeep is brought to the Oncology Center and, after changing into a hospital gown, is positioned on a treatment table with her arms over her head. The technologist adjusts the linear accelerator head for optimum aim and then moves behind a shield. A whirring noise from the machine indicates that radiation is being delivered, and Sundeep remains motionless for a few minutes until the tech tells her to relax. The process is repeated from a few different angles, which helps localize the radiation effects to the target area, with the goal of killing any cancer cells that might remain. The radiation is more damaging to rapidly growing cancer cells than to normal cells, but some damage still occurs, sometime causing side effects such as fatigue, loss of appetite and a sunburn-like rash in the area. Sundeep's treatments are repeated daily for several weeks and are monitored by x-rays and blood tests.

Some tissues will selectively absorb particular radioactive materials, in which case (if there is a tumor in that particular tissue) relatively low concentrations of the material can be injected intravenously; the patient□s body then concentrates the substance in the target tissue where it can deliver effective doses of radiation until it dissipates. An example of this is the thyroid gland□s ability to concentrate iodine, including its radioactive isotopes. Obviously, this method doesn□t require a radiation therapy machine, but many of the same precautions in handling the radioactive material are required.

AKA □(none).

Related devices □**PET scanners (237)**.

Where found □ diagnostic imaging departments, special radiation therapy clinics.

Positron Emission Tomography (PET) Scanners

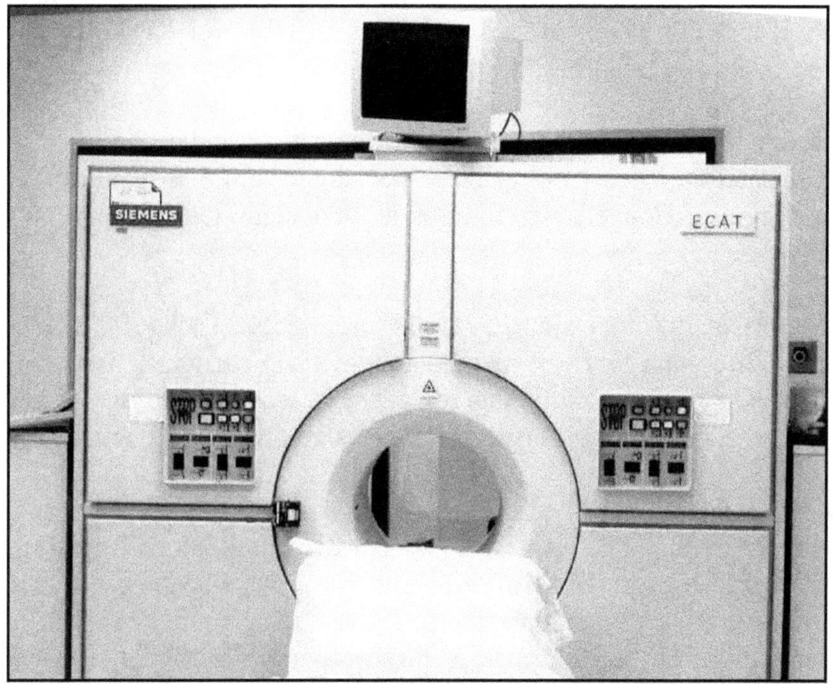

Overview □It can be important to know which areas of the body are active metabolically in determining disease or injury conditions in a patient. Since specific compounds are involved in certain metabolic functions, a means of identifying the location and rate of uptake of these compounds will give information about metabolic activities in the tissue or organ in question.

Function □ Various molecules utilized in metabolic activity within the body can be □labelled□ with radioactive elements that either replace the normal atoms of that same element within the molecule or attach themselves to the molecule in such a way that chemical activity is effectively unchanged.

The resultant molecules are produced in a huge, high□tech machine called a cyclotron, and are referred to as □radiopharmaceuticals.□ These radioactive atoms are then carried through the body along with the whole molecules and are concentrated within organs or tissues that utilize these molecules and are currently active

One example of such a molecule is fluorodeoxyglucose, which acts like normal glucose and is absorbed by any tissue in the body that is active metabolically. This is particularly useful in the brain, where tumors, injury sites, or areas involved in mental processes typically are more active than other nearby areas.

A second radiopharmaceutical is radioactive iodine, which is concentrated in the thyroid gland, especially in tumors or abnormally active regions. Conversely, iodine is less concentrated in abnormally inactive areas.

There are many other such radiopharmaceuticals, each of which is specific to certain types of metabolic activity in particular tissues or organs. They are used to help diagnose disease conditions in the target areas, or to perform research studies involving those areas.

Once the radiopharmaceutical has been concentrated in the target tissue, the actual PET scan can be performed. Radioactive atoms give off positrons in the form of gamma-rays, which can be detected by a device called a gamma camera. By arranging as many as 180 of these gamma-ray detectors in a circular pattern around the target area, gamma-ray activity can be measured. Combining signals from the various detectors and processing with a computer system gives "slice" images, which are colored artificially to show different degrees of metabolic activity in the image area. Each color assigned to the image by the computer corresponds to a particular level of activity; this makes it easy to differentiate between active and inactive regions.

<u>Mammograms for the Masses – Sundeep – Diagnostic Imaging III</u>

*Once Sundeep is feeling better following the radiation treatments, her doctor suggests to her and her family that some tests should be done to assess the progress of her Alzheimer's. He schedules a PET (Positron Emission Tomography) scan, which will give a good indication of any structural changes in her brain related to the disease. This can aid in both counseling and in planning drug and physical therapies that may help alleviate some symptoms or slow their progress. The PET scanner is located in the Diagnostic Imaging department and looks somewhat like an **MRI (229)** or **CT (214)** machine, with a narrow table on tracks and a large box with a round opening that the table, with patient, can slide through.*

A technologist injects a radioactive chemical into Sundeep's bloodstream and in an hour or so this chemical is concentrated in the active areas of her brain. The molecules of the chemical emit particles called positrons, which are detected by the machine and the results processed and analyzed to produce 3-dimensional images of the brain showing the areas of greater and lesser metabolic activity. The distribution of activity helps to diagnose the cause of dementia, with Alzheimer's disease showing a distinctive pattern. The chemical is depleted after a short time and disappears from the body. After the procedure is completed, the table slides Sundeep out of the chamber. The technologist helps her to her feet and an aide assists her in getting dressed so that her son can take her home.

Some PET scan systems can take a series of adjacent slice images and combine them to give a three□dimensional view.

Images are viewed on a video display and can also be stored or printed for later examination.

<u>Application</u> □ The radiopharmaceutical chosen for the particular study is administered to the patient intravenously. After a pre□

determined time, which varies with each type of examination, the patient lies on a moveable table, which slides them into the detector ring. Movements of the table are controlled by the operator and/or the computer system to position the patient in order to obtain the desired images. Images may be obtained in a series of slices to produce a 3□D picture, and several exposures may be taken over time to observe changes in metabolism. Patients may find the enclosed interior of the unit to be claustrophobic, something the operators need to discuss beforehand and be aware of during the procedure.

Radiation produced by the chemicals involved is relatively low□ level, and the molecules either decay to harmless levels in a short time, or they are excreted by the body, or both. Since operators are potentially exposed to more radiation than individual patients, they must take adequate precautions to avoid overexposure.

AKA □PET scanner, PE scanner.

Related devices □**CT scanner (214)**, **MRI scanner (229)**, **room x–ray equipment (241)**.

Where found □ diagnostic imaging departments, specialized facilities, mobile units.

Room X-ray Units

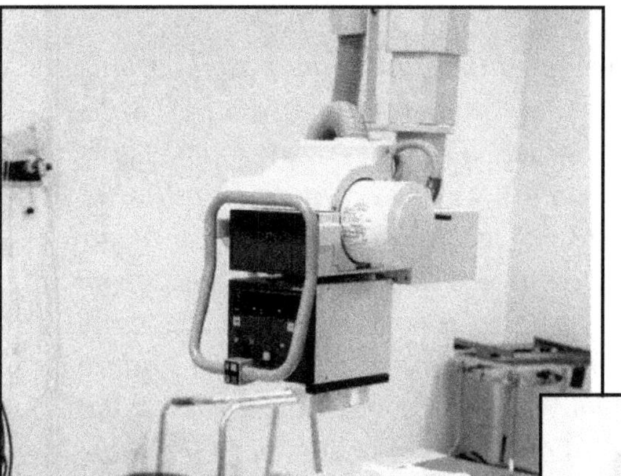

Overview – X-rays of the appropriate power will penetrate tissues. If an appropriate detector is placed on the opposite side of the body from the source of the x-rays, a "shadow" image is obtained which can give vital information about various structures within the body, since different body parts and tissues block the x-rays to a greater or lesser degree.

Function – By focusing a high-energy beam of electrons onto a spinning metal disc, the atoms of the metal can be excited to a point where they give off x-rays, an extremely high frequency form of electromagnetic radiation. Other examples of electromagnetic radiation are light rays, infrared or heat radiation, and radio signals.
The most common means of detecting and recording the images produced by an x-ray machine is silver-halide-based photographic film. This film is similar to everyday film used in cameras, but is generally much larger. It is optimized for x-ray exposures rather than light exposures, and it is very fine grained so that maximum detail can be seen in images.

<u>Accidents Happen – Felipe – Diagnostic Imaging II</u>

Another trip to the hospital, this time for x-rays of his fractures. Felipe changes into a hospital gown and waits uncomfortably until he is called in to the x-ray room. He is helped onto a hard x-ray table with just a tiny foam pillow to make it more comfortable. A technologist drapes a heavy lead apron over Felipe's hips to shield his testicles from potentially harmful x-rays and turns on a light in the x-ray head above the table. The collimator light casts a square with dark cross-hair shadows to help aim the x-ray beam. The tech uses a hand-held controller to adjust both the table position (and Felipe along with it) and the position of the x-ray head. The head can move up and down, forward and back, and side to side, as well as being able to rotate. When everything is right, the tech steps behind a leaded-glass wall, asks Felipe to keep perfectly still, and presses a button on the control panel to trigger the exposure. There is a noise from the overhead device and Felipe is told he can relax. The procedure is repeated a few times to get images of Felipe's various injuries. This x-ray system is digital, meaning that the images are detected electronically and stored in a computer system, rather than using film that would have to be developed and processed. The images are instantly displayed on a video monitor in the control area, and are also made available on the hospital's ***PACS (232)*** *(Picture Archiving and Communication System) so that authorized users such as radiologists and Felipe's personal physician can view them from anywhere there is a PACS terminal.*

Electronic components act to focus the x□ray beam at the plane of the film, and thus care must be taken to place the film and the x□ray source at the correct distance from one another.

Since the x□rays themselves cannot be seen, a visual system of aiming is used, with a light shining from the same point as the x□rays and making a shadow of cross□hairs. This part of the unit also has adjustable edges so that exposure can be limited to the specific target area.

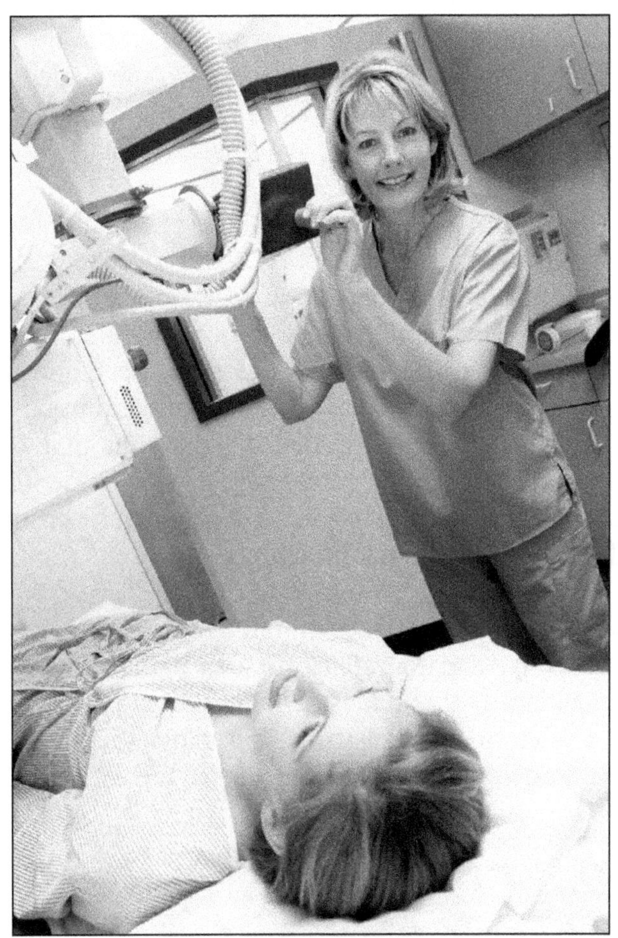

X–ray unit being positioned.
Modified from Shutterstock, Inc, www.shutterstock.com, with permission

Adjusting the power and time of the x□ray emission controls exposures. Power is measured in units called kilovolt□amps, or kVA. Different tissue densities and thickness, and varying requirements for detail and speed of exposure, determine these parameter settings.

Certain structures can be better seen on x□rays if a material that blocks the rays is placed into spaces within the body. Examples of this include a liquid form of barium which the patient may drink to help define parts of the upper digestive tract, or which may be given by enema when the lower parts of the digestive system are being investigated. Radiopaque dyes may be administered intravenously to show either blood vessels or the urinary system (after the dye is removed from the bloodstream by the kidneys).

Some x□ray units have mechanisms to automatically and rapidly change several film cassettes, in order to follow the progress of the barium or dye mentioned above as it moves through the patient□s body. Others have a roll of film, as in a movie camera, to record a greater number of frames (though in a smaller format).

Excessive exposure to x□rays can be harmful, especially to reproductive organs, and so patients are normally draped with flexible lead aprons and/or sheets to limit exposure to the target area. Staff members use this equipment over long periods of time and so must take precautions to avoid overexposure. Lead aprons are worn if they must be in the vicinity of the patient during exposures, otherwise they move behind a leaded shield for the time of exposure. Film badges are worn which can help evaluate the total dosage received over a period of time, and if levels reach certain threshold levels, staff may be reassigned for a while.

<u>Application</u> □ Patients are asked to remove any clothing from target areas of the body, and to replace it with a thin gown in order to minimize blocking of the x□rays. They are then placed in a position (either on a table or standing) that will allow the best view of the target, and distances and areas to be exposed are set.

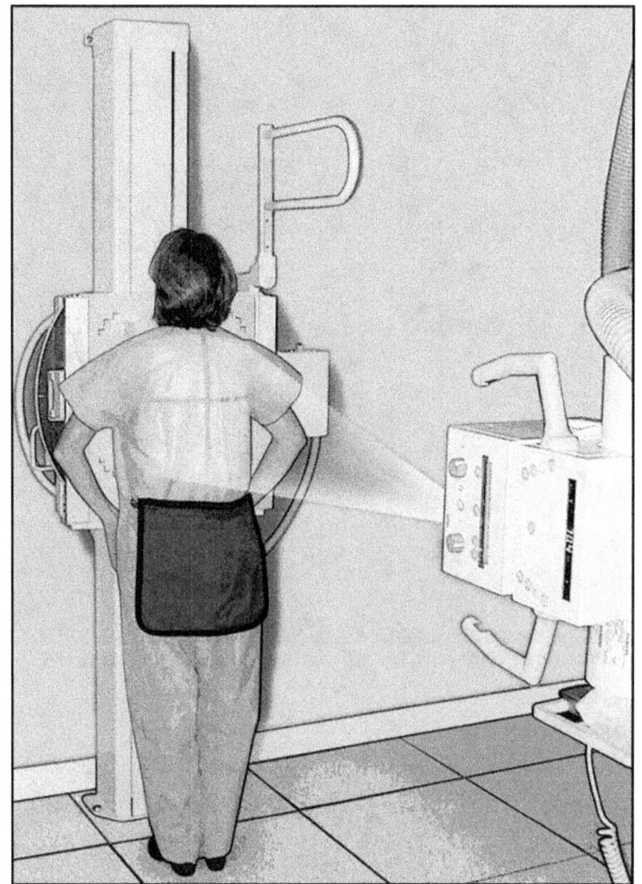

Wall x–ray unit, used mainly for chest examinations.
Public domain image.

Since exposure times are often measured in relatively large fractions of a second, or sometimes even multiple seconds, the patients must remain still during exposures. If the target area is in or near the chest, the patients are asked to hold their breath for the exposure.

Barium is usually administered before the x-ray procedure starts, though it may be given while making exposures if, for example, swallowing actions are to be examined. Radiopaque dyes are usually injected immediately before x-rays are taken; pre-injection images may be taken for comparison purposes.

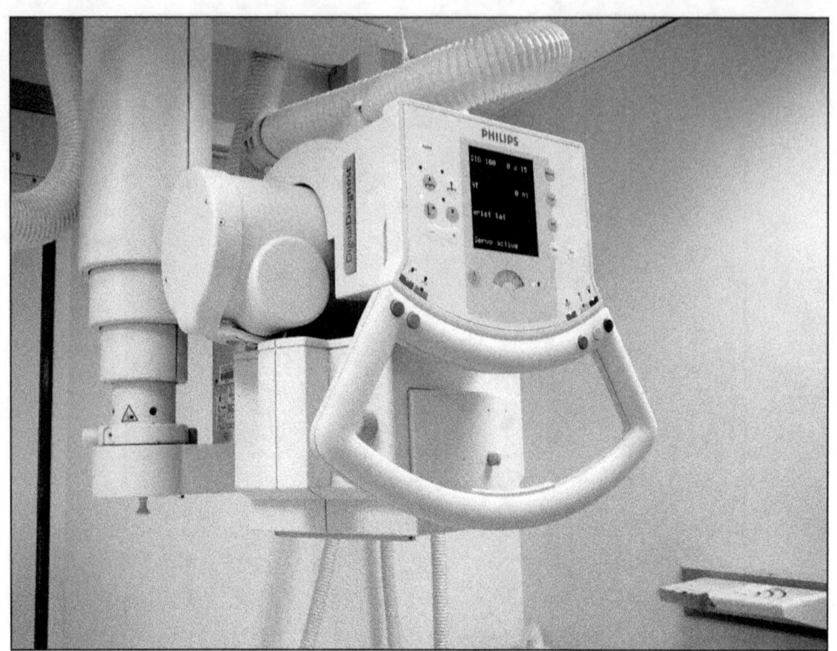

X–ray unit head with controls for adjusting position and angle.

<u>AKA</u> □radiography units.

<u>Related devices</u> □ **mobile C–arms (212), dye injectors (222), CT scanners (214).**

<u>Where found</u> □ diagnostic imaging departments, mobile x□ray trailers

Chapter 12 – General Hospital Areas and Miscellaneous

Equipment Descriptions

Following are more detailed descriptions of equipment found in many areas of the hospital.

The types of medical devices described in this section are found throughout a typical hospital, in many different areas. Some of the devices such as **stethoscopes (327)** are simple, while others, such as **ECG machines (270)** or **IV pumps (289)**, are complex and highly technical. Some special devices are also included in this section.

Alternating Pressure Mattresses

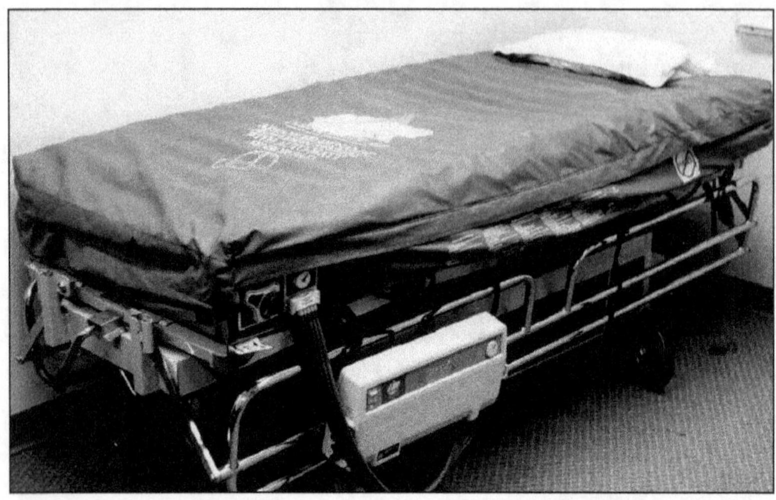

Overview □ Patients with limited mobility are often subject to bed or pressure sores, as they are unable to shift their position to allow blood to flow to all areas that come in contact with the bed. While staff can provide changes in position, this isn□t always practical, and, during the night, it might disturb the patient by repeatedly interrupting sleep.

Function □ Alternating pressure mattresses have many separate sections, usually in two alternating groups, which can be inflated independently. By first inflating one group, then partially deflating it and inflating the second group, the mattress never is in firm contact with a given point on the patient for an extended period of time. The cycle time of the mattress is generally fixed at several minutes, as a compromise between comfort and effectiveness. Mattress pressure can be adjusted between preset limits to accommodate different patients and situations. Most systems can also be set to a non□alternating, or static, mode, in which all sections of the mattress remain inflated at the selected pressure.

The pumps for these systems have low and high pressure alarms, and the mattresses have valves that allow for rapid deflation in case this is necessary (for example, to allow CPR to be performed). The valves can also be closed off completely so that the mattress remains inflated while the pump is removed or unplugged, such as when the patient is being moved to a different area. The low□pressure alarm is inactive for several minutes after the pump is first turned on to allow for initial inflation.

Because the pumps are used for long periods close to the patient, they must be designed to be as quiet as possible.

Function □ The patient is placed on the deflated mattress, which is then inflated by the pump. Pressure and mode are set once the mattress is fully inflated.

AKA □pillow pumps, pressure mattresses.

Related devices □**electrical hospital beds (277)**.

Where found □ areas of the hospital where patients are confined to bed for long periods, such as extended care, burn, or palliative care units.

Aspirators

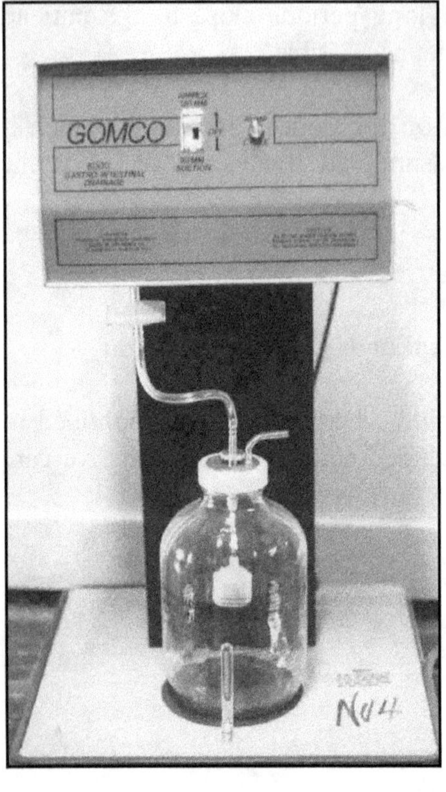

Overview □ In emergency situations, the patient□s airway must be cleared of fluids that might block airflow.

Function □ An aspirator is simply a suction pump that provides vacuum to a tubing system that connects to a specially designed tip that is inserted into the patient□s throat to remove fluids. The tip has openings that help prevent intake of larger objects and are less likely to be blocked by surrounding tissue than would be a single, larger opening.

The glass or plastic reservoir between the pump and the patient serves two purposes: to collect the fluids drained from the patient; and to even out the air flow in the system by acting as a vacuum reservoir.

Other important components of the system include: a vacuum gauge to indicate the amount of vacuum available (and also give an indication that the system is set up correctly □ a low reading may mean a leak); a vacuum level control mechanism, usually a knob; a filter system that helps to keep fluids from entering the pump and also to help prevent harmful materials from being sent into the air with the pump exhaust; and an overflow device to shut the system off if the reservoir becomes full of fluid. The overflow device can be a simple float valve, or a switch mechanism that depends of the weight of the reservoir to turn off the vacuum.

Pumping for the system can be accomplished by an electrical pump (either AC or battery□powered) directly associated with the rest of the components, or by a central pump that connects via a plumbing system to vacuum "outlets" (of course they are actually "inlets") at each bedside or treatment station. Self-powered systems are more portable, but central systems make for less clutter at the bedside.

Fluids collected by aspiration systems are non-sterile and must be treated appropriately.

Application – The pump is turned on and suction level adjusted, then the suction tip is applied to the area to be drained. Care must be taken not to damage tissues with excessive suction.

AKA – suction units, suctions, Gomcos (after a manufacturer).

Related devices – **gas regulators (285)**.

Where found – most areas of the hospital.

Bladder Scanners

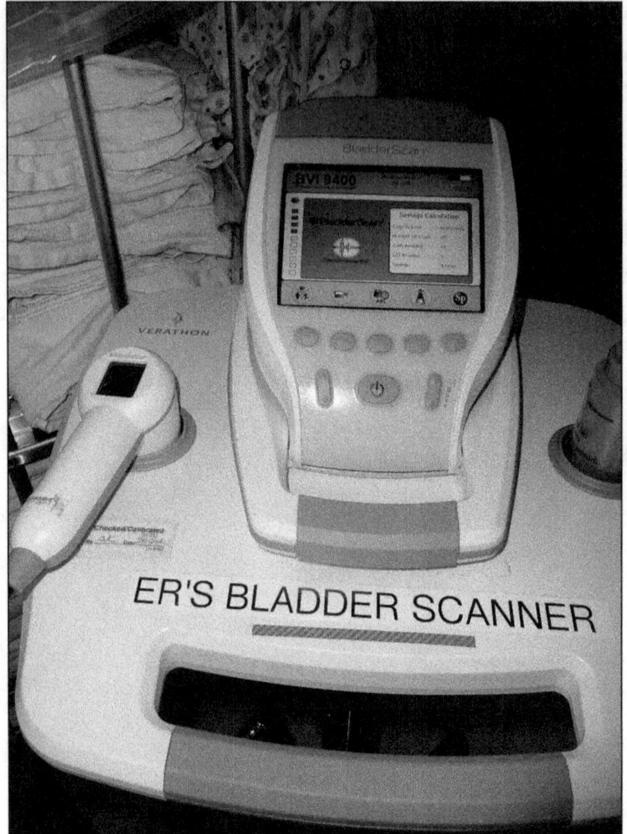

A bladder scanner, with the ultrasound head on the left.

Overview It is sometimes difficult to measure urine output to determine fluid intake and output balances, which can be important in evaluating a patients condition. Also, incomplete bladder emptying can be both a symptom and a cause of medical problems. For these reasons, a simple and quick means of measuring bladder volume is useful.

Function A bladder scanner is a small, portable and dedicated ultrasound machine. It consists of ultrasound scan heads and connecting cables, an analysis computer system, a data entry keyboard and a video display. The principle of operation is the same as that of other diagnostic ultrasound machines, but it is specifically designed to optimize scanning the bladder, and the analysis computer system can detect the bladder and generate an accurate measure of the volume of urine it contains. The video screen displays both the ultrasound image and text information of the bladder volume.

Application □ As with other ultrasound machines, gel is applied to the patient□s lower abdomen to increase sound wave transmission. The ultrasound probe is pressed against the skin over the bladder area and moved around until the unit detects the bladder and calculates its volume. Scans may be repeated to ensure an accurate reading is obtained.

AKA □(none).

Related devices □**ultrasound machines (217)**.

Where found □most areas of the hospital, as needed.

Capnographs

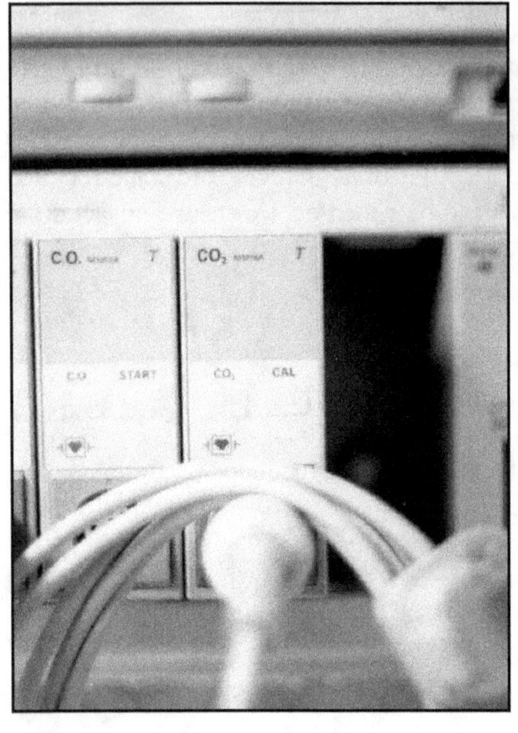

Overview □ In many medical situations, it is important to know how much carbon dioxide (CO_2) is present in the exhaled breath of the patient.

Function □ A capnograph, which can be either a stand□alone unit or a module of a multi□function monitor, measures values by passing part of the exhaled air through a small chamber with glass sides. By passing precisely controlled beams of infrared light through the chamber and measuring the output, the CO_2 content can be determined. The percentage is then displayed as a numeric value and/or as a graph on a display or recorder. If the capnograph is part of a monitoring system (either a module or a built□in component), the values may be stored over time to provide tabular or graphical displays of data which show changes over time.

Application □The capnography sensor is applied to the measurement window, which is usually in line with a ventilator or breathing tube. Because of the sensitivity of the measurements, the sensor must be calibrated before each use, and at specific intervals while in use. A pair of chambers is provided which have specific CO2 content, and the measurements can be adjusted to match these values. A calibration factor, specific to that particular sensor, may be marked on the calibration portion of the sensor; if so, this value is entered into the system at a specific point in the calibration process.

Once the sensor is calibrated, measurements can commence.

AKA CO2 analyzers, exhaled CO2 analyzer, endtidal CO2 monitors.

Related devices **oxygen analyzers (305), point of care blood analyzers (318), ventilators (334), physiological monitors (314).**

Where found critical care areas of the hospital.

Cast Cutters

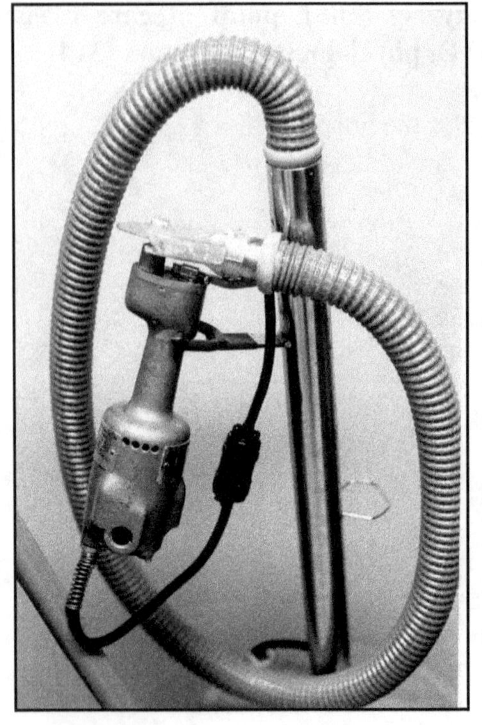

Overview □ When it is time to change or remove a cast, the material (usually either plaster or fiberglass) must be cut. It is too hard and thick to cut with scissor□like devices, and because the patient□s skin is very close underneath, conventional□type saws or knives are too dangerous.

Function □ Cast cutter saws use a round, saw□toothed blade which is oscillated by the saw, rotating it a few degrees and then back very rapidly. The teeth are only moderately sharp, and, since skin is elastic, if the oscillating teeth should strike it, they merely push it back and forth without cutting. When the blade is applied to the hard, brittle cast material, it cuts through.

Application □ Cutting a cast with a cast saw is simply a matter of turning the unit on and applying it to the part of the cast to be cut. Since it is noisy (and appears more dangerous than it is), and produces clouds of dust, patients need to be informed about the procedure in advance.

The dust from either type of cast material can be hazardous if inhaled, and is also very messy if spread around the room. Cast cutters often come with a vacuum attachment that sucks the dust from the cutting location before it can spread.

AKA □ cast saws.

Related devices □ (none).

Where found □ outpatient clinics, emergency rooms.

Cryosurgery Units

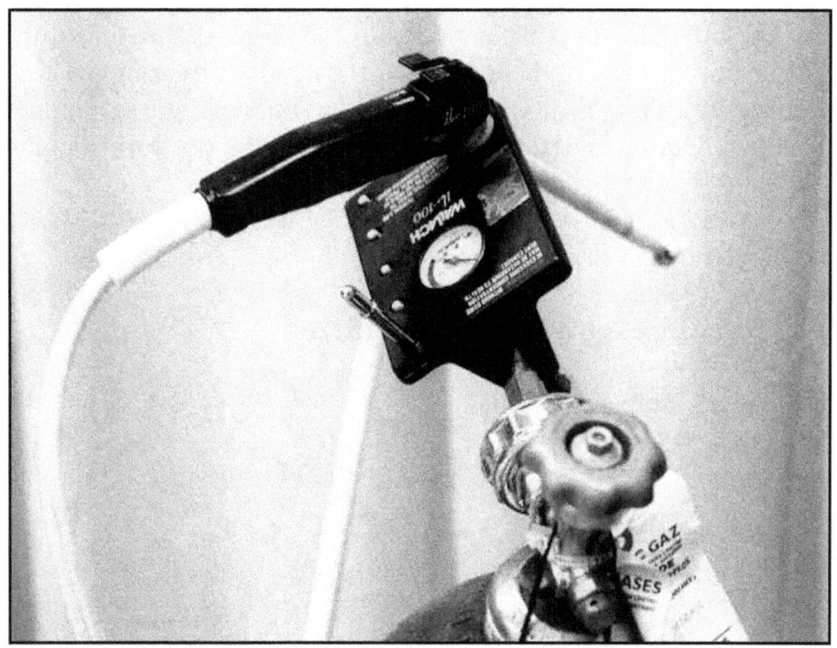

Overview — Small skin abnormalities are often removed for clinical or esthetic reasons. Cutting the skin often results in considerable bleeding and opens the possibility of infection. By freezing the tissue concerned, the cells will die and eventually be sloughed off without an open wound forming.

Function — While some situations requiring freezing may be handled by a simple swab soaked in liquid nitrogen pressed against the tissue, other circumstances require more control and longer application times. A cryosurgery machine uses the controlled expansion of a compressed gas to produce extreme cooling in a small metal tip, which can then be applied to the target tissue. Tips used are of various shapes and sizes, depending on the situation. Gases most commonly used are nitrous oxide and carbon dioxide; since both of these are potentially harmful (especially nitrous oxide), the units must be used in well-ventilated areas; preferable is to have the expended gas exhausted to the outside. The gas can be routed through the probe in such a way as to defrost the instrument at the end of the procedure.

Application □The operator depresses a control to release gas through the probe tip, continuing until the tip is well cooled (indicated by a coating of frost and "smoke" □ wisps of freezing water vapor □ around the tip). The tip is then applied to the target tissue, for a time determined by the size of the target and the depth of freezing desired. Additional gas may be used to keep the tip cold during longer applications. Defrosting is necessary to prevent the tip from sticking to the target tissue when treatment is finished.

AKA □cryo units.

Related devices □**electrosurgery units (51)**.

Where found □outpatient clinics.

Defibrillators

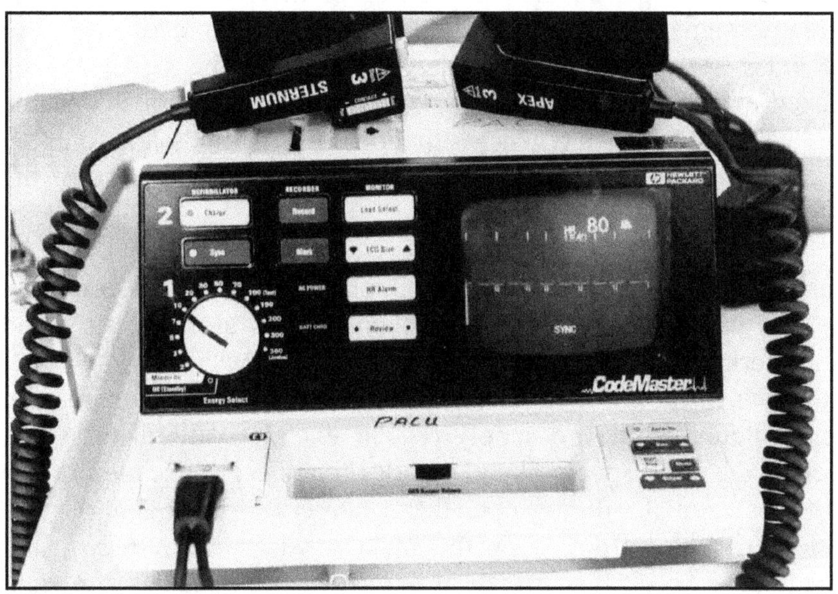

Overview — The contraction of the heart is controlled by electrical signals, which must be of the correct size, timing, and distribution to cause coordinated and effective pumping. Many factors can disrupt these signals, such as blood electrolyte and/or gas levels, body temperature, various drugs, damage to the heart muscle or to the conductive pathways that distribute the signals, and physical or electrical shock. When the heart no longer beats effectively, blood flow is compromised, and serious harm or death can result. Note that the heart may continue to beat in some fashion, but not effectively (that is, it fibrillates or is in fibrillation), or the heart may cease to beat at all (asystole, “flat line”). Whatever the cause, it is essential that proper function be restored as soon as possible. This may be accomplished by medication, by physical intervention such as CPR or body temperature adjustment, or by applying an electrical signal to the heart that will restart or re-coordinate (de-fibrillate) its contractions. A defibrillator is a device that supplies such corrective signals.

For a more detailed discussion of arrhythmias, see Appendix C, p. 392.

Function – Defibrillators may act on the heart directly, with electrodes applied to the cardiac tissue, or indirectly, with electrodes (called paddles) placed on the exterior of the patient's chest. The corrective signal, or shock, required is much, much greater when the electrodes are external, since a large portion of the signal will be blocked or redirected by the tissues between the electrodes and the heart itself. In most emergency situations, it is not possible to apply the electrodes directly to the heart, so most defibrillators are of the external type.

Internal defibrillators can be either implantable, in which case they must be capable of determining when shocks are necessary and administering them automatically, or manual, in which case the size and timing of the shock is determined by the operator. Most manual internal defibrillators are simply regular external defibrillators with specially designed spoon-like electrodes for direct application to the heart (for example, during open-heart surgery). These defibrillators must be capable of delivering the small-sized shocks required, and most have a circuit that detects when the internal paddles are being used to prevent the selection of higher shock levels.

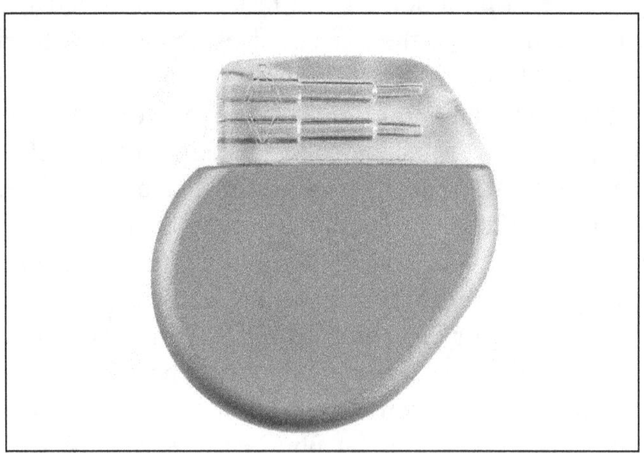

Implantable defibrillator module.
Modified from Inmagine Corp, www.123rf.com, with permission.

Implantable defibrillators use wire electrodes that are embedded in the cardiac muscle at the appropriate location. They measure the ECG signal and analyze it to determine its characteristics. If these characteristics fall into a class that has been designated as abnormal but correctable, they will automatically administer an appropriately-sized-and-timed shock to re-establish proper cardiac function. This is different from implantable pacemakers, which apply smaller signals in order to maintain proper rhythms. Generally, a pacemaker is used when the degree of damage to the heart that requires corrective action is less, whereas an implantable defibrillator is used when there is greater damage and more extensive intervention is required to restore proper function.

External defibrillators may also be automatic; this is usually a feature of a machine that can also be used in manual mode.

Manually□controlled external defibrillators have some means of detecting and displaying and/or analyzing the ECG signals from the heart. This may be done directly through the paddles, or through separate ECG electrodes. Using separate electrodes generally produces more accurate ECG signals, but it takes time to apply them, and so the paddles themselves are used in more urgent situations. When separate electrodes are used, they must be located so as not to interfere with the optimum placement of the paddles. If the paddles are placed on top of the ECG electrodes, the shock can be reduced in effectiveness and/or burns can result to the patient□s skin. Units often have a visual indicator of paddle contact quality.

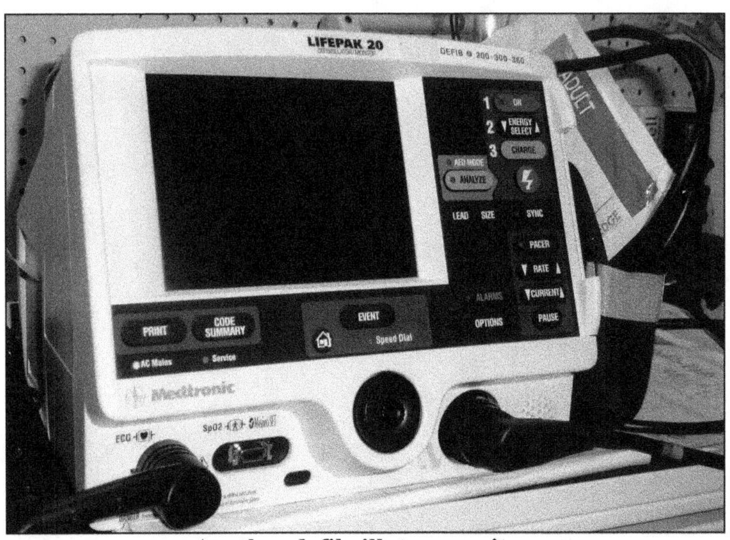

Another defibrillator–monitor.

Controls for the defibrillator include energy selection level, charge initiation, and discharge. The discharge buttons are usually a pair, one on each paddle handle, which must both be depressed to cause a discharge. Charge initiation and sometimes even energy selection controls may also be located on the paddles, as well as on the front panel.

These units have some kind of display of the ECG signal. This may be a simple visual or audible indicator of each beat, but usually it is a graphic display of the ECG waveform. Along with the graphic display, there may also be an audible beat indicator, whose volume can be adjusted or turned off. There is often a paper recorder that prints the signal and usually indicates the point at which the shock is administered and its size, as well as the date and time, which can be important for later medical analysis or legal considerations. The recorder often will have a memory function which allows it to print out several seconds of ECG signal from before the time the shock was applied, which gives a better picture of the event as a whole.

More and more public areas have very simple defibrillators that can be operated by almost anyone who can read. These automatic external defibrillators, or AEDs, perform ECG analysis and determine the level and timing of shocks. The operator simply has to apply the defib pads and activate the unit.

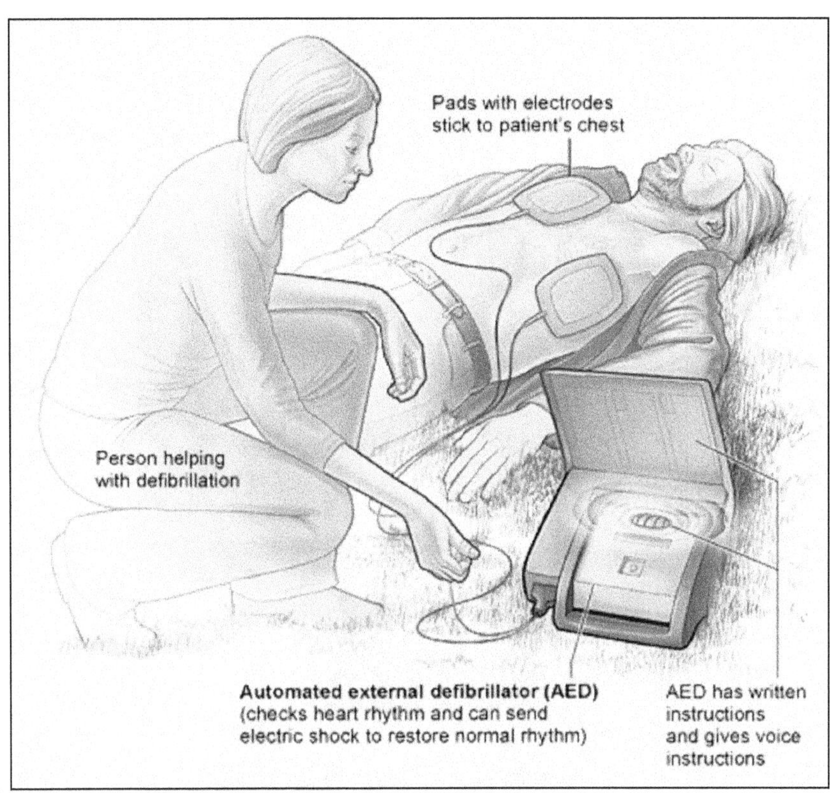

An automatic external defibrillator in use.

Courtesy of the National Institute of Diabetes and Digestive and Kidney Diseases, National Institutes of Health.

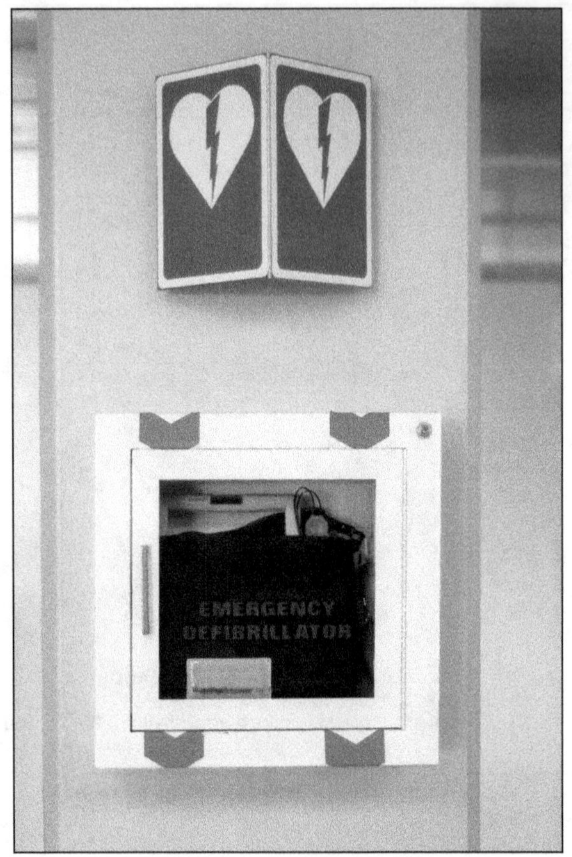

AED mounted on a wall.
Modified from Inmagine Corp, www.123rf.com, with permission.

Defibrillation may be required to correct other abnormalities of the cardiac rhythm. The most common of these is when the atria of the heart are fibrillating but the ventricles are beating normally (atrial fibrillation or afib). In this case, the shock must be applied at a very precise time in relation to the ventricular beats. Since this would be almost impossible for a human operator to time correctly, defibrillators are often equipped with circuitry to detect the ventricular beats and apply the shock at the next correct time after the operator depresses the shock (or discharge) buttons. This procedure is called synchronized cardioversion. Since the proper timing requires an accurate ECG signal, the defibrillator will not enter this mode unless ECG electrodes are applied and used.

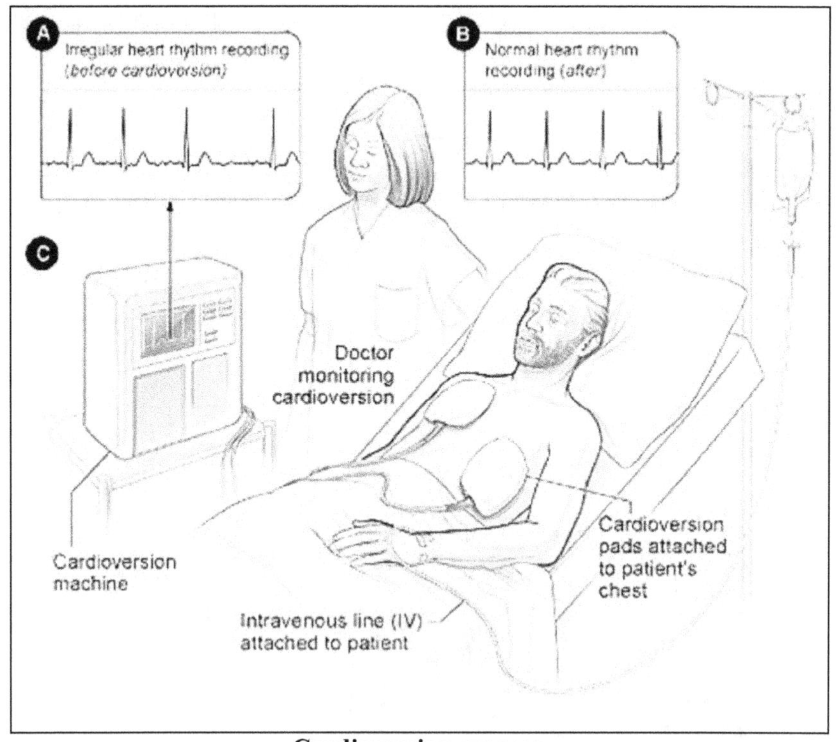

Cardioversion process.

Courtesy of the National Institute of Diabetes and Digestive and Kidney Diseases, National Institutes of Health.

The mode is normally called □sync□ (synchronized), and there is usually a light flashing and/or tone sounding to indicate its selection. There is usually a □marker□ signal placed on top of the normal contraction signals so that the operator can determine whether the timing is correct.

Because they are often used in emergency situations, defibrillators often have internal batteries that can provide power for all functions.

Defibrillators may have other functions built in, such as **pulse oximetry (320)** (SpO2), in order to help caregivers better assess the condition of the patient.

<u>Application</u> □ Once the need for defibrillation has been established, the patient must be at least minimally prepared. The patient must be placed in a safe position, ensuring that the defibrillator paddles can make good contact with the correct areas of the chest wall. Conductive materials such as saline, blood, and ECG electrodes must be clear of the site. The team leader then decides on the optimum

energy setting (though it may be selected by another team member). If a synchronized cardioversion is to be performed, that function must be selected. A button is pressed to start the unit charging, and a tone often sounds to indicate that this is happening. Another tone signals that charging is complete, and then (usually after notifying the other team members first) the operator presses the discharge buttons, which causes the shock signal to be delivered to the patient. The ECG signal of the patient is then observed to determine whether the treatment was successful. If not, the energy level may be increased and the procedure repeated.

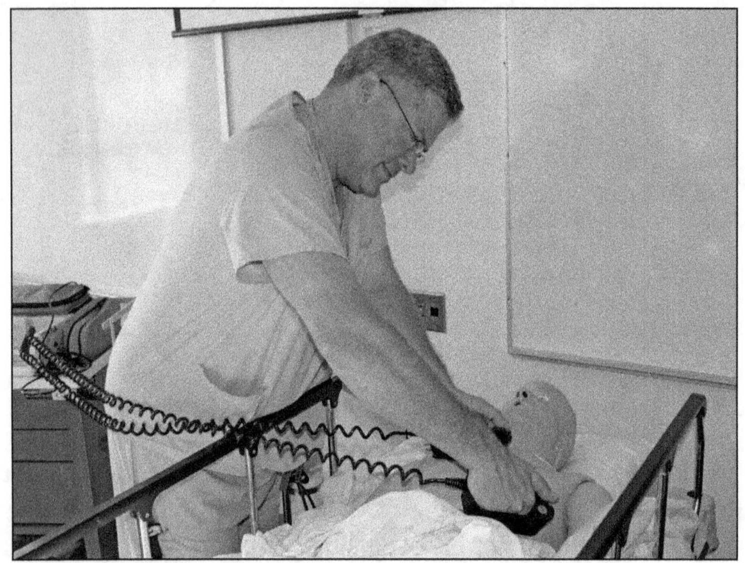

Defibrillator in use, in this case on a test dummy.

Because the shock delivered by a defibrillator is quite large, and because the signal may travel to other parts of the body than the heart, where it may cause sharp contractions of muscles, the patient may twitch rather violently when the shock is delivered. This means that appropriate measures must be taken to prevent injury to the patient or to attending staff.

AKA defibs.

Related devices **pacemakers (25)**, **pulse oximeters (320)**, **physiological monitors (314)**.

Where found critical care areas, general areas of the hospital on crash carts.

Electro□Convulsive Therapy (ECT) Units

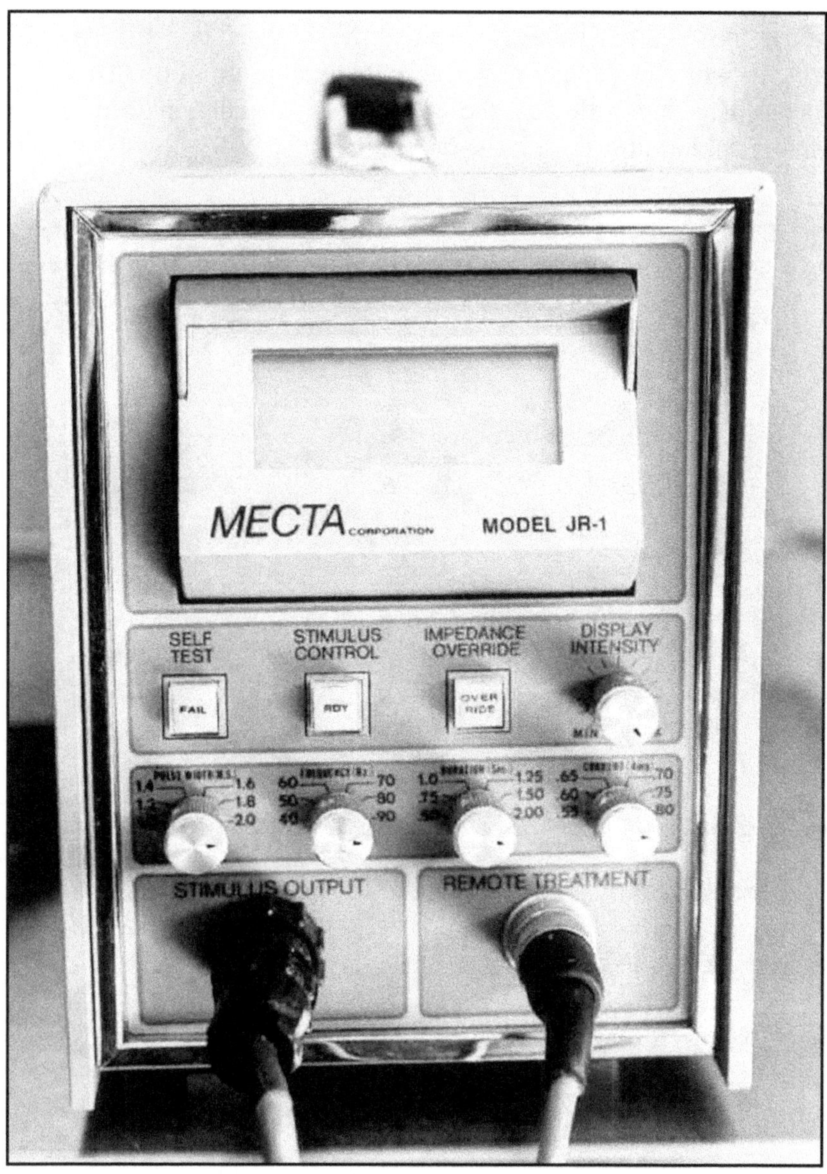

Overview □ Certain psychiatric conditions seem to respond well to the administration of a controlled electrical shock to the brain.

Function □ An Electro□convulsive Therapy (ECT) machine provides precisely shaped and timed signals (both parameters under control of the operator) via special electrodes placed on the patient's scalp.

Application Since these electrical signals can cause powerful muscle contractions in other parts of the body, and for patient comfort, the patient is anesthetized or heavily sedated prior to the treatment, which is usually only a few minutes in duration. To watch for possible side effects, the patient is usually placed on a physiological monitor during the procedure.

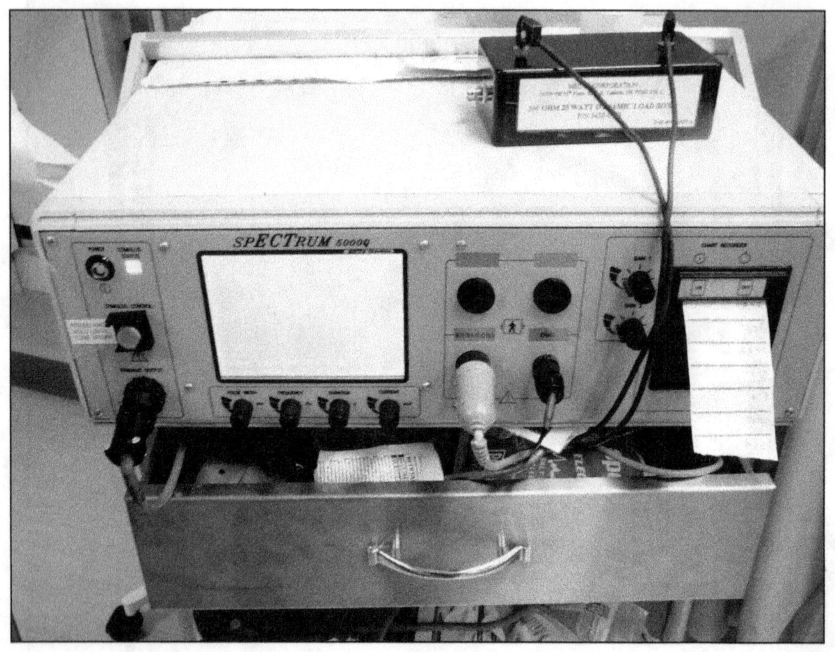

AKA shock therapy units.

Related devices EEG machines, physiological monitors.

Where found specialized outpatient clinics, postanesthesia recovery areas, operating rooms, psychiatric special procedure rooms.

Heart Attack! – John – ECT

Even though the bypass surgery went well and the pacemaker is functioning properly, John becomes depressed. His doctors try various medications and psychotherapy with little effect, and so they decide to try shock treatment. John is admitted to hospital as a day-care patient and is made comfortable in bed. He is given a sedative and his psychiatrist explains the procedure. Electrodes are placed on either side of his head, near the temples, and are held in place by an elastic strap. ECG monitoring electrodes are connected to his chest and both types of electrodes are connected (through special connectors that prevent them being mixed up) to an ***electro-convulsive therapy (ECT) machine (267)****, which is able to provide the necessary electrical signal to the head electrodes as well as monitor ECG. John's vital signs are checked, and then he is injected with drugs to put him to sleep and also to partially paralyze his muscles. This is to prevent severe muscle contractions when the ECT shock is administered; such contractions could cause injury to John as well as to staff members. When all is ready, the operator triggers the ECT machine and a series of electrical pulses are delivered through the electrodes on John's head. The pulses are up to about 225 volts and 750 milliamps, and are designed to produce the most beneficial psychological results with minimal side effects. During shock delivery, staff closely observes John's toes to see if they twitch. This indicates that the shock was delivered successfully; if there is no twitch, the shock was not delivered or was not strong enough. The procedure may be repeated, and once the psychiatrist is satisfied with the results, John is disconnected from the machine and brought out of anesthesia. He is kept under observation for a few hours before being released.*

Electrocardiograph (ECG) Machines

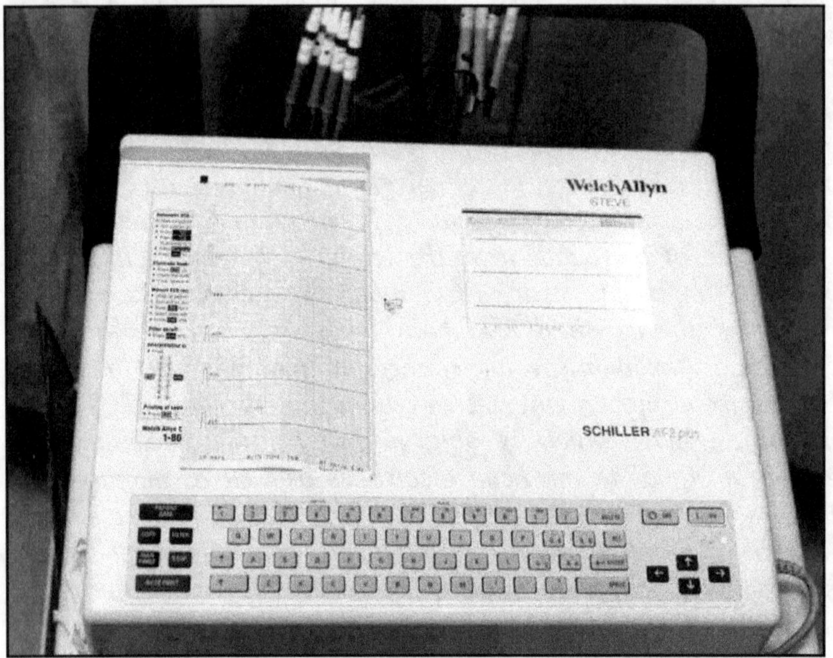

Overview □ When a patient might have cardiac problems, caregivers need the most accurate indication of the functioning of the heart possible.

Function □ One means of providing an indication of cardiac function is with the ECG machine, which makes precise measurements of the heart's electrical activity from several different perspectives, by using an array of electrodes (usually either five or twelve) placed in carefully selected positions on the patient□s chest. The circuitry of the machine then translates these signals into a graph and prints them out on chart paper, with one trace for each of several combinations of electrodes (or □leads□). Since the signals are very small (measured in thousandths of a volt), compared to much larger electrical interference signals, the circuitry must be very sophisticated to provide useful results.

Most newer ECG machines provide annotations on the chart, giving lead labels, time and date, patient information, etc. Some provide precise values for various measurements of the ECG signal, and some also give a possible interpretation of any abnormalities present in the signals. The more complex machines usually have some kind of display screen and a keyboard for entering information. Some have data ports for connection to computer systems and/or to allow sending the results through a modem to a remote location.

Electrodes are usually either an adhesive patch with a conductive area in the center, or a silver cup with a rubber suction bulb that literally sucks the cup onto the patient's skin. The suction type are used with a conductive cream and are quicker and easier to apply and remove; adhesive electrodes are less obtrusive and stay in place better for longer term applications.

Most ECG machines have batteries that allow them to be used when access to a power outlet is difficult; many also have data storage so that records can be printed out at a later time, since they are often used in the midst of an emergency situation and need to be removed from the scene as quickly as possible.

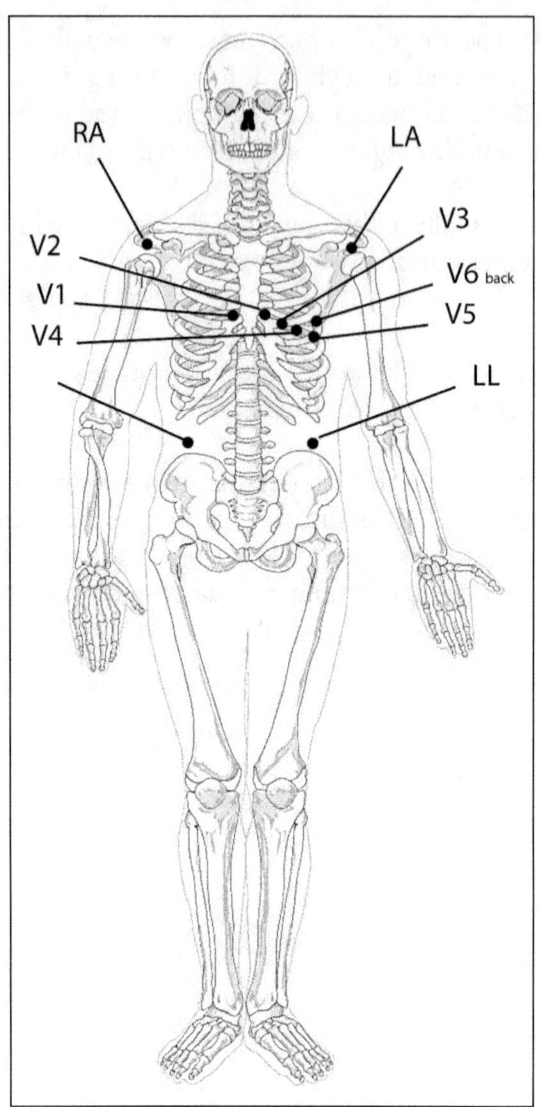

12–lead ECG electrode placement sites.

<u>Application</u> The patients skin is prepared for electrodes by shaving the sites (if necessary) and then cleaning the surface thoroughly. Natural or artificial oils on the skin can reduce contact quality, but the salts in the skin increase conductivity, so gentle physical abrasion of the skin is preferred over soap and water or alcohol cleaning. Electrodes are then applied; accuracy of placement in the prescribed locations is critical for obtaining the best results. Most systems allow the operator to view the signal before making a recording; when the set up is complete, a recording is initiated. This

usually only takes a few minutes, though some situations call for recordings made over a longer period of time.

AKA □ electrocardiographs, EKG machines (from the German spelling of the term), EKGs, ECGs, 12 leads, ECG/EKG recorders.

Related devices □ **physiological monitors (314)**, **ambulatory ECG recorders (166)**, **stress test machines (184)**.

Where found □ units are usually mobile and can be taken to any area of the hospital where patients might have cardiac problems, but are usually seen in emergency wards, intensive care units, post anesthesia recovery areas, or cardiology rooms.

Electroencephalographs (EEG)

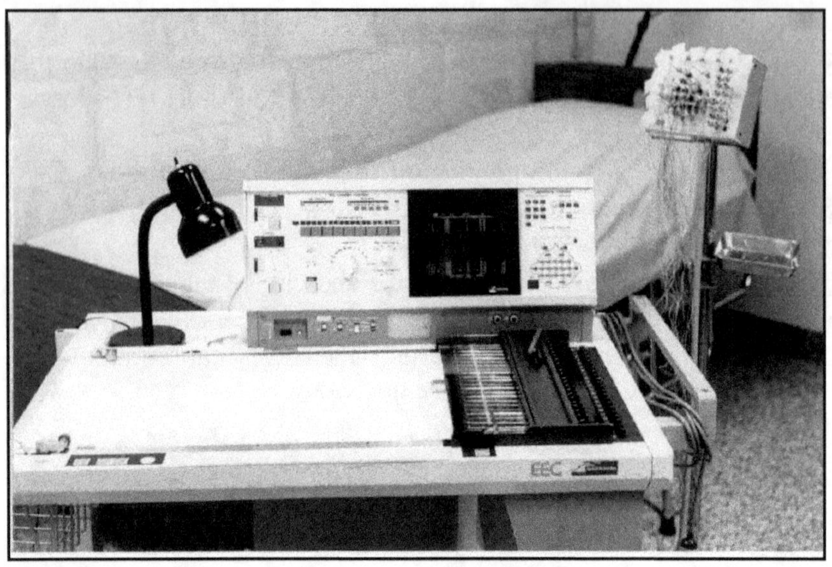

Overview □ Electrical activity in the brain can give important information about its function and possible disease conditions.

Function □ By taking signals from a large number of electrodes on specific points on the patient□s scalp, amplifying and processing these signals, and then comparing and combining the various signals and analyzing the results, the electroencephalograph can present a recording of the signals that originate from various points within the patient's brain. The recording can be printed out on a chart, or recorded electronically for later examination. Most EEG machines incorporate a means of providing various stimuli to the patient, such as light flashes or sounds, which can then be related to changes in the electrical signals from the brain.

Application □ Electrodes are applied to the patient□s scalp according to a pre□defined pattern. Depending on the complexity of the analysis being performed, different numbers of electrodes are used. The operator checks connection quality and then proceeds with the test. The patient may simply lie quietly, or stimuli (such as sounds or light flashes) may be delivered. The timing of these stimuli is recorded so any changes in brain waves in response to the stimuli can be found.

EEG tests may be quite long, especially if relatively rare brain activity events are being studied. Portable EEG recorders have been developed that allow the patient to move around while measurements are being taken.

AKA □EEG machines, brain wave machines.

Related devices □**ECG machines (270)**.

Where found □special areas, laboratories.

Level of Consciousness Monitors

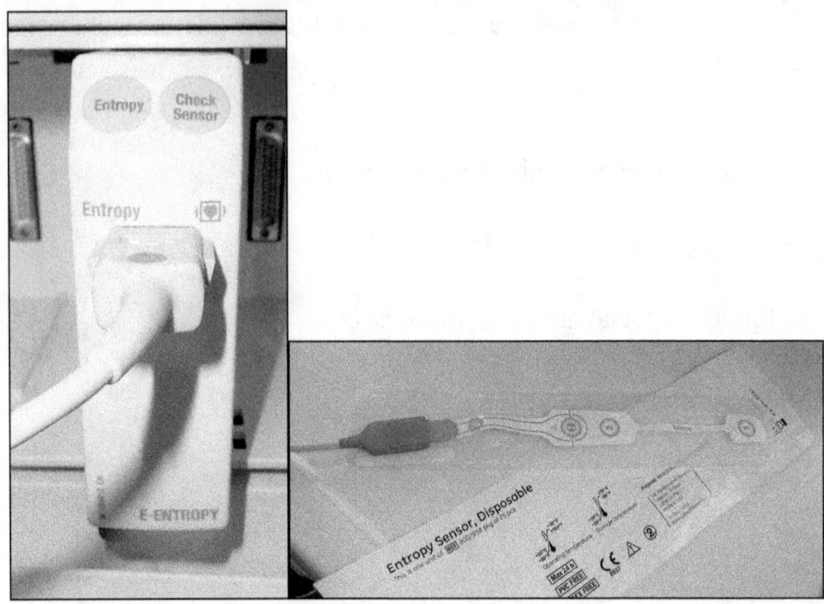

A level of consciousness module in an anesthetic machine (left) and an electrode for the unit (right).

A very specialized type of EEG measurement and analysis system is now often used to measure the level of consciousness in patients. This can be important in general anesthesia, where a balance between too shallow and too deep unconsciousness it important. It can also be critical in evaluating and monitoring patients in traumatic or induced comas. The systems collect and analyze specific portions of EEG data and, based on extensive research, provide a numerical value to indicate level of consciousness. Some systems refer to this as the BiSpectral, or BiS, index.

AKA □BiS monitors.

Related devices □**EEG machines (274)**.

Where found □ICUs, ORs, ERs.

Electric Hospital Beds

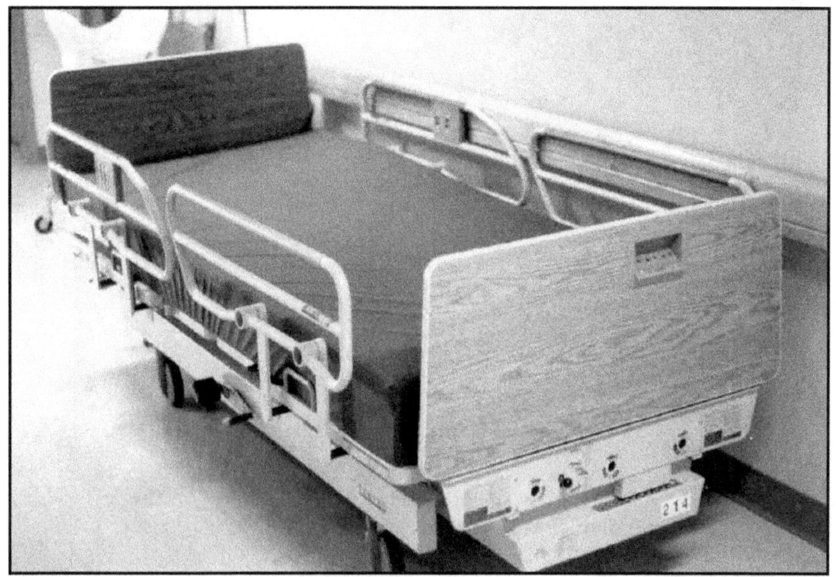

Overview □Hospital patients need to be able to change their position in order to be as comfortable as possible, especially if they are in bed for long periods of time. It is useful if the patient can adjust the bed to become more comfortable; it is also valuable to staff to have the patient make position changes unassisted.

Function □ Electric hospital beds have a comfortable, flexible mattress, and a frame and mechanism to allow for a variety of patient positions. Controls activate motors that raise or lower the whole bed, the head, the feet, and the hips independently (within ergonomic limits); these controls are usually placed both on a pendant or stalk so that the patient or a bedside attendant can use them, and at the foot of the bed for attendant control. Sometimes duplicate controls are on the bed rails on either side of the mattress. There is usually a lockout switch so that caregivers can prevent the patient from activating the controls, if this is necessary.

The whole unit is on wheels, which can be locked to prevent movement when necessary. Rails on either side of the bed can be raised or lowered, often in multiple positions, to help prevent the patient from falling out of bed. As with all hospital beds, the mattress is covered with an impermeable material to aid in cleaning.

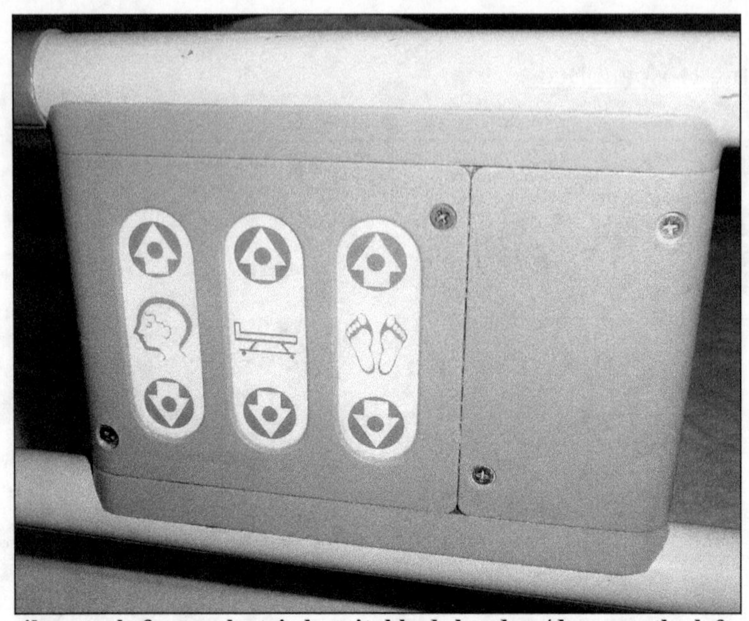

Bed rail controls for an electric hospital bed; head up/down on the left, whole bed up/down center and feet up/down on the right.

Application □The bed is adjusted to suit the patient□s comfort and/or treatment situation.

AKA □power beds.

Related devices □**Birthing beds (89)**.

Where found □general patient wards.

Electronic Probe Thermometers

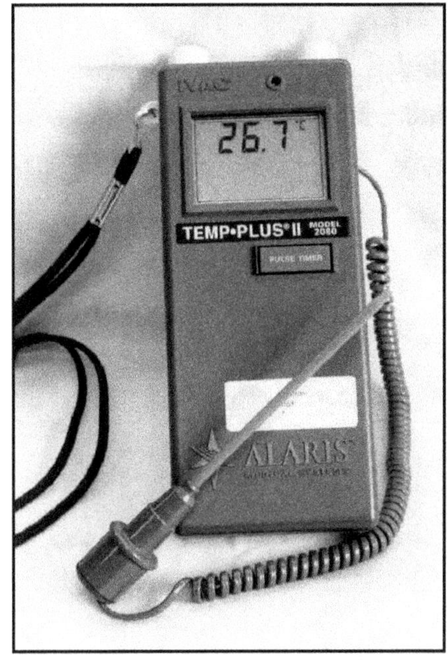

Overview □ Body temperature is a critical vital sign.

Function □ Probe thermometers use a tiny electronic device to measure the temperature of the body part to which they are applied. The temperature is then displayed on a digital read□out, which may be on a small, hand□held box or on the screen of a larger, multi□function monitor. Hand□held units usually have the sensor on the end of a thin rod, which can be placed under the tongue, under the arm, or rectally. To ensure patient safety, there are separate, color□coded probes for oral and rectal use, and the probes are covered with a smooth, tough disposable cover which is changed for each patient. Often, there is a timer in the hand□held part which beeps when the temperature reading has had time to stabilize, or the unit can be set to continuously measure the patient's temperature. For longer□term monitoring, sensors on a small, flexible wire are available; these can be placed on the patient and not interfere too much with movement.

Units usually have a switch to select between Celsius (Centigrade) and Fahrenheit degrees.

Probe thermometers are often built in to **physiological monitors (314), infant resuscitators (105) and infant incubators (100).**

Application □ A clean cover is placed on the probe, and it is applied to the patient. After an appropriate time, the temperature reading is recorded, the probe is removed, and the cover discarded.

AKA □ electronic thermometers, digital thermometers, probe thermometers.

Related devices □ **tympanic thermometers (332), physiological monitors (314).**

Where found □most patient care areas of the hospital, but because most ICU and OR multifunction monitors have built□in thermometers, they may not be used in these areas.

Examination Lamps

Overview In evaluating the condition of a patient, it is important to be able to see clearly.

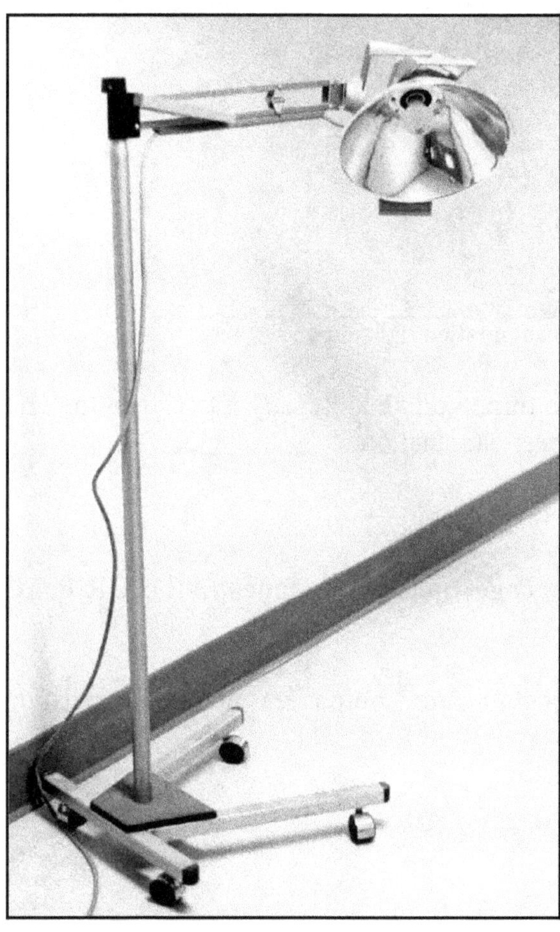

Function Proper observation requires a light source that can easily be placed in a variety of positions, and which provides bright illumination, with no coloration that might obscure clinically significant details such as tissue color. Since the examination lamp may be used for extended periods, it shouldn't give off excessive amounts of heat. They may be ceiling or wall mounted, or on a moveable stand. Most are line powered, though some smaller units have batteries. Some have intensity adjustments.

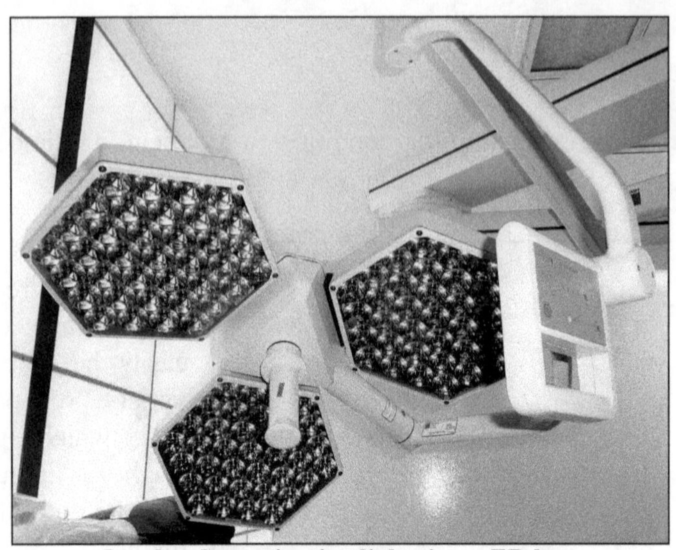

Overhead examination lights in an ER bay.

Application The light is turned on and intensity is set, then the unit is positioned to give the best illumination.

AKA lamps, lights.

Related devices **oto–laryngo–ophthalmoscopes (301)**, **OR lights (64)**.

Where found emergency rooms, outpatient areas, examination rooms.

Feeding Pumps

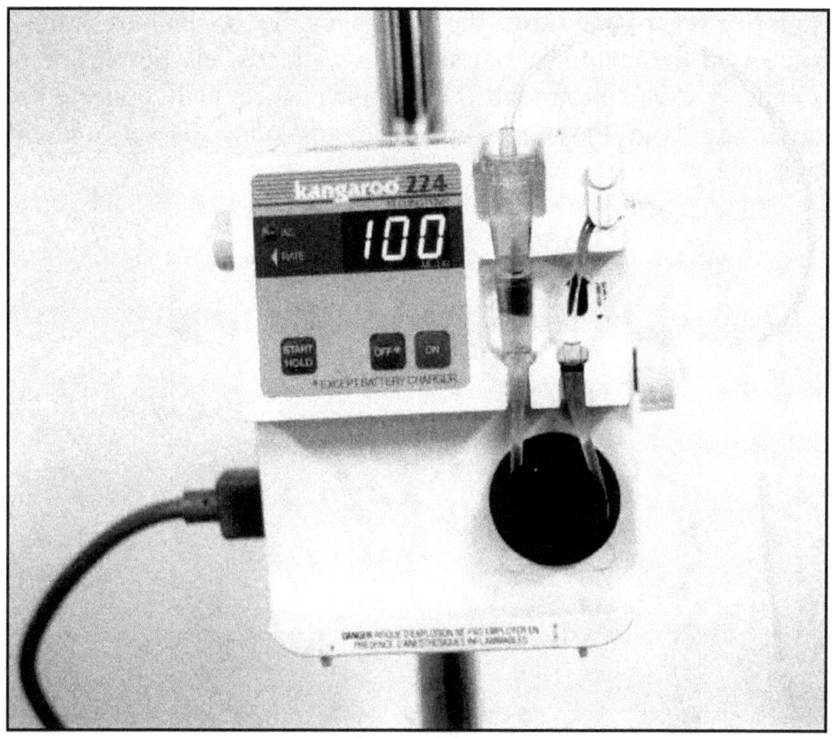

Overview — For a variety of reasons, a patient may not be able to swallow food adequately. In such cases, food must be administered through a tube inserted into the stomach. Obviously, the food has to be liquid, and as such liquids are generally quite thick, they may not flow easily enough to pass through the tube by gravity alone.

Function — Feeding pumps provide pressure to make the liquid food flow through the feeding tube and into the patient's stomach. The most common mechanism for these pumps is a wheel, around part of which an elastic section of tubing is stretched. Cylindrical roller bearings at intervals around the wheel compress the tubing as the wheel rotates, squeezing the fluid in the tube in a peristaltic wave. This pushes the liquid food through that section of tubing and toward the patient, while at the same time drawing more food from a reservoir. Pumps generally have controls that allow flow rate and desired volume to be set, and have some method of signalling when the set volume is reached. They often have a means of detecting blockages, and alarms for when this occurs.

Application □ Use of feeding pumps is relatively straightforward. Once the feeding tube is inserted into the patient□s stomach (usually through one nostril and down the esophagus, but sometimes through an incision in the abdomen and stomach wall), the elastic portion of the tubing is stretched around the pumping wheel and connected to the food reservoir. Flow rate and required volume is set, and the pump is started.

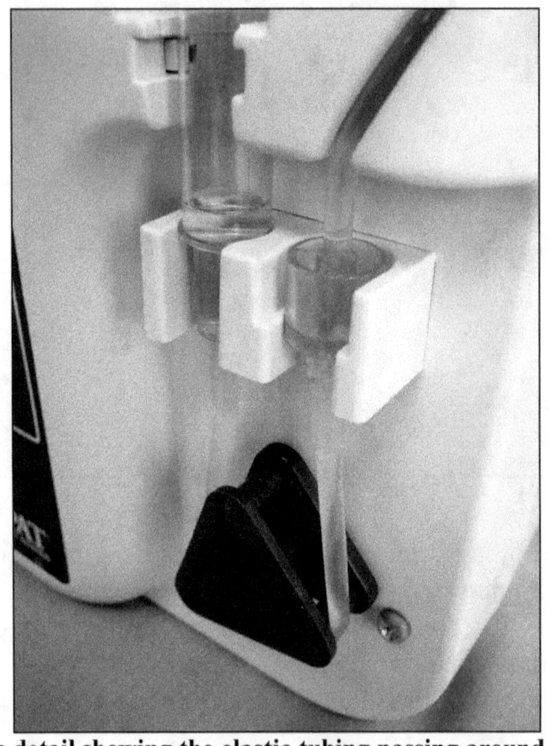

Feeding pump detail showing the elastic tubing passing around the triangular pump head..

AKA □ enteral feeding pumps, Kangaroo pumps (after one large manufacturer□s model name).

Related devices □**Intravenous pumps (289)**.

Where found □ most areas of the hospital, extended or continuing care units.

Gas Regulators

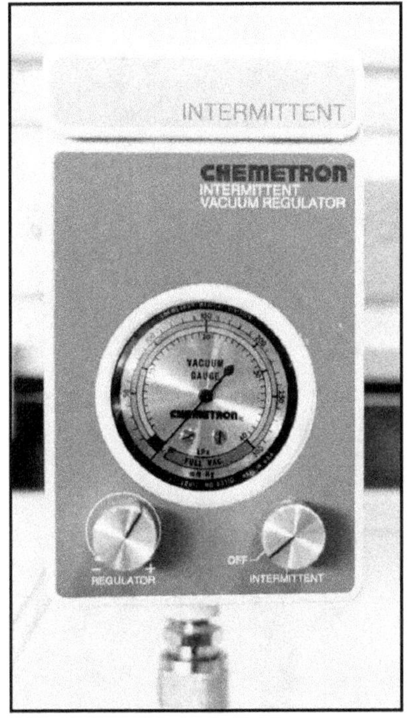

Overview □ A variety of gases are used in routine patient care, particularly air (both supplied as compressed air and removed as vacuum) and oxygen. Some areas also might have nitrous oxide available.

In all cases, the gases are supplied by a source with a certain, relatively□high pressure. The source may be local, such as a smaller pressurized cylinder or portable suction pump, or remote, from much larger pressurized tanks or a central vacuum pump.

This pressure is usually too great to apply directly to patients, so some kind of gas regulator must be used.

Function □ Gas regulators are usually mechanical units that employ bellows and/or needle valves to control pressure and flow, and usually they have indicators for both of these parameters. The indicators may be dial gauges or digital displays. For flow readings, a small ball may be used in a tapered, marked tube; the gas flows up the tube and the ball rises to a height proportional to the flow rate. Units have controls (usually knobs) to control the flow and/or pressure, and may have alarms to indicate high or low pressures.

Gas regulators may be built in to other devices, such as infant incubators and resuscitators, anesthetic machines, insufflators and ventilators.

Application □ Units are used to adjust the flow rate and pressure required for the specific situation.

AKA □ Oxygen or O2 regulators/gauges/meters, air regulators/gauges/meters, vacuum regulators/gauges/meters, suction regulators/gauges/meters, flow regulators/gauges/meters, pressure regulators/gauges/meters.

Related devices □**oxygen analyzers (287)**, **aspirators (250)**.

Where found □all patient care areas.

Glucometers

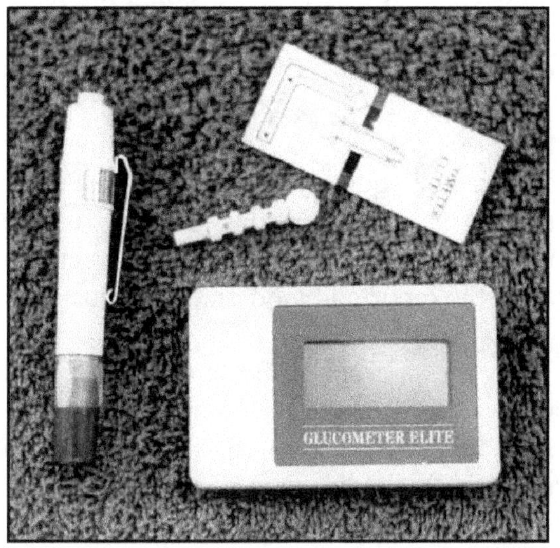

Overview □ For patients with diabetes, and sometimes in other situations, it is important to be able to determine blood glucose levels.

Function □ Devices for measuring blood glucose are small, reliable, accurate, and simple enough to be used by patients themselves, though of course medical caregivers use them as well. The devices rely on a chemical reaction in which glucose in the blood causes a color change on a small paper or plastic strip. A small drop of blood is applied to the strip, and, after a pre□set time (usually signalled by the testing device), the strip is inserted into a port in the unit. Electronic circuitry measures the color change of the strip and from this data, determines the blood glucose level and displays it on a screen.

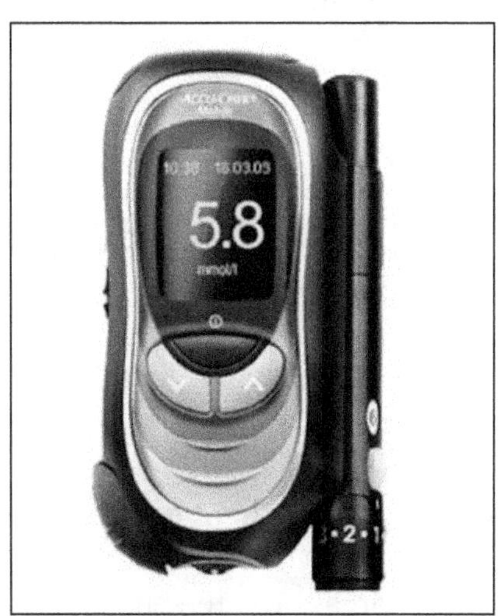

Glucometer.

Accu□Chek® products imagery courtesy of Roche Diagnostics Canada.

Because of the critical nature of this test, glucometers must be very accurate and stable. They have means by which the user compensates the unit to each batch of test strips, to account for slight variations from batch to batch. They also have calibration strips, which have precisely controlled colors, to check for proper operation.

Blood glucose levels can change quickly following meals or exercise, and measurements must be made with this in mind. Factors such as timing and type of food or drink taken and patient activity level must be noted, along with the reported blood glucose values.

Application □ The unit is prepared and calibrated, and then a small blood sample is taken, usually from a lancet prick on a finger. The blood drop is placed on a strip from the same batch as the calibration strip, and the unit timer started. When the time is up, the strip is placed in the measuring slot, and the blood glucose level is recorded.

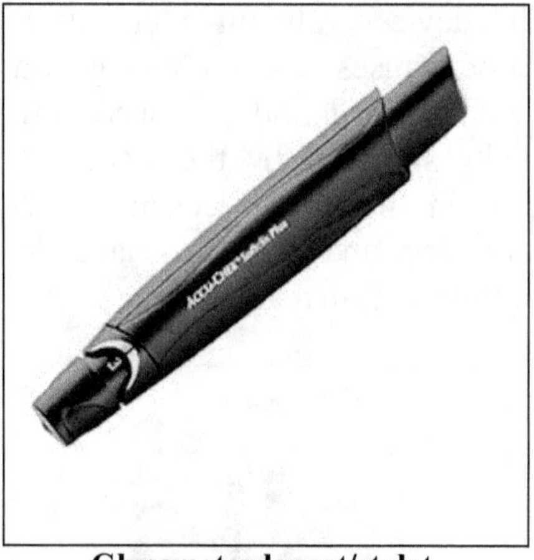

Glucometer lancet/stylet.

Accu□Chek® products imagery courtesy of Roche Diagnostics Canada.

AKA □ blood sugar analyzers.

Related devices □ **Point of care blood analysis systems (318)**.

Where found □ most areas of the hospital, outpatient clinics, patients□ homes.

Intravenous (IV) Pumps

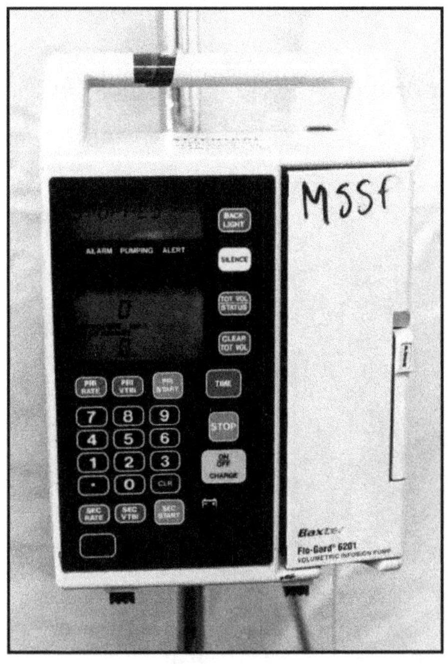

Overview □ Medications, blood, or fluid often must be delivered into a patient's bloodstream at an exact rate for a relatively long period of time. In the □old days□ caregivers had to measure how fast the liquid was dripping and calculate the rate, adjusting the flow often. The intravenous pump makes this much easier by pumping the fluid in a controlled and accurate manner.

Function □ There are several different techniques of pumping. One of the most common is "peristaltic," in which either a set of "fingers" or some rollers on a drum squeeze the fluid tubing, one after another, pushing a wave of fluid through the tube. Because the tubing is precisely manufactured, the speed at which the pump operates determines the flow rate of the fluid. The other common pumping method uses a cassette that fits into the pump and is compressed by a piston. The size of the pumping chamber in the cassette is very precise, and, by varying the frequency of compression, the flow rate can be controlled. This method is generally more accurate than the peristaltic method. With either method, an internal computer calculates and displays the flow rate, and also the total volume to be infused, how much has been infused, and how much is left.

Pumps have very accurate sensors which can detect air bubbles in the line and stop the pump, sounding an alarm before the bubbles can get past the pump and into the blood stream. They also can detect blockages, either before or after the pump.

Application □ After establishing an intravenous line, the tubing or cassette is carefully inserted into the pump. Infusion rate and total volume to be infused are set, and the pump is started. Some pumps can be programmed to pump at one rate for a set time or volume, and then change to another rate. For example, when two different doses of different medications are being given at once, the smaller dose is pumped first, then the other.

Also, some pumps can control two or more different fluid lines at the same time.

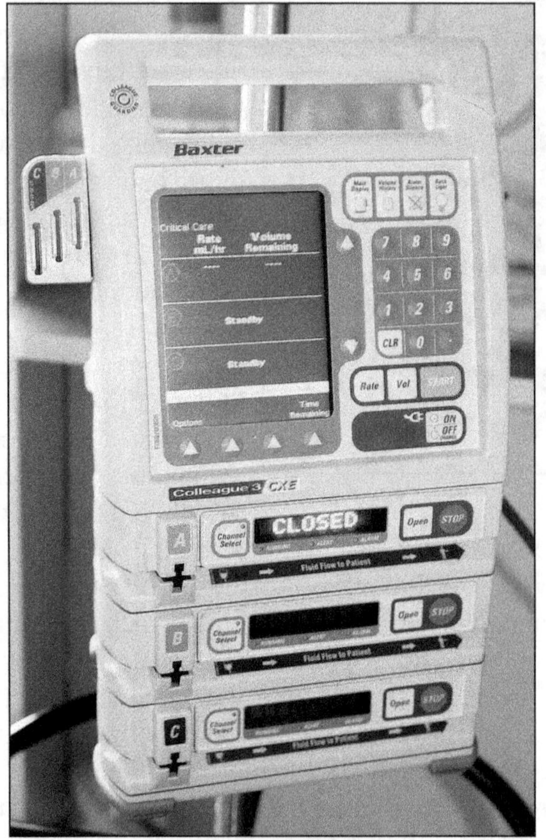

Three channel IV pump.

Most pumps have an internal battery that allows all functions to continue when the pump is unplugged from the AC wall outlet, allowing the patient to go the washroom or to be moved to other areas or even a different hospital without interrupting pumping.

When the pump has delivered the programmed volume, an alarm sounds and a visual indicator is displayed. The alarm function may be interfaced with a nurse call system to alert personnel who may not be in the immediate vicinity. Usually, the pump continues to deliver a very small amount of fluid in order to prevent blood from clotting over the tip of the intravenous needle or catheter; this is referred to as a □keep vein open□or KVO mode, and is usually accompanied by an intermittent tone.

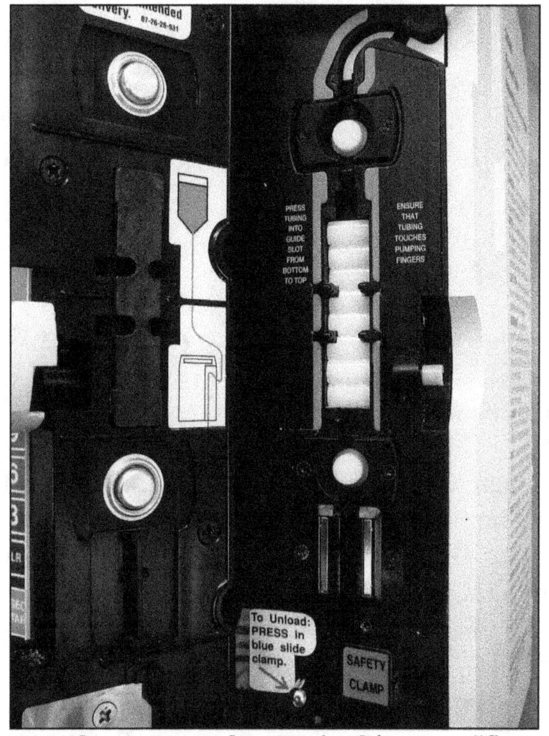

IV pump door open to show peristaltic pump "fingers."

Because tubing or cassettes may wear and/or become deformed with continued use, possibly affecting flow accuracy, they must be replaced regularly, in accordance with manufacturers recommendations.

AKA □ IV pumps, IVACs (after one of the first manufacturers of such pumps), infusion pumps.

Related devices □ **patient–controlled analgesia pumps (311), syringe pumps (329), feeding pumps (283).**

Where found □most areas of the hospital.

Intubation Assist Devices

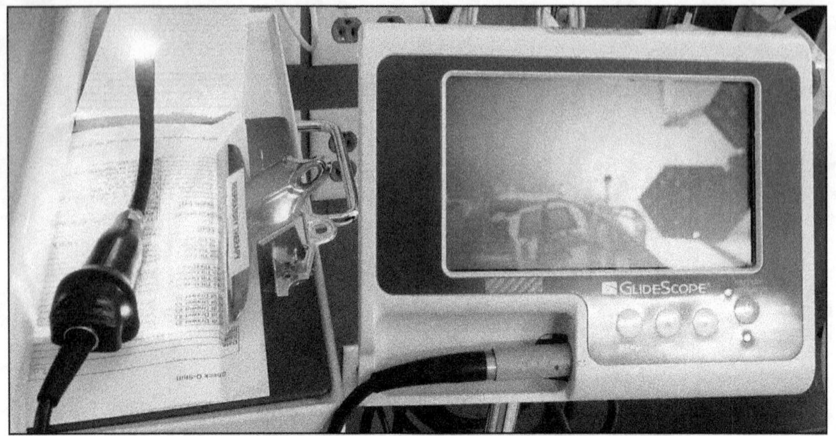

Note the laryngoscope part on the left with LED illumination, and the image from the scope displayed on the screen.

Overview □When it is necessary to put an endotracheal tube in place (such as for ventilation or general anesthesia), it is sometimes difficult to guide the tip into the trachea; incorrect placement can result in compromised breathing, brain impairment and even death if not corrected in time.

Function □ The intubation assist device is essentially an electronic **laryngoscope (301)**, and consists of a smooth, curved blade that is used to press the tongue out of the way and allow better access to the trachea, a fiber optic channel embedded in the blade to provide both light and imaging, a light source and a small color video screen to display images.

Application □ The blade is inserted into the patient□s mouth and positioned to depress the tongue and provide access to the trachea, which is readily visible on the video screen. The tip of the endotracheal tube is then passed through the mouth and to the tracheal opening, where it can be safely guided into the trachea while being observed on the video screen. Once the tube is successfully placed, the blade is withdrawn.

AKA □(none).

Related devices □**ventilators (334)**, **anesthetic machines (47)**, **laryngoscopes (301)**.

Where found □ intensive care units, emergency departments, operating rooms.

Invasive Pressure Monitors

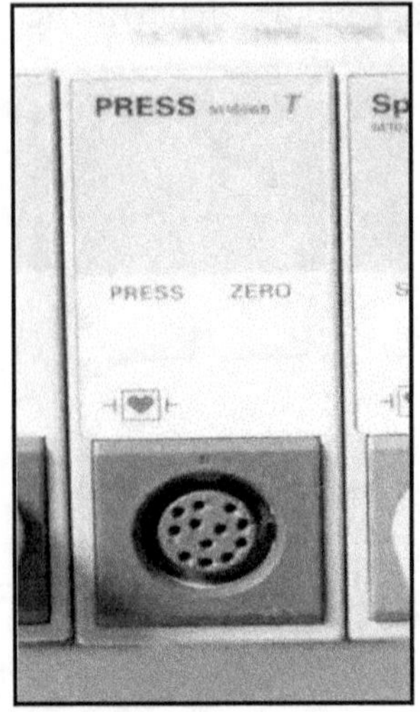

Overview □ It is often important to know pressure values within the patient□s body. This is most commonly the pressure in limb arteries, but can also include blood pressures in the venous system, at various points of the arterial system close to the heart, or cerebrospinal fluid pressures in the skull or spinal column. Blood pressures are pulsatile, and the maximum (systolic), minimum (diastolic), and mean pressure values are also important.

Blood pressure can be measured at the limbs non□invasively by **NIBPs (296),** but this method is susceptible to errors, it is not continuous, and it cannot give values for anything but limb arterial pressure.

Function □ By introducing a catheter with an electronic pressure transducer at its tip, exact measurements of pressure can be made continuously, at whatever point the catheter is positioned. Transducers are small and can be guided from a convenient insertion point to various locations within the circulatory system, either by simply watching the pressure values and knowing the typical measurements from various locations, or by viewing the catheter and vessels with x□rays.

Because of the continuous nature of these pressure measurements, a waveform of the values can be displayed on an associated monitor; the shape of the wave signal can be significant as well as the various pressure values. Systolic, diastolic, and mean values can be displayed; many monitors also record measurements over time so they can be displayed in tabular or graphic form. High and low alarm levels can be set, sometimes for systolic, diastolic, and mean values independently.

Pressure transducers are sensitive and must be calibrated prior to each use; they must also be □zeroed□ regularly by exposing them to atmospheric pressure in order to compensate for slight variations.

Invasive blood pressure monitors are almost always a module or component of a **physiological monitoring system (314).**

Application □ A catheter with pressure transducer is established in the vessel or chamber to be monitored. The system is zeroed and calibrated as necessary, and measurements begun.

AKA □pressure monitors, BP monitors.

Related devices □ **physiological monitors (314)**, **NIBPs (296)**, **cardiac catheterization units (169)**.

Where found □ critical care areas, operating and post□op recovery rooms, some special units (e.g., cath labs).

Non-invasive Blood Pressure (NIBP or NBP) Monitors

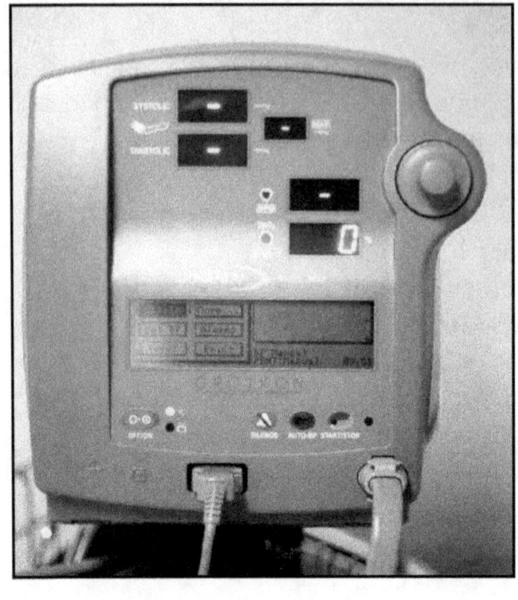

Overview — A patient's blood pressure is a vital measurement for diagnosis. When absolute accuracy is needed, and/or monitoring will be over an extended period, and/or when continuous, instantaneous measurements are required, a catheter is inserted into the patient's blood vessels, and pressure is measured directly by an attached transducer. This invasive technique is often not desirable, however, and is generally impractical to take blood pressure readings manually at frequent intervals over an extended period of time.

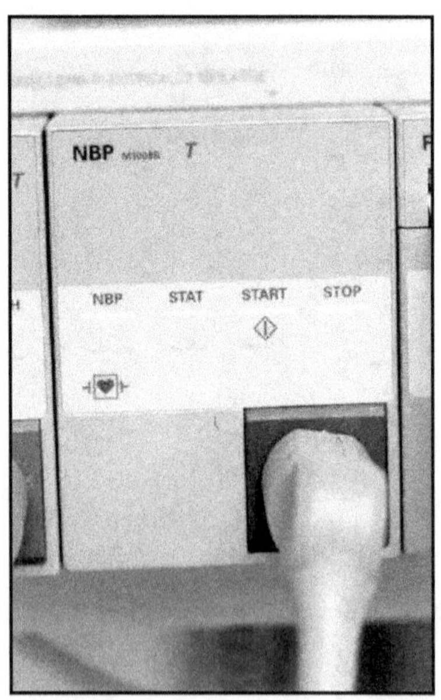

Function — Non-invasive blood pressure monitors (NIBPs) allow blood pressure measurements to be made automatically.

Most NIBP systems use a technique similar to that of manual blood pressure measurement. An inflatable cuff is placed over the patient's limb (usually the arm but sometimes the thigh). The cuff is inflated until arterial blood flow is occluded and then pressure is slowly released while monitoring the return of partial and then complete blood flow. The cuff pressure at which partial flow commences is equivalent to the systolic blood pressure, while the point at which complete flow is restored is equivalent to the diastolic pressure.

Two basic types of NIBPs are in common use. In one, a microphone placed near the patient's artery, usually under the inflatable cuff, determines the presence or absence of blood flow. Associated electronic circuitry processes the sound signals and analyzes the resulting waveforms to determine the systolic and diastolic points.

The second type of NIBP measures small variations in air pressure within the cuff caused by blood pulsing within the patient's arm. The pattern of these variations is used to determine blood pressure measurements.

In both systems, readings may be initiated by the operator, or may occur at regular intervals, the timing of which is determined by the operator. There is some kind of display for results; systolic and diastolic values may be displayed alternately in a single window, or they may each have separate displays. Mean pressure may be calculated and displayed as well.

Some systems have a "stat" button, which causes the machine to take several measurements in quick succession. Many also have programmable alarm limits to notify staff when pressures are too high or too low. Another common feature is a recorder module, which allows printouts of results, along with the time they were taken, and sometimes a graph of pressure trends over time.

A new technology uses motion of the blood vessel wall to determine pressures, and will allow continuous, instantaneous blood pressure measurements, without requiring the insertion of a catheter.

NIBPs may be stand-alone, they may be built into devices that also measure ECG and/or SpO2, or they may be modules in a general physiological monitoring system.

Application – An appropriately-sized cuff is selected and applied to the patient's limb. Measurement interval is selected, and the unit is started. A blood pressure measurement is taken and the values are displayed. Measurements are repeated automatically at the selected intervals.

Cuff size and placement are important for accurate readings.

Note that, because of the nature of the measurement process, values obtained by NIBP units may be different than those from manual or invasive measurement. Pressure values do not necessarily correspond exactly to absolute values within the blood vessels; however, they are accurate enough for most purposes and give a very good indication of trends in measurements over time.

AKA BP machines, Dinamaps (after one of the common early models), NBPs.

Related devices **physiological monitors (314)**, **invasive pressure units (294)**, **sphygmomanometers (325)**.

Where found most areas of the hospital.

Ophthalmic Lasers

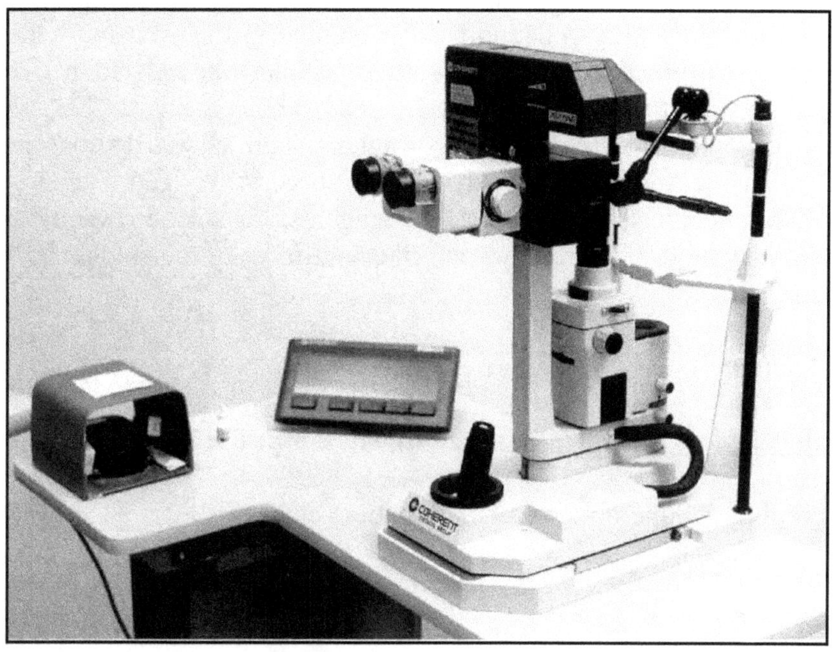

Overview □ Various ophthalmic conditions such as astigmatism and myopia cause difficulties for the patient and must be resolved if possible. Corrective lenses provide adequate focusing improvement in most situations, but they may be unsuitable for some patients either for aesthetic reasons or for physical limitations or specific job requirements. Surgically reshaping either the cornea or the whole eye may produce satisfactory results.

Function □ Ophthalmic lasers allow surgeons to reshape the cornea to correct focusing problems. Specifically□selected light wavelengths, power levels, and application methods allow the cornea to be reshaped without incision, resulting in greatly shortened procedures and healing times. Precise control of the laser□s action is vital to produce optically accurate curvatures and surface.

Application □ The patient is positioned with chin and forehead resting on supports, to help maintain a precise position during treatment. The ophthalmologist views the target structures on the eye with the microscope portion of a slit lamp. After setting power and duration parameters, and aiming using a targeting beam, the

treatment beam is triggered. Results are examined, and treatment continues until the final goal is attained.
Because laser beams may cause damage to the retina, either through direct exposure or by reflection, all personnel in the area must use proper eye protection, and adequate signs must be posted in the vicinity to warn that lasers are in use.
There is some concern that disease agents such as viruses may be present in the smoke produced by laser surgery. To guard against possible infections caused by these agents, a smoke evacuator system may be used to remove and filter out most of the smoke from the surgical site.

AKA (none).

Related devices **surgical lasers (70), slit lamps (322)**.

Where found operating rooms, outpatient clinics

Oto/Laryngo/Ophthalmoscopes

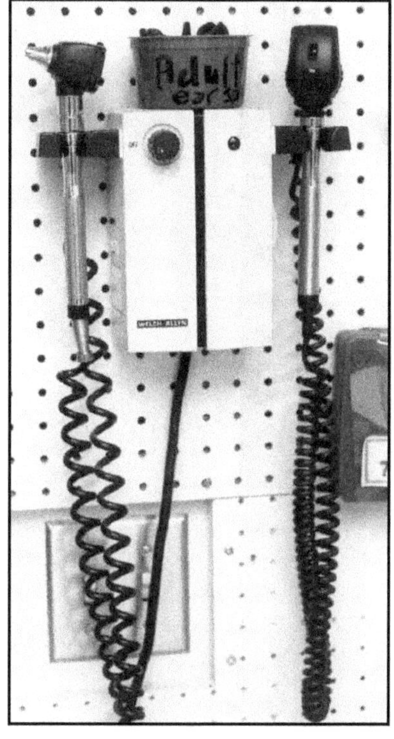

Overview □ The ear (oto), throat (laryngo), and eye (ophthalmo) are body parts that often require close examination. To do so effectively, equipment must provide bright, adjustable lighting that can illuminate the subject while allowing a clear view.

Function □ Otoscopes typically have a tapered tube that can be inserted into the ear canal, with a magnifying lens (sometimes interchangeable for various magnifications) over the large end. Light is supplied by a small bulb in a handle that is either battery□ or AC□powered. The light in most otoscopes is channelled from the bulb into the ear by a set of optical fibers embedded within the viewing tube, so that the light emerges in a ring around the end of the tube, thus providing light without interfering with viewing.

Some otoscopes use a simpler arrangement, with a bulb shining directly down the tube and blocked from view by a shield. This shield, of course, obstructs the field of view somewhat. Disposable covers are usually used to help prevent the spread of infection from one patient to another.

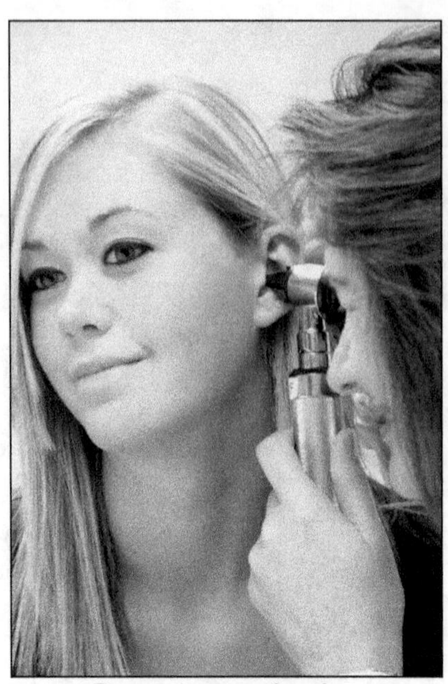

Otoscope examination.
Modified from Inmagine Corp, www.123rf.com, with permission.

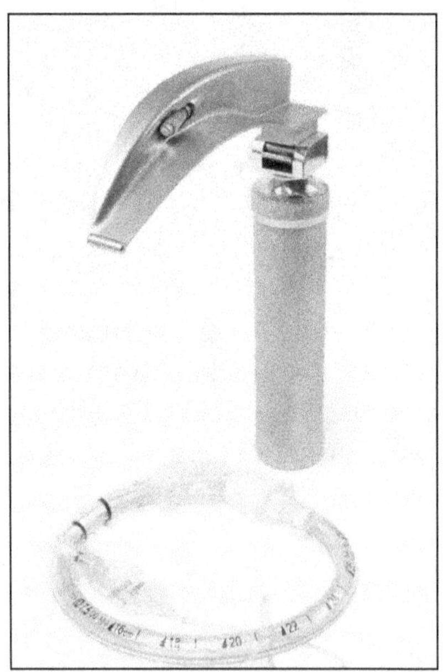

Laryngoscope and endotracheal tube.
Modified from Shutterstock, Inc, www.shutterstock.com, with permission.

Laryngoscopes need a means of holding the soft tissue in the patient's mouth (mainly the tongue) out of the way for viewing other structures. They are usually equipped with a curved metal blade for this purpose. The blade has rounded edges and is made of metal so that it won't break if the patient inadvertently bites down. A bright light (either a bulb or the end of an illuminated fiber optic channel) is placed at the base of the blade to illuminate the area being viewed. Laryngoscope blades must be sterilized between patients.

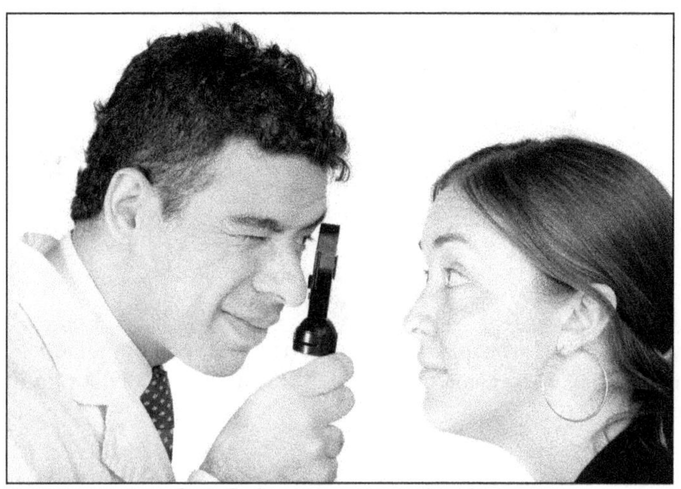

Ophthalmoscope examination.
Modified from Inmagine Corp, www.123rf.com, with permission.

Ophthalmoscopes have a bright light source as well, but since structures of concern in the eye are generally smaller than those in the ear or throat, ophthalmoscopes have lenses of various powers to aid in observations. Some eye conditions are visualized better with colored light, so filters are often available for the observation light. In addition, some situations require a narrow line of light to illuminate the eye, so mechanisms are provided to make such lines, usually of various widths.

OLO scopes can be powered with rechargeable or disposable batteries, or they may be connected to a power supply fed from a wall outlet. Since they are required for many emergency cases, the units in the ER are often wall mounted and line powered, so that dead batteries are not a problem.

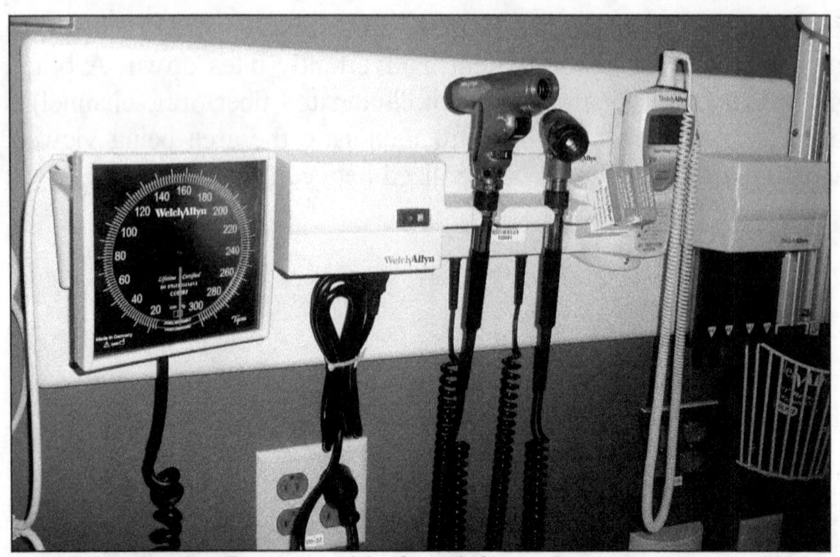

An ER bay headwall set–up, with (from left) a sphygmomanometer (325), an ophthalmo/otoscope, an electronic probe thermometer (279) and a dispenser for otoscope covers.

<u>Application</u> □Scopes are used to examine the body part in question.

<u>AKA</u> □ear/throat/eye scopes.

<u>Related devices</u> □**slit lamps (322), intubation assist devices (292)**.

<u>Where found</u> □most areas of the hospital

Oxygen Analyzers

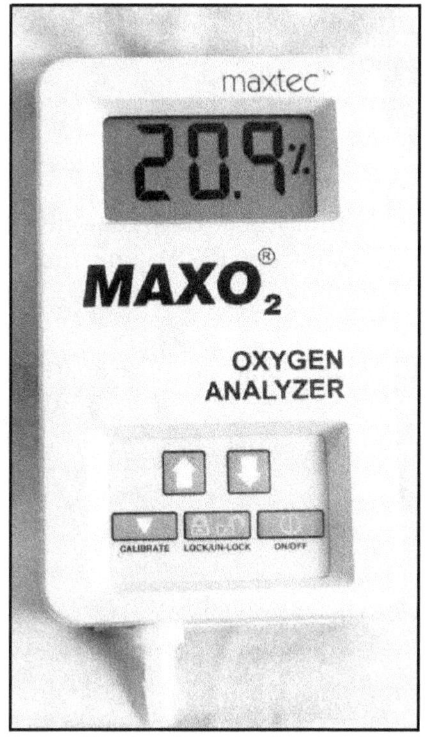

Overview □ Whenever the needs of the patient for oxygen (O2) are different than normal, it is necessary to determine the percentage of oxygen being delivered. This is particularly true for premature infants, as both too much and too little oxygen can be detrimental.

Function □ Oxygen analyzers measure and display O2 levels. They may have alarms that can be set for both high and low levels, and, as they are often battery powered, there is usually a low battery indicator.

Most oxygen analyzers work by directing a small amount of the gas being delivered to a patient onto a cell. This cell uses the oxygen present in a chemical reaction that varies with O2 concentration; the reaction produces a voltage, which can then be processed and measured to determine the specific O2 percentage.

Because the chemical reaction varies with factors such as temperature and the age of the cell, the system must be calibrated frequently to ensure correct readings. Calibration consists of exposing the cell to 100% oxygen and adjusting the display to match, and then returning the cell to room air, which is very consistently 21% oxygen. If the display shows 21% after settling, the system is ready for use; if not, it must be recalibrated, and if correct calibration is not possible, the cell must be replaced.

Oxygen enters the cell through a thin membrane, which must be clean and undamaged for proper functioning.

Since the absorption of oxygen by the patient can be affected by many variables, it is often valuable to monitor blood oxygen levels (SpO2) while oxygen is being administered.

Application The unit is calibrated, and the sensor is placed in a location where it is exposed to the air to be monitored.

AKA O2 analyzers, O2/oxygen monitors.

Related devices **oxygen concentrators (307), gas flow regulators (285), infant incubators (100), SpO2 monitors (320), anesthetic machines (47).**

Where found nurseries, pediatric wards, intensive care areas, operating rooms.

Oxygen Concentrators

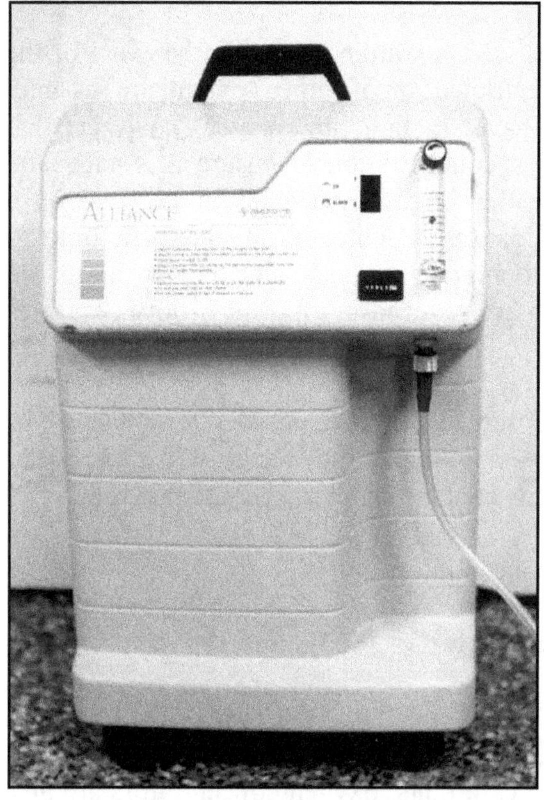

Overview □ Some patients may be located in areas where there is no wall outlet to supply oxygen.

Function □ In certain situations, an oxygen concentrator must be used. These devices utilize the fact that special resin bead materials absorb nitrogen; since nitrogen composes about 79% of air, and oxygen almost all of the remaining 21%, if the nitrogen can be removed, almost pure oxygen will remain.

Obviously, no material can absorb an infinite amount of anything, so oxygen concentrators use two sets of resin beads, placed in canisters called sieve beds. A system of valves, hoses, and pumps causes room air to flow through one sieve bed, which removes the nitrogen. The resulting oxygen is then delivered to the patient, at a rate set by the caregiver. When the first sieve bed is near to maximum capacity, flow is switched to the second sieve bed. Then air is flushed in a reverse direction through the first sieve bed, which removes the built□up nitrogen and vents it harmlessly back into the atmosphere. When the second bed is full, the system switches back to the first bed and the process starts again while the second bed is back□flushed. A small pressure tank near the outlet of the system maintains constant flow to the patient during switchovers.

Because these units operate for long periods of time and are providing vital oxygen, they must be very reliable. They will typically operate for several thousand hours before requiring service.

Another design consideration, since they are used at the patient□s bedside 24 hours a day, is that they are quiet, and considerable effort is put into silencing the mechanisms as much as possible.

Oxygen concentrators must have a warning alarm in the event of the flow of gas becoming restricted or if other potentially harmful conditions arise. Some have a built□in oxygen analyzer that measures the output oxygen concentration to ensure it is adequate, though most units require that an external analyzer be used on a scheduled basis to test for this. Generally, if the flow rate is maintained, the system is operating properly and oxygen levels are adequate. If the sieve beds are reduced in efficiency, flow decreases and the flow alarm sounds.

Application □ The unit is turned on, and, after a few cycles, the oxygen flow rate is adjusted to meet the needs of the particular patient. The line is then connected to the delivery system in use.

AKA □oxygen units, O2 concentrators.

Related devices □ **oxygen analyzers (305)**, **gas regulators (285)**, **pulse oximeters (320)**.

Where found □ some hospital areas where wall oxygen is not available, such as extended care units; oxygen concentrators are also often used in patient□s homes.

Patient Lifts

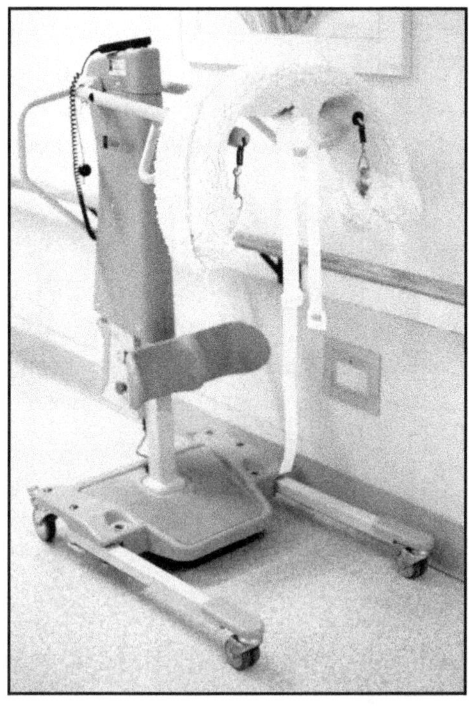

Overview □ Patients who are unable to move themselves must be lifted regularly, for treatments, baths, bedding changes, and transfers to wheelchairs, among other reasons. Caregivers who are involved with these movements must be careful to avoid injury to the patients or to themselves, especially if there are not enough people available to safely move the patients manually.

Function □ Patient lifts, as their name implies, are designed to help with such patient transfers.

Generally, lifts consist of a metal frame with an arm that can be extended over the patient, a sling or platform that can be slipped under the patient which is then attached to the overhead arm, a base that fits under the patient□s location to allow lifting without overbalancing, and some mechanism to raise the arm once the patient is secured. There are wheels to allow the lift to move around, and locks on the wheels to keep it steady while the patient is being raised or lowered.

Some lifts have the ability to move the patient horizontally with respect to the base, but this must be limited to within the balance area of the base.

Lifting is accomplished by a manually□operated lever/jack mechanism or a battery□powered electric motor. With electric lifts, there must be provision to lower the patient manually should the motor or battery fail.

Lifts must be designed with adequate stability to prevent tipping, so the bases must be quite long and wide. Also, there should be some mechanism to prevent attempts to lift patients who are too heavy for the capacity of the lift, such as an alarm or a mechanical lock-out.

Some lifts incorporate a scale in their design, so that staff can keep track of the patient's weight.

Application – The patient is maneuvered onto the sling or chair portion of the lift. Care must be taken not to twist or pinch the patient. The sling or chair connects to the lift arm, then the mechanism to lift the patient is activated. Once at the appropriate level, the patient is then moved to the desired location and lowered carefully.

AKA – lift chairs.

Related devices – **infant scales (108)**.

Where found – most areas of the hospital, especially extended care units and spinal cord injury units.

Patient□controlled Analgesia (PCA) Pumps

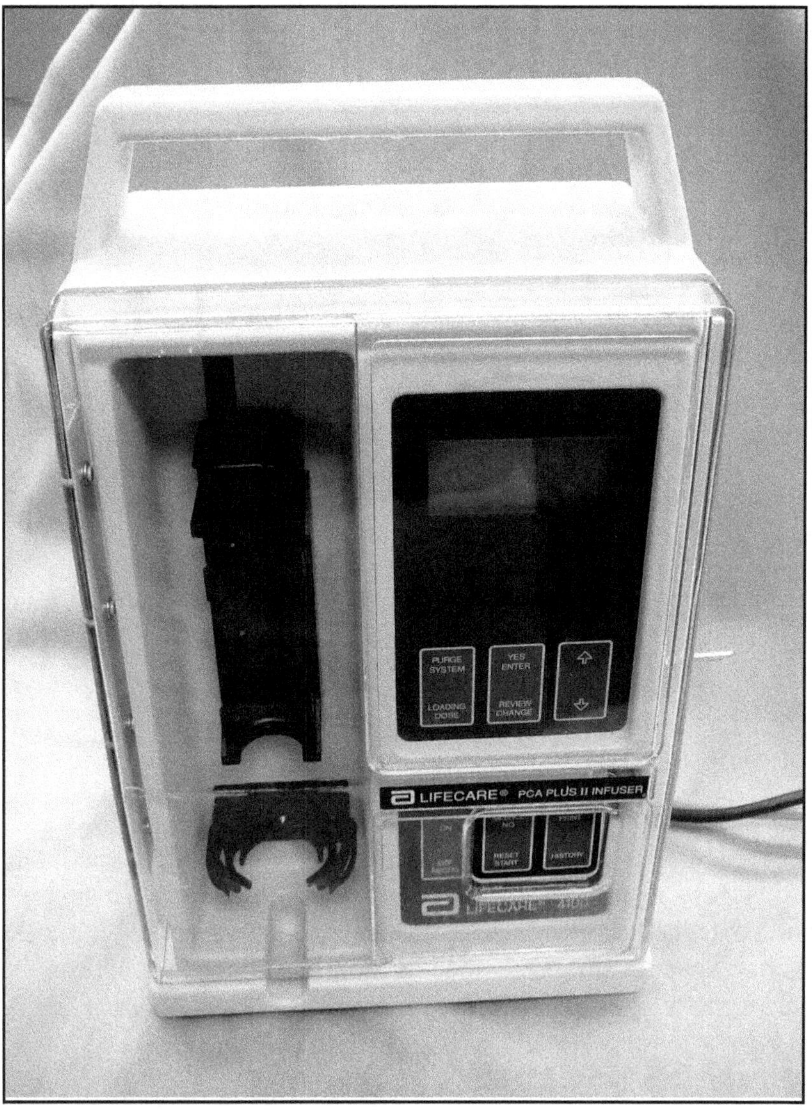

Overview □ When patients are experiencing ongoing pain, either from surgery, injury, or disease, intravenous analgesia requirements are variable and subjective. Giving the patient some control over when dosages are administered both allows them better control over their pain and allows nursing staff to attend to other duties.

Function □ A Patient□Controlled Analgesia Pump allows patients to control their own painkiller administration. To help prevent abuse of analgesic drugs, the solutions are usually packaged by the hospital pharmacy in sealed glass cartridges. These cartridges contain a piston and delivery port that is compressed by the pump mechanism to deliver the solution. This mechanism is precisely controlled to ensure accurate dose delivery.

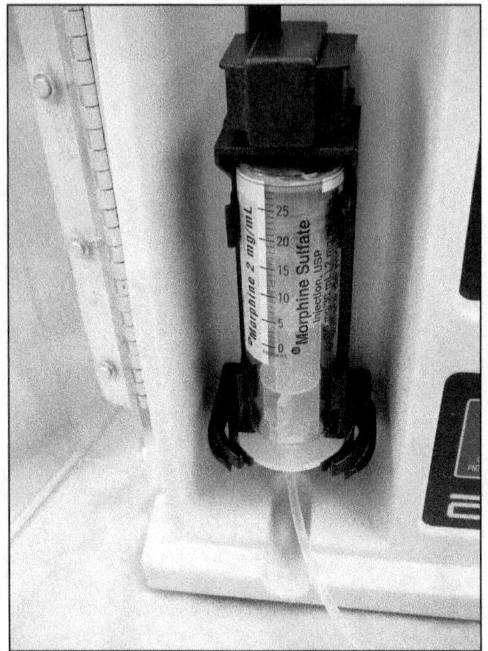

PCA pump drug cartridge.

Pumps can be programmed for continuous delivery rates, maximum total dosages, maximum patient□controlled dosage and maximum patient□controlled dose frequency. Most units have pre□programmed values for specific drugs at specific concentrations, which can be selected directly, thus avoiding some potential calculation errors.

Most controls are located behind a lockable panel.

<u>Application</u> □ An intravenous line is established, and staff sets the various parameters so that harmful dosages cannot be delivered. The control panel is then locked, and the patient is given a cable with a push□button on the end, which, when pressed, causes the pump to deliver the pre□set dosage of medication.

<u>AKA</u> □PCA pumps.

Related devices □**IV pumps (289), syringe pumps (329)**.

Where found □ post□operative recovery areas, palliative care units, burn units, other patient areas where pain management is necessary.

Physiological Monitors

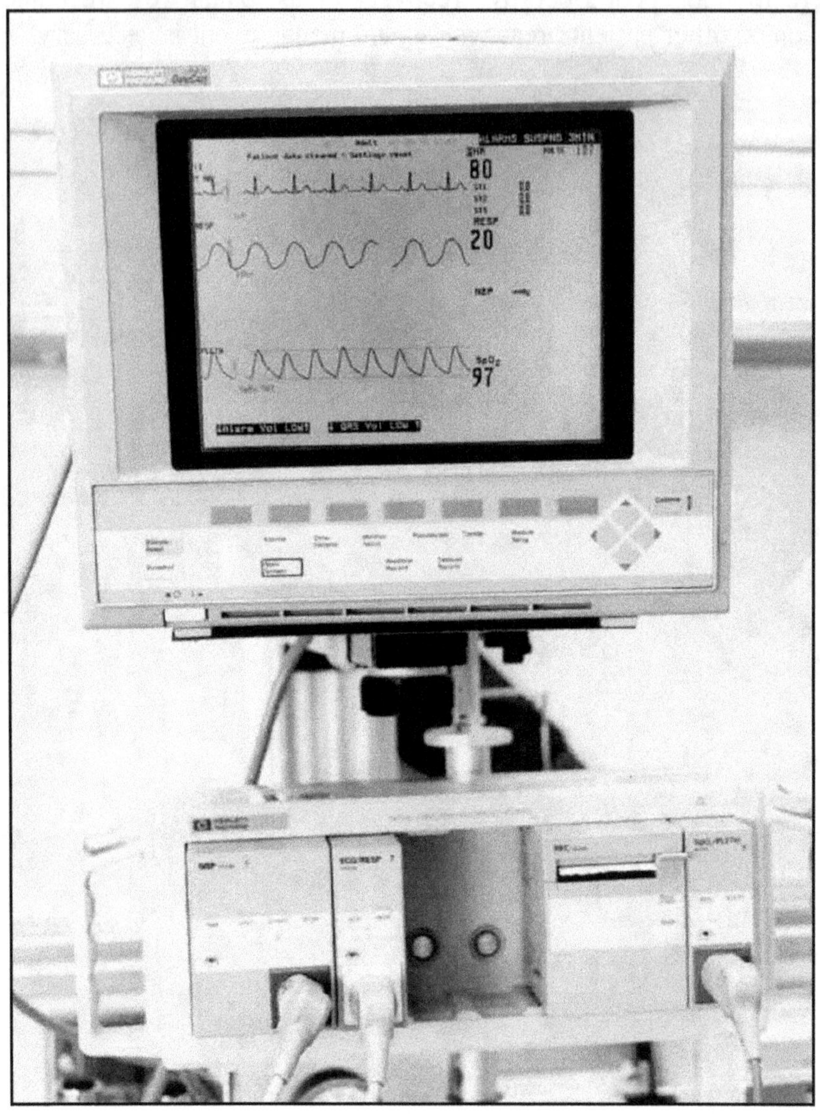

Overview □ Patients in serious condition must have their vital signs monitored continuously.

Function □ Physiological monitors bring a number of different critical measurements together, so that a comprehensive picture of the patient□s condition can be obtained. The number of parameters measured is different for various situations, and monitors are designed to meet these different needs.

There are two general formats of physiological monitors: configured, in which the unit is built with various measurement capabilities and cannot be changed; or modular, in which various modules that measure different parameters can be added or removed as needed. Configured monitors are typically more compact and less expensive; modular monitors are more flexible in terms of the types of measurements they can perform, and have the advantage that, if a particular module fails, it can simply be unplugged and exchanged with another in minutes.

Monitors can measure ECG, respiration, temperature, blood oxygen saturation (SpO2), blood pressure (either non-invasively or invasively), other pressures (such as intra-cranial or spinal), temperature, cardiac output, exhaled carbon dioxide levels (capnography), blood carbon dioxide saturation, and blood chemistry (POC blood analysis). In addition, monitors may be able to interface with other devices such as ventilators and nurse call systems. They may have a recorder module included, or they may connect to a central monitoring system and/or patient charting system.

The display portion of a monitor shows the results of the various measurements, either as a graph or as a numerical value, or both. Monitors can usually display a number of different parameters simultaneously, and can store values even when they aren't displayed.

Most parameters monitored can be set up so that an alarm sounds if the values go beyond certain pre-determined levels; these alarm levels are set to generic values when the monitor is turned on, but can be changed depending on individual circumstances. Alarms may be audible or visual or both, and they may be set to initiate a recording, signal a central monitoring station, or trigger a nurse-call system.

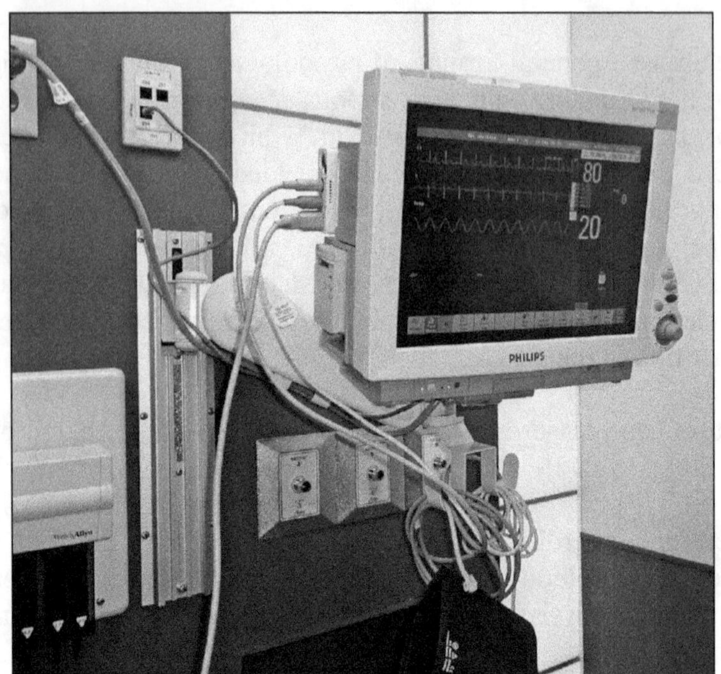

Wall mounted physiological monitor.

Monitors may record various measurements, which can later be called up as tables or graphs so that changes can be tracked more easily; some systems allow marking of specific events, such as physical activity or medication administration, so that these can be correlated to measurements. Tables and graphs may be available for print-out on a built-in recorder or on a larger-format printer at a central station.

Some monitors have a built-in battery so they can continue to function if there is a power failure or during patient transport.

<u>Application</u> – Monitor application is complex, and varies from one model and/or manufacturer to another. A user's manual and/or experienced operator must be consulted before setting up a monitor.

Generally, the various sensors to be used are applied to the patient, calibrations are performed as necessary, alarm levels and other situation-specific parameters are adjusted, and monitoring commences.

AKA □ ECG monitors, bedside monitors, monitors, multiparameter monitors, patient monitors, cardiac monitors.

Related devices □ **ECG recorders (270), SpO2 monitors (320), NIBP monitors (296), invasive pressure monitors (294), capnographs (254), defibrillators (259), central stations (29), probe thermometers (279), point of care blood analysis systems (318), level of consciousness monitors (276).**

Where found □ intensive care areas, emergency rooms, operating rooms, special treatment areas.

Point of Care (POC) Blood Analysis Systems

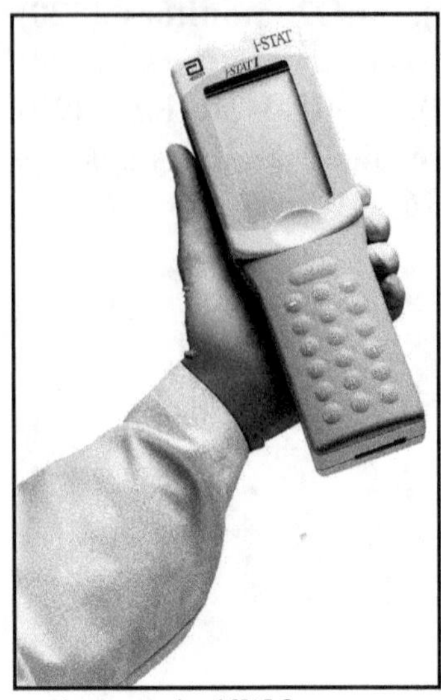
Image courtesy i-STAT Corp.

Overview □In order to provide the most timely and effective treatment of patients, caregivers need to be able to assess their condition as completely as possible. An important aspect of this assessment is the patient□s blood chemistry. Levels of blood gases (especially oxygen and carbon dioxide), electrolytes (sodium, calcium, potassium), and other components (urea, hemoglobin) can fluctuate rapidly in response to injury or disease processes or as a result of medications or other therapies, such as oxygen administration or temperature control. In the past, determination of blood chemistry involved calling a technologist to take a sample, having the blood drawn, sending to the laboratory, having the analysis performed, obtaining a list of measurements, and returning the list to the patient□s bedside.

While in many cases this is an adequate process, critical patients need to have blood chemistry results available more rapidly in order to ensure the most effective treatment.

For more information on blood chemistry, see Appendix D, p. 392.

Function □ Point of care analysis systems have been developed to meet the need for quick results. Generally, they take one of two forms: a stand□alone unit with its own display screen and printer; or a module that connects to a physiological monitor, in which case the monitor display and recorder are used.

The function of these systems depends on specially designed cartridges (specific to one or sometimes two or three blood components), into which a small blood sample is placed. Chemicals within the cartridge are applied to the sample, and the ensuing reactions produce an electrical signal, which can then be measured by the main unit; this signal correlates to the particular blood component being analyzed. The results are displayed on a screen and printed out; results may be tabulated for a printout or graphed so that changing values can be tracked.

A number of different cartridges must be kept on hand, in specific environmental conditions, and the systems must be carefully quality□controlled to ensure proper measurements. The range of measurements is somewhat less than can be obtained from a full laboratory analysis, but blood samples required are much smaller (a few drops that can be taken from a finger prick, as opposed to a syringe full from a blood vessel for lab testing) and results are available much more quickly, usually within a few minutes of the sample being taken. Also, if the blood analysis unit interfaces with the patient monitoring system, measurements can become part of the overall patient vital signs record, allowing a more complete view of their current and past condition.

Some new systems can analyze a more limited range of blood chemicals using a high□tech tip on an in□dwelling catheter, producing even faster measurements without the need to take blood samples at all.

Application □ The unit is calibrated, and then a cartridge is selected, depending on the values to be measured. A small blood sample is obtained, usually from a finger□prick, and is applied to the cartridge, which is inserted into the measuring port. After a pre□set time, the measured values are displayed.

AKA □ POC systems, blood analysis units, chemistry analyzers.

Related devices □ **physiological monitors (314)**, **SpO2 monitors (320)**, **ventilators (334)**, **capnographs (254)**, **blood glucose analyzers (287)**.

Where found □ intensive care units, emergency rooms, operating rooms.

Pulse Oximeters

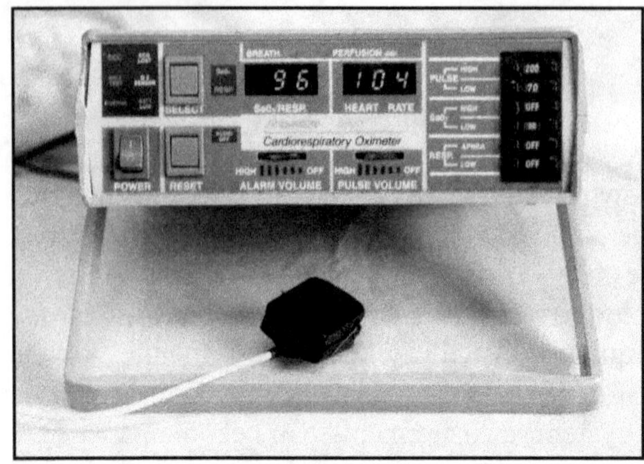

Overview □ Many disease conditions can reduce the amount of oxygen present in a patient□s blood. Physical effects of low oxygen levels may not been apparent until after the optimal time for intervention, therefore a means of measuring oxygen content (or oxygen saturation) of the blood is important.

Function □ A pulse oximeter measures the amount of oxygen in the patient's blood by sending both red and infrared light beams through tissue, and measuring how much of each is transmitted. Blood in the tissue transmits light differently depending on its oxygen saturation levels; by comparing the values for infrared and red light transmission, the unit can calculate oxygen percentage saturation.

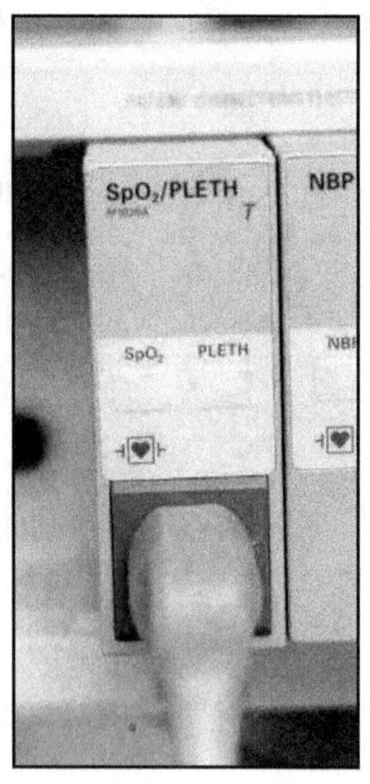

Most oximeters also give a read□out of pulse rate, in beats per minute. Some have a tone that sounds with each pulse beat, which may change in pitch depending on the oxygen concentration. Some may also have alarms for high and low oxygen levels and pulse rates; the alarm levels may be fixed or adjustable, though adjustable alarms are usually only used in more critical settings.

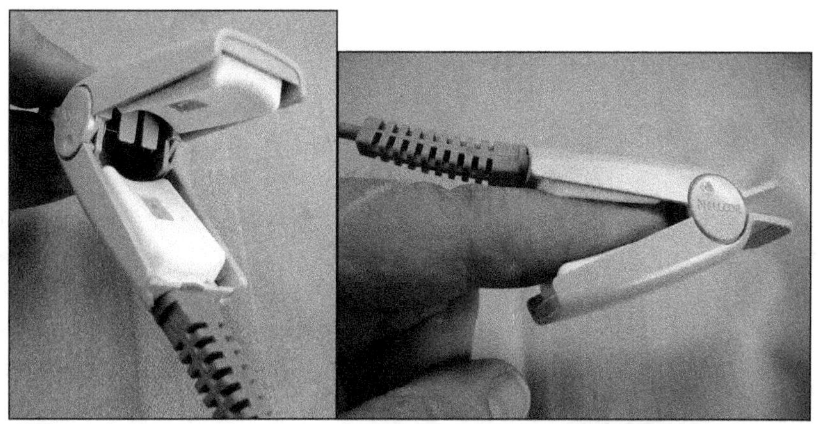

Pulse oximeter probes, open showing sensors and on a patient's finger.

<u>Application</u> □ A sensor, either wrap□around or clip□on, is placed on a small part of the body that has good blood flow, such as a finger, toe, or earlobe. The sensor has an emitter that produces the red and infrared signals, and a receiver that picks up what is left of each after they pass through the tissue. The unit then processes the measurements and gives a digital readout of the saturation value.
Pulse oximeters may be stand□alone, or integrated into units such as **physiological monitors (314), defibrillators (259), fetal monitors (95)** or **vital signs monitors (338).**

<u>AKA</u> □ O2 (oxygen) sat meter, sat meter, oximeter, pulse□ox, SpO2 meter, SaO2 meter.

<u>Related devices</u> □ **oxygen analyzers (305)**, **physiological monitors (314)**, **oxygen concentrators (307), vital signs monitors (338)**.

<u>Where found</u> □ most areas of the hospital.

Slit Lamps

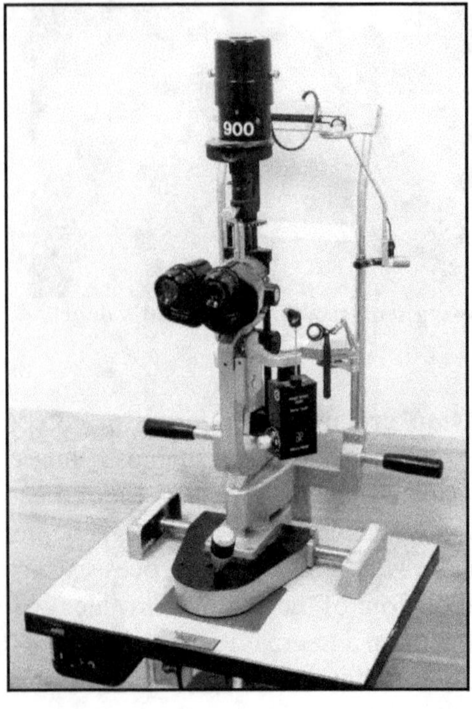

Overview □ The structure of the eye, both internal and external, must be clearly visible during certain examinations and surgical procedures. Since many of the structures involved are small, magnification is also important.

Function □ A slit lamp is a combination light source and microscope. The light source can be focused to give a very narrow line, or slit, of high□intensity light, which aids in defining the curvatures and surfaces of ocular structures. A binocular microscope gives the operator a three□dimensional view of the areas being examined.

A camera may be attached to the microscope so that photographs can be taken.

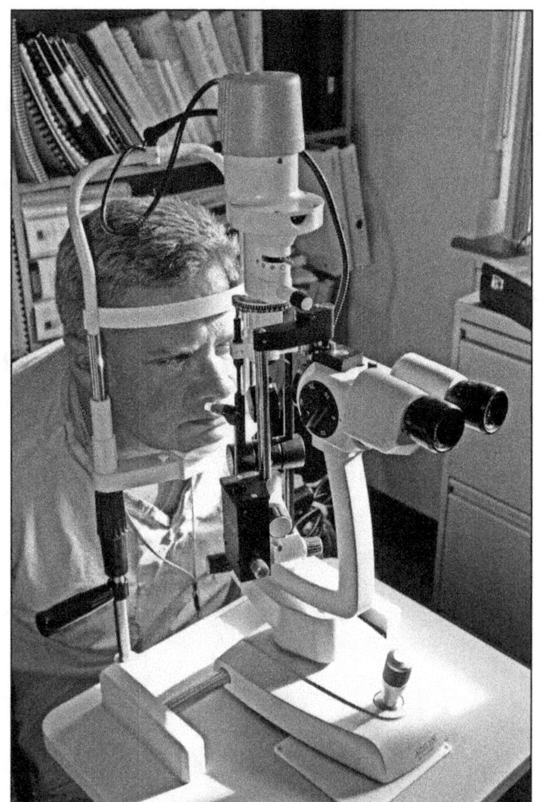

Slit lamp in use.

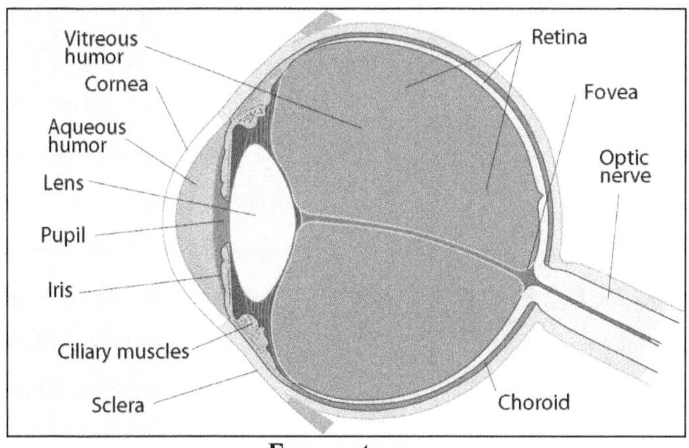

Eye anatomy.

Modified from Shutterstock, Inc, www.shutterstock.com, with permission.

Application Fluorescein dye stains the outer surface of the eye, causing the eye to fluoresce under certain lighting conditions. Dye is sometimes applied to the patient's eye prior to a slit lamp examination in order to highlight various features of the eye. The patient places the chin in a cup□shaped device and rests the forehead against another curved support; this helps to reduce any motions that may interfere with examination or treatment. The operator then adjusts the shape and intensity of the light beam, and proceeds with the examination or treatment, viewing the illuminated eye through the microscope.

AKA □(none).

Related devices □ **operating microscopes (68)**, **ophthalmic lasers (299)**.

Where found □ specialized clinics, outpatient departments, emergency rooms.

Sphygmomanometers

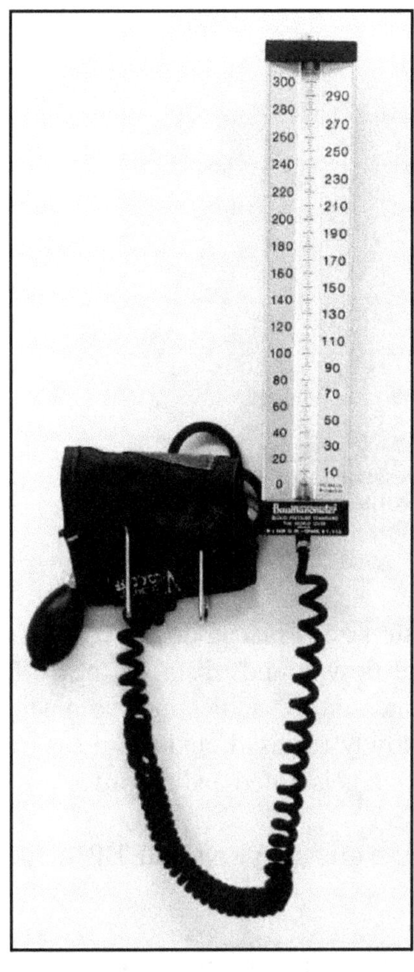

Overview □ Blood pressure is a critical vital sign.

Function □ An indication of blood pressure can be made using a sphygmomanometer, which consists of an inflatable cuff, a stethoscope, and a pressure gauge, or manometer. The cuff is placed around the patient's limb (usually the upper arm, but sometimes the thigh or other parts), and is normally held in place with attached Velcro strips. A rubber bulb is used to inflate the cuff while the practitioner listens to pulse sounds in an artery distal to the cuff. When not occluded, there is little noise from the artery. When the cuff pressure reaches diastolic pressure, a sound is produced by the alternate starting and stopping of blood flow. This continues until the cuff reaches systolic pressure, at which point the sound ceases again because there is no blood flow at all.

Pressure is indicated by either a graduated mercury column, a mechanical dial, or a simple electronic pressure indicator.

It is usually easier to determine the points where sounds start and stop when the cuff is being deflated by opening a valve, as the drop is smoother than the rise under pumping and there is no interference from the pumping itself.

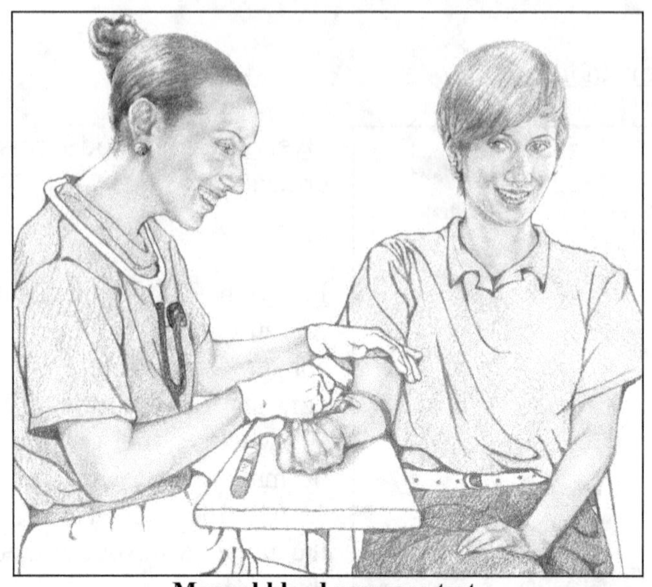

Manual blood pressure test.
Courtesy of the National Institute of Diabetes and Digestive and Kidney Diseases, National Institutes of Health.

Application □A cuff of the appropriate size is placed on the patient□s limb. The practitioner listens to blood flow sounds distal to the cuff, and the cuff is inflated until sounds stop, indicating complete occlusion of the artery. Pressure is slowly released, and the pressure at the beginning and ending of flow sounds is noted and recorded.

AKA □ BP cuff, BP unit, blood pressure units, manual BP units, pressure cuff.

Related devices □ **non–invasive blood pressure monitors (296)**, **invasive blood pressure monitors (294)**, **stethoscopes (327)**.

Where found □ most patient care areas of the hospital. Since many areas will have electronic blood pressure units, the manual ones might not be used much there, though they will usually be in place if needed.

Stethoscopes

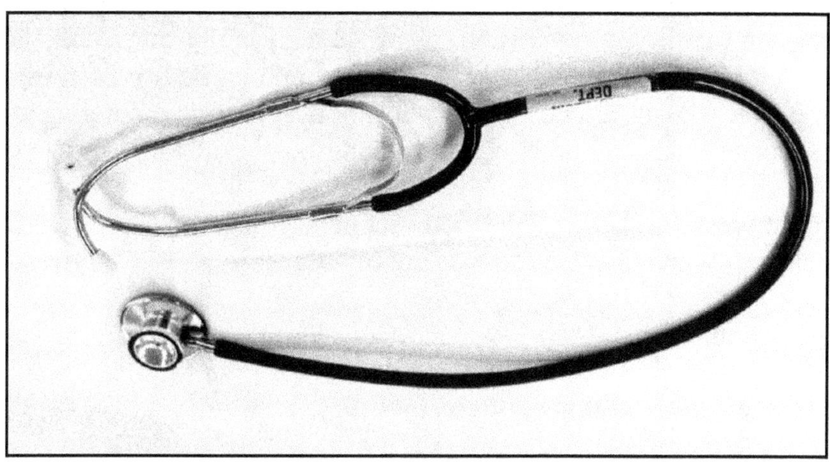

Overview – In many circumstances, sound is important in determining the state of a patient's health. Heart beat, lung condition, blood flow, gastrointestinal function, and fetal health, among others, are all parameters that produce sounds that can aid in diagnosis.

Function – The stethoscope is one of the oldest of medical devices, the earliest being simply a cone that magnified sounds and carried them to the physician's ear.

Most modern stethoscopes still operate on this principle, though refined and perfected. A cup- or bell-shaped part picks up sounds from within the body. The end of this part may be either open or covered with a diaphragm, which helps to transmit sounds in some circumstances. Some stethoscopes have two different-sized cups for different situations. The sounds are then carried by hollow tubes, divided by a Y, and carried to each ear. Some units have disposable earpieces, especially if more than one person regularly uses them.

Electronics technology has allowed the stethoscope to become more sensitive and precise, though, of course, an electronic version will be more expensive (and usually less durable) than its mechanical counterpart. Electronic stethoscopes use a microphone to pick up sounds. The microphone may be in a bell-housing, as with mechanical stethoscopes, or the microphone element may be applied directly to the patient. In the latter case, a gel may be used between microphone and skin to help increase sound conduction and reduce outside interference. The signal from the microphone is amplified and filtered, then fed to a small speaker which may be open so that more than one person can listen, or inside a structure much like the Y and earpieces of mechanical stethoscopes and carried to both ears of the practitioner. Electronic amplification also allows filtering of extraneous signals and precise volume control.

Application □The head of the stethoscope is placed on the patient□s skin near to the area whose sounds are of interest.

AKA □steth.

Related devices □**fetal heart detectors (93)**.

Where found □most areas of the hospital.

Syringe Pumps

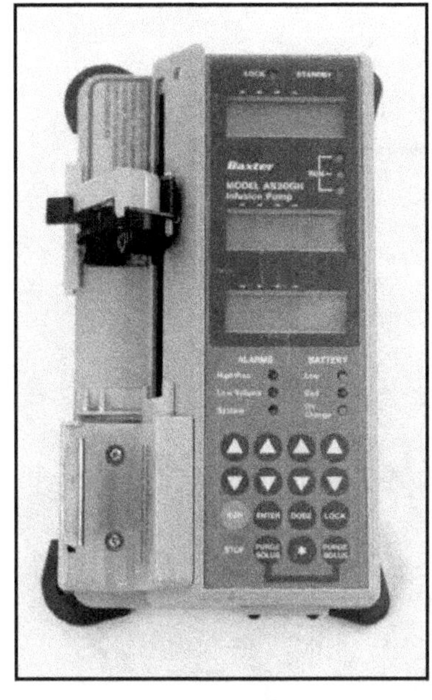

Overview □ Some intravenous medications must be delivered in relatively small quantities but in very accurate dosages.

Function □ In such cases, a syringe pump is often used. These devices consist of a motor and drive system, into which a standard hypodermic syringe is fitted. The motor presses the plunger of the syringe, delivering the medication according to the rate and dosage information programmed by the operator. Syringe pumps are sometimes used in ambulatory situations, such as for pain medication, chemotherapy, or chronic conditions requiring small quantities of medication, such as insulin.

Application □ An intravenous line is established, and a syringe is loaded with the medication to be delivered and placed into the cradle of the pump. Flow and dose parameters are set, and the pump is started.

AKA □(none)

Related devices □**IV pumps (289)**, **PCA pumps (311)**.

Where found □ operating rooms, critical care areas, palliative care units.

Tourniquets, Automatic

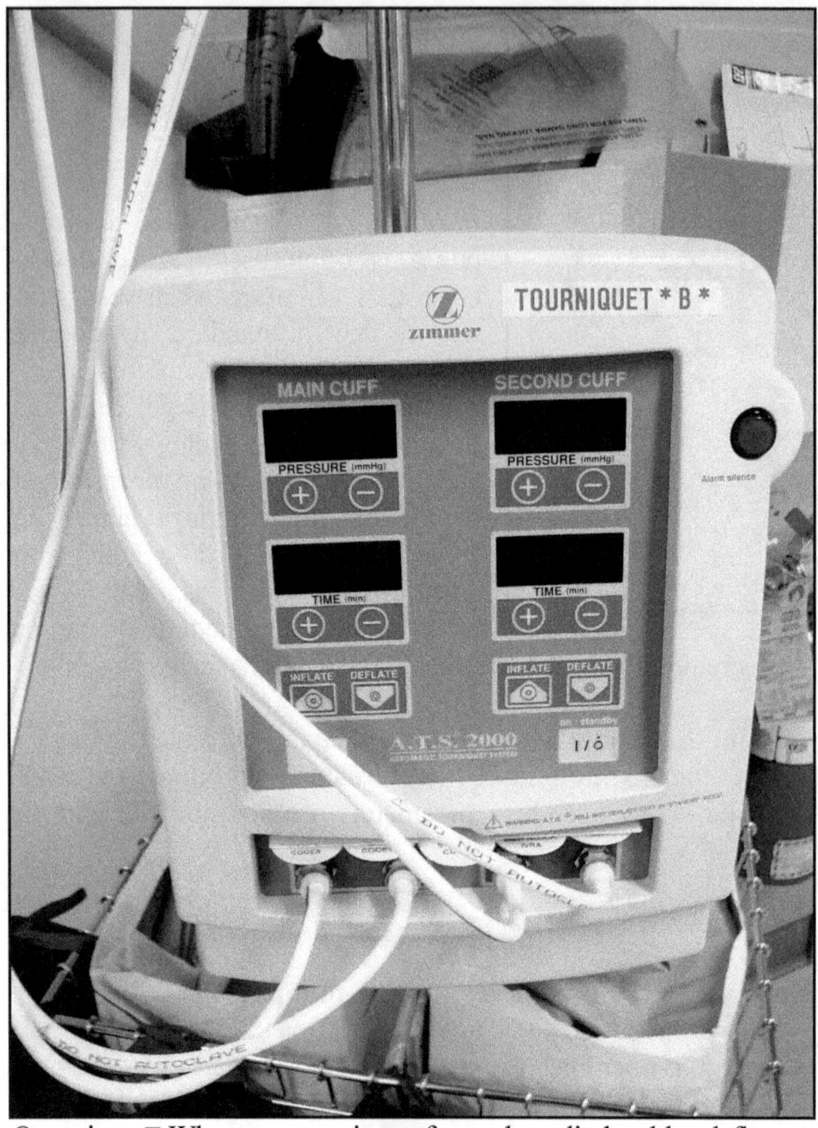

Overview □ When surgery is performed on limbs, blood flow to the surgical area can be problematic, both obscuring the field of view and contributing to patient blood loss.

Application □ Automatic tourniquets incorporate pumps and timing mechanisms that can be programmed for inflation pressure and inflation/deflation cycle timing. Many systems have two independent mechanisms to allow for placement in two different locations.

Pressure must be released occasionally to allow adequate blood flow to the area.

AKA □none

Related devices □n/a

Where found □operating rooms, outpatient surgery, emergency

Tympanic Thermometers

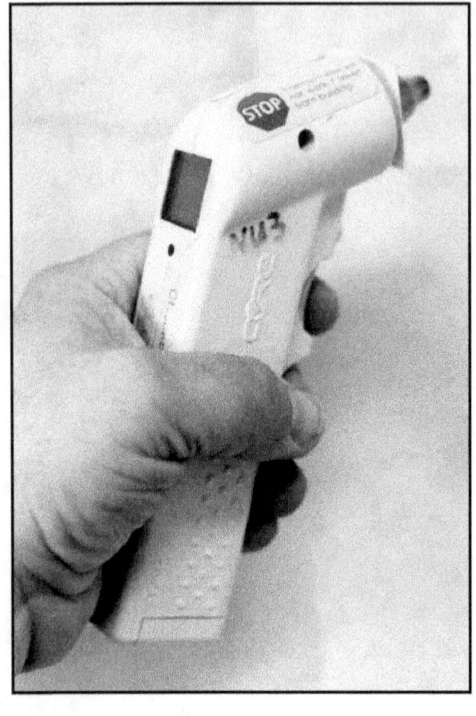

Overview □ Medical caregivers need to know the patient's internal temperature, and want to be able to measure it quickly, with minimal discomfort to the patient.

Function □ A tympanic thermometer does this by measuring the infrared (heat) radiation of the eardrum (or tympanic membrane, which is where this device gets its name). This is usually very close to internal temperature.

Application □ After applying a disposable cover (which goes over the tip to help prevent the passing of material from one patient to another, and also to keep the tip clean), the sensor of the device is inserted into the patient□s ear canal; it is important, though sometimes difficult, to have the sensor pointing directly at the eardrum. Otherwise the temperature of the wall of the ear canal is measured, which may be different than the actual core temperature. When the probe is positioned correctly, a button is pressed to initiate a reading; when the measurement stabilizes (sometimes indicated by a sound), the value is displayed in either Centigrade or Fahrenheit degrees. This technique requires some practice to produce useful results.

It should be noted that these devices compare the temperature of the target with that of an internal heat source. Therefore, the unit must be near room temperature to function properly. Also, the clear □window□ at the end of the sensor must be clean; any obstruction affects accuracy.

AKA □infrared thermometer, IR thermometer.

Related devices □**electronic probe thermometers (279)**.

Where found □Most areas of the hospital.

Ventilators

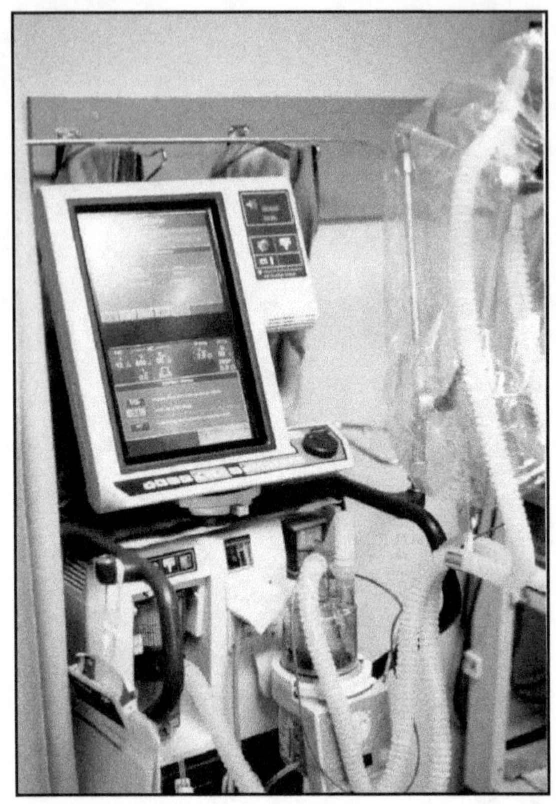

Overview – In response to disease conditions or trauma, the ability of a patient to breathe may be reduced or non-existent. In these cases, ventilation must be provided artificially, either through mouth-to-mouth means, via a “breathing bag” which is pumped by hand, or by a mechanical ventilator. For situations where artificial ventilation is required for more than a few minutes, a mechanical ventilator is preferred.

Function – Ventilators range from relatively basic devices that simply provide a properly-timed boost in air pressure to assist patients in drawing air into their lungs, up to very complex units with a number of variable parameters, built-in compressors and oxygen blenders, monitoring and alarms systems, and battery back-up power.

The goal of all systems is the same: to provide adequate ventilation to the patient, while minimizing harm to their lungs and associated structures. Minimizing harm is especially important in situations where ventilation may be required for periods of days, months, or years.

Most full-featured ventilators can operate in a variety of modes, depending on the needs of each patient.

Breaths may be delivered by the ventilator at a pre-selected rate; when the patient goes too long without taking a breath unassisted; or whenever the patient makes an effort at drawing a breath (within set limits).

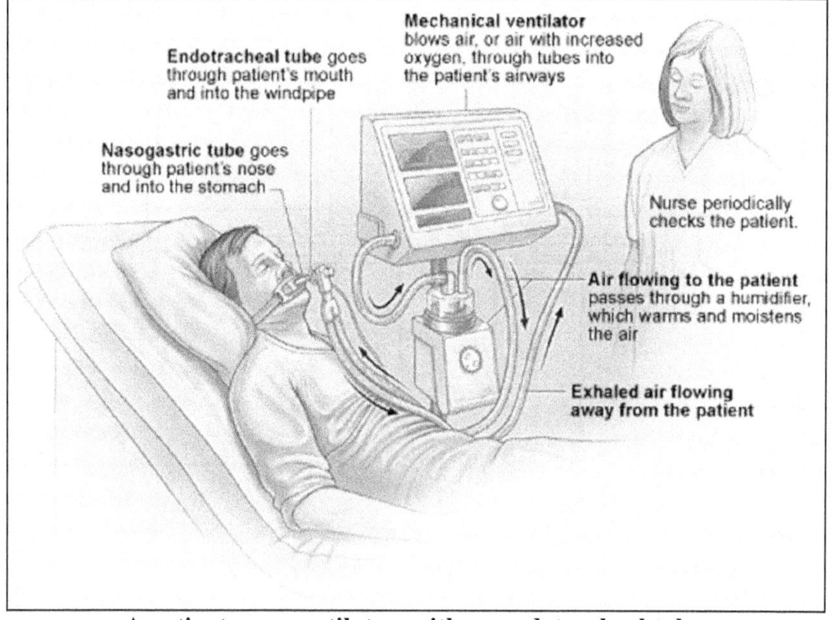

A patient on a ventilator, with an endotracheal tube.

Courtesy of the National Institute of Diabetes and Digestive and Kidney Diseases, National Institutes of Health.

Since ventilation is obviously a critical factor, ventilators must be designed to be highly reliable, in both normal and emergency situations. Ideally, they should be able to continue to function if line power or wall oxygen pressure should fail, and should have redundant critical components to minimize the risk of failures. Alarms must also be reliable, and must be designed so that they cannot be turned off.

When a patient is being ventilated, it may be important to monitor the **oxygen content (305)** of delivered air, **blood oxygen concentration (320)**, and **expired CO2 levels (254)**. These functions may be performed by separate devices or by ones integrated into the ventilator; CO2 levels are usually measured by a separate device. All of these functions may be performed by a **physiological monitor (314)**; some such monitors can interface with the ventilator, allowing for recording of ventilation parameters and integration of alarms into a **central monitoring system (29)**.

Application Ventilator function is very complex and critical, and varies greatly from one model and/or manufacturer to another. An experienced operator must be consulted during set up and use.

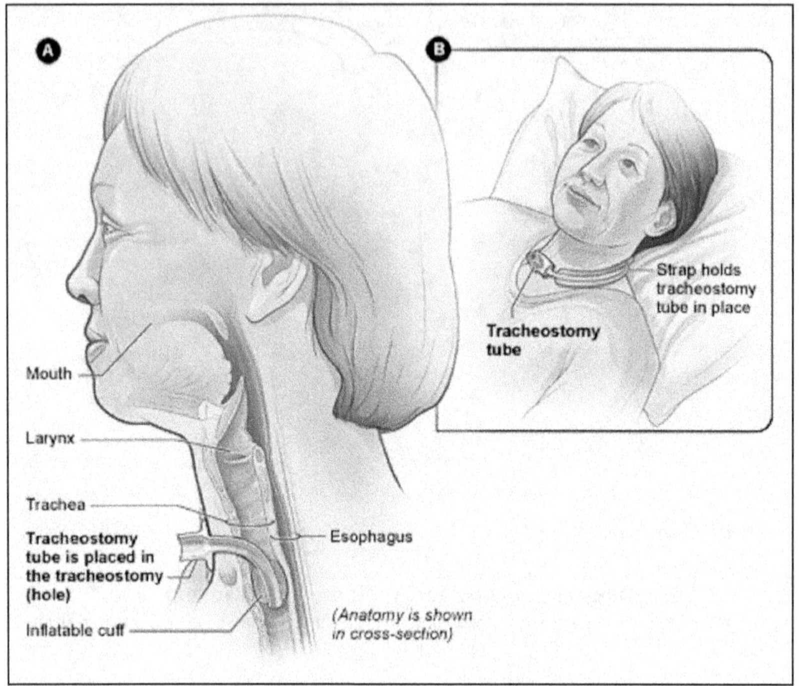

Tracheostomy tube placement,
Courtesy of the National Institute of Diabetes and Digestive and Kidney Diseases, National Institutes of Health.

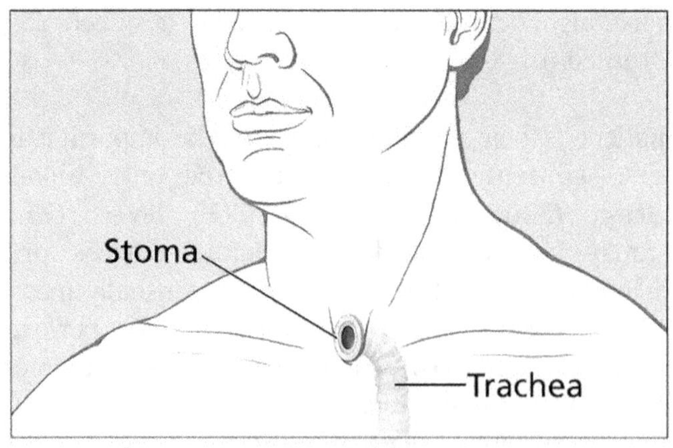

Tracheostomy.
Public domain image.

Generally, an airway is established, either with an endotracheal tube or via a tracheostomy, and then the ventilator is connected. A **laryngoscope (301)** or an **intubation assist device (292)** is used to help place the endotracheal tube. After setting the various parameters to suit the patient, the unit is turned on, and it begins to breathe for the patient.

AKA □vents, respirators, breathing machines.

Related devices □ **oxygen analyzers (305)**, **capnographs (254)**, **intubation assist devices (292)**, **physiological monitors (314)**, **pulse oximeters (320)**.

Where found □critical care areas.

Vital Signs Monitors

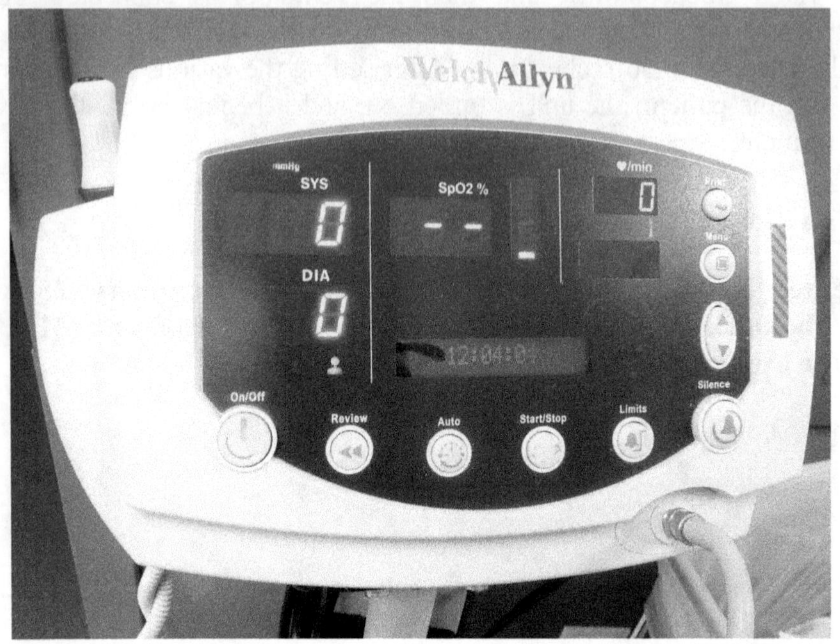

Overview □ As part of routine nursing care, vital signs including blood pressure, temperature and pulse rate are taken and recorded on a regular schedule, the records of which then form part of the patient□s chart. Ever increasing demands on nursing staff time as well as the need for accurate, repeatable results, make an automated method of taking theses measurements desirable. Patients often do not need the full monitoring capabilities of a **physiological monitor (314).**

Function □ A vital signs monitor is a portable device that incorporates one (but usually at least two) or more sections to measure and display vital signs, such as **temperature (279), non–invasive blood pressure (296)** and **blood oxygen saturation/ pulse rate (320)**. Units may also include a strip chart recorder that can print out numerical data for the measurements taken plus date and time, and possibly graphs of measurement trends. Systems can be set to take a single sample of each measurement, or to take measurements at regularly defined intervals. They are usually mounted on a wheeled stand for portability.

Application The components of the system are used just like the individual devices.

AKA (none).

Related devices **Physiological monitors (314), electronic probe thermometers (279), non–invasive blood pressure monitors (296)** and **pulse oximeters (320)**.

Where found most areas of the hospital.

Appendix A – The Hospital

All hospitals, from the smallest to the largest, share a common organizational structure, since they all have the same objectives: to care for patients. Some of the departments described may be combined in a smaller hospital, or diversified in a larger hospital. Also, since certain hospitals are specialized, they may not include all the departments found in a general hospital.

Hospital departments

Medicine

The medical department of a hospital consists of physicians and physicians-in-training.

General practitioners and specialists can admit and discharge patients, and are in charge of their care, determining what medications are required and what tests and diagnostic procedures may be needed. They perform physical examinations, review vital signs and patient conditions, interpret test results and decide on the best course of treatment for each patient. Various specialists may be involved in the care of a patient depending on the complexity of their case.

Some GPs perform surgery, though specialist surgeons handle the majority of surgical cases.

Medical specialties include dermatology (skin and related structures), cardiology (heart and circulatory system), emergency medicine, family medicine, geriatrics (older patients), laboratory medicine, neurology (brain and nervous system), obstetrics and gynecology, oncology (cancer), otorhinolaryngology (ear, nose and throat), pathology, paediatrics, psychiatry, radiology and urology (kidneys, bladder and related organs).

Most physicians maintain a practice outside the hospital, but some are directly employed by the hospital, usually radiologists and pathologists.

Medical residents are MDs training for a specialty, and sometimes actually reside in the hospital, though this is less common that it once was. Most hospitals provide a quiet room with a bed where resident doctors can catch a bit of sleep between shifts.

Interns are medical school students who are working in a hospital for a relatively short time in order to gain clinical experience. An MD, often one of the residents, always supervises them.

Many hospitals now employ Physician Assistants, who are able to perform many of the routine functions of physicians such as conducting physical exams, ordering tests and prescribing medications, under the general supervision of a physician.

There is generally a Chief of Medical Staff for the facility and, depending on the size of the hospitals, various medical departments may each have a department head.

Nursing

Most of the nursing staff in hospitals is made up of registered nurses (RNs) or licensed practical nurses (PNs, LPNs or various other terms), as well as nursing aides (also sometimes called orderlies, patient care aides, and other terms.) Together, the nursing staff members are the people who provide most of the direct care to patients. RNs have the highest level of responsibility, while aides have the lowest and LPNs in between.

Nurses often specialize in areas such as ORs, maternity, psychiatry, geriatrics, oncology or paediatrics. There is an increasing trend towards longer training periods for nurses, particularly RNs, with many programs now consisting of four years of study instead of the traditional two. Nurses are usually expected or even required to participate in continuing education programs. The various medical departments of the hospital have head nurses or nurse clinicians, and many have a staff member who is focused on organizing and implementing education for fellow nurses.

Many hospitals, as well as other sectors of the health care system, are increasingly utilizing nurse practitioners. These are RNs who have undertaken extra training and are given expanded responsibilities, including performing physical examinations, making disease diagnoses and prescribing medications. Their focus is usually patient wellness, education and prevention. Nurse practitioners often specialize in specific areas of medicine such as family health, neonatology or oncology among many others.

Administration

Managing the overall operation of a hospital is the function of Administration. Depending on the definition of the term, administration may include, in addition to direct administrators: the financial department including accounts payable and receivable; human resources; purchasing; and stores. Stores may include shipping and receiving as well.

Administration is responsible for organizing and coordinating the staff and facilities of the hospital, ensuring that patients receive the best possible care while also operating the system within a reasonable budget. They also represent the hospital to the public and to various funding bodies and other outside agencies such as insurance companies and professional organizations.

Clinical support

The clinical support portion of a hospital includes a wide variety of large and small departments, these include:

- Cardiology, responsible for taking and organizing ECG records. These may include **12 lead ECGs (270)**, **stress tests (184)**, **ambulatory ECG monitoring (166)**, **plethysmography (173)**, and others. Cardiology is sometimes a sub‑department of the clinical laboratory.
- Respiratory, responsible for maintaining and sometimes operating **patient ventilators (334)**, **anesthetic machines (47)**, **oxygen concentrators (307)**, **suction units and gas regulating devices (285)**, among others. RTs (respiratory therapists or technologists) may also run a respiratory rehabilitation program for people with acute or chronic respiratory problems, and they may be in charge of systems such as **pulmonary function analyzers (180)**. They may be specialists for intubating patients, or for drawing blood for gas analyses.
- Diagnostic imaging (DI) or radiology was once simply the x‑ray department, but its role has expanded along with the technology used. Basic **x–rays (241)** are still used frequently, but more complex systems are available such as **CT (214)** (computerized tomography), **MRI (229)** (magnetic resonance imaging), **PET (237)** (positron emission tomography) scans and nuclear medicine scans. **Ultrasound machines (217)** can produce good images of soft tissues with less potential cell damage than x‑rays. DI technologists, who are often specialized for the various imaging modalities, operate imaging equipment. Radiologists (who are MDs) interpret results and prepare reports on the findings, as well as supervising some of the imaging procedures or performing some of the more complex procedures.
- The clinical or medical laboratory analyzes blood and tissue samples from patients and provides reports on their findings. Laboratory technologists, often specialized, perform lab work and a physician pathologist supervises the lab. The lab has various sub‑departments.

- Pathology is concerned with disease effects. Histopathology studies diseased tissues, while cytopathology focuses (often literally, using microscopes) on disease-related cells.
- Microbiology studies various disease-causing organisms, with subsets of bacteriology, virology, parasitology and mycology (fungi). Tissue and blood samples may be examined directly for such organisms, or they may be cultured in special incubators for further testing.
- Hematology is involved with blood, testing for various parameters such as counts of the various blood cells and coagulation measurements. Hematology usually also looks after the collection, storage and distribution of blood and blood products for transfusions.
- Biochemistry handles samples from patients, testing for specific chemicals, using very high-tech computerized and automated analyzers.
- The hospital morgue may be a part of the lab, administratively though usually not physically. Deceased patients are taken to the morgue for autopsy, if required, and storage until family can make funeral arrangements. Morgues may maintain samples of organs for research or legal purposes.
- Some manufacturers offer point-of-care testing devices that can analyze blood samples for a wide variety of values right at the bedside, integrating the results into the patient record being generated by physiological monitoring. This provides immediate results, which can be very important in critical cases, and represents a merging of direct patient care and laboratory functions.
- Lab work may involve long time periods for testing, or a very short turn-around time may be required, for example if blood gases from a patient need to be analyzed in order to determine an urgent course of treatment. Tissue samples may need to be examined and reported on during the course of surgery, so that the surgeon can determine if further intervention is required.

- Dietary departments coordinate with nurses and physicians to ensure that specific dietary needs of individual patients are being met. This requires an in-depth knowledge of nutrition and how various foods affect the health of patients with different diseases or conditions.
- Rehabilitation services include physical (or physio) therapy and occupational therapy. This work is aimed at maximizing the recovery of motion and function for patients after surgery or a course of disease. A variety of methods is used, including supervised exercises, heat or cold therapy, range of motion work, ultrasound and other technologies, and massage and manipulation.
- Many hospitals have a spiritual care department, providing direct support to patients, family members and staff, or coordinating such support from outside sources, or simply providing quiet spaces within the hospital for those wishing to pray or contemplate.
- Biomedical Engineering is responsible for the support of the patient care electronic equipment in the hospital. Some Biomed departments also look after such things as **electric patient beds (277)**, **gas and suction regulators (285)** and **patient lifts (309)**, as well as clinical laboratory equipment. Departments are often divided into clinical and imaging sections, with clinical looking after such devices as **physiological monitors (314)**, **defibrillators (259)**, **infant incubators (100)** and **IV pumps (289)**, while imaging takes care of the **x–ray (241)**, **CT (214)**, **MRI (229)** and **ultrasound (217)** equipment. Biomed may be involved in the evaluation of potential new equipment, and also on-going training of nursing staff in the most effective use of equipment. Equipment repair, preventive maintenance and performance testing are functions of Biomedical Engineering.

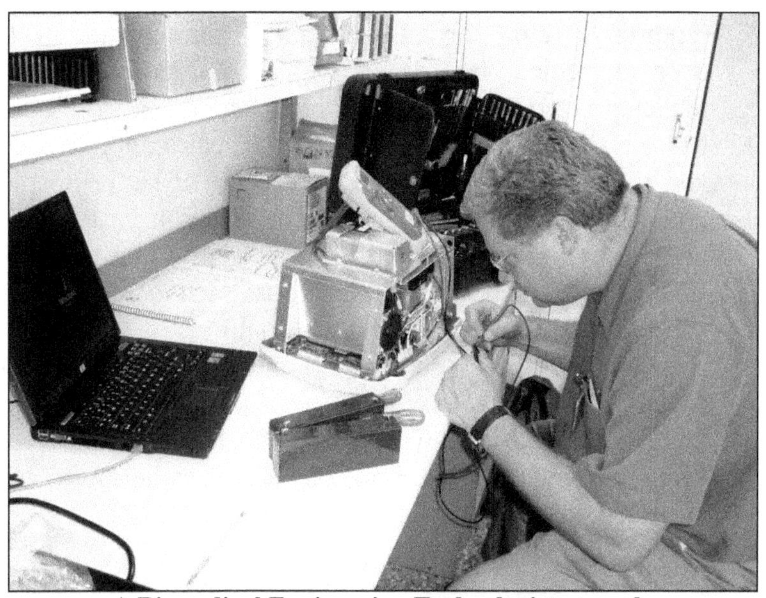

A Biomedical Engineering Technologist at work.

- Infection control staff may be part of the clinical laboratory, but certainly work closely with the lab. Hospital patients are especially vulnerable to infections, and staff are often exposed to potentially harmful pathogens, so it is critical that sufficient precautions be take to minimize these risks. Infection control staff work to ensure that both nursing and support staff are thoroughly trained in infection control procedures, that infection control protocols are adequate and that they are followed, and that hospital facilities are clean and meet current standards. They coordinate with nursing, housekeeping, laboratory and central processing.
- Prosthetics departments are usually found only in larger or specialized hospitals, where patients need to be fitted with custom artificial arms, legs or other body parts. These parts may by simple and for cosmetic purposes only, or they may be more functional. Some facilities are working with mechanical limbs that are controlled by the patient's remaining muscle activity or even brain waves.
- The medical records department provides critical legal documentation of the course of treatment of patients in the hospital. It includes their demographics, medical history, details of their medical condition, charts of vital signs and medications administered, tests and treatments performed, and results of these tests and treatments. Each country

requires specific formats, procedures and materials to be used in medical records, as well as storage conditions and the length of time that the records must be kept.

- Most hospitals have a library of medical texts and journals, and they have access to the collections of larger hospital or university libraries. The Internet provides a vast amount of professional resources for hospital staff to utilize. Library staff collects and organize material, and assist other staff members in finding and using material.
- Patients and family members are often placed in difficult social or emotional circumstances due to the illness or injury involved, and social workers in the hospital help them to deal with these issues, as well as acting as liaison to outside agencies and facilities.

Facility support

Any large building or collection of buildings, including a hospital, requires a team to keep everything running and to meet the physical needs of the occupants.

- Plant services, or physical plant, or building maintenance, provides for the structure and mechanical operation of the hospital. Heating, ventilation and air conditioning, plumbing, electrical wiring and lighting, alarm systems, hospital beds and **patient lifts (309)** are all maintained by plant staff. They may also look after emergency power generators and medical gas systems. Trades people such as plumbers, electricians, carpenters and painters may be part of the plant services staff, to do repairs and some new installations. Larger construction project are usually contracted to outside companies, working in coordination with plant services.
- Security is a vital part of hospital operations, both for staff and patients and visitors. Security staff provides surveillance and protection, and help to ensure that the building and its occupants are safe and that theft and vandalism are prevented.
- Housekeeping keeps the facility clean, taking care of garbage removal, room and floor cleaning, washroom maintenance and cleaning of special areas such as operating rooms. Housekeeping may include laundry services, but this may also be contracted to an outside company.
- Food Services provides nutritionally balanced meals to hospital patients, working with dieticians and medical staff to ensure that any special needs are met. Food services staff may also operate employee and visitor cafeterias and snack bars, though these are often contracted out.
- Information Management/Information Technology/ Information Services/Data Processing/ □Computers□ are all various terms for the department that provides, operates and maintains the computer systems of the hospital. These systems are used for both non□patient care functions such as financials, education, personnel and e□mail, as well as patient care functions including logging patient data from monitors and lab tests, ADT (admission, discharge and transfer) and patient charting. Information Management is responsible for the selection and installation of software packages, and

interfacing the main hospital computer system with various specialized medical computer systems, as well as the Internet.

- Volunteers are an important part of any hospital, with services ranging from simply visiting with patients, to operating carts with snacks and magazines, to running gift shops and organizing fund□raising activities.

Outside agencies

Hospitals interact with a variety of organizations and agencies in the course of operation.

- Government regulatory bodies such as the Food and Drug Administration in the US, the Health Products and Foods Branch of Health Canada and the Medicines and Healthcare products Regulatory Agency in the UK, set standards which medical devices and medications must meet before thy can be used for treating patients. These bodies carry legal authority, and it is incumbent upon the device or medication manufacture to prove that their products meet requirements. The regulatory bodies also perform their own tests to confirm compliance.
- A number of non-governmental organizations exist to perform tests on medical devices. They may have their own standards for equipment, and many levels of government and health care organizations such as individual hospitals or Health Maintenance Organizations use these standards in developing specifications for equipment purchases. Some of these testing and safety organizations include Underwriters Laboratories, the Canadian Standards Association, ECRI (formerly the Emergency Care Research Institute), the American National Standards Institute, the Association for the Advancement of Medical Instrumentation, ASTM International (formerly the American Society for Testing and Materials), and the International Electrotechnical Commission.
- Operating a hospital requires a huge range of supplies and equipment, and all the vendors of these things must be dealt with in an economical, efficacious and ethical manner.
- Most hospitals rely to a greater or lesser degree on funding from various charities, fund raising groups or the donations from individuals or organizations. Some of these may be branches of the hospital, or they may be independent. In any case, ethical guidelines must be in place to deal with the groups properly.
- Various professional organizations such as the American, Canadian and British Medical Associations have some influence over hospital staff, and their concerns must be taken into consideration.

- Many hospital employees are members of unions, and as such, their unions must be dealt with in regards to negotiating contracts and resolving grievances.
- Government health agencies, Health Maintenance Organizations, other medical or liability insurance companies, the Armed Forces, police departments, and Workers Compensation Boards all may contribute towards the costs of hospital patient care, and as such, they have a greater or lesser degree of influence on how those costs are managed.

Selected Hospital Medical Units

Every hospital provides a different range of services, some of which are common to almost all facilities and others that may only be offered in specialized hospitals. Generally, larger hospitals offer a wider range of services, although a small hospital in a relatively isolated area may provide a more complete range than a similar□ sized suburban hospital, where specialty services are readily available in nearby city facilities.

This is by no means a comprehensive list of clinical units and services, but serves as an example of what a relatively full□featured general hospital might offer

Addiction Treatment □ providing emergency treatment of patients in addiction crises, support and treatment during the withdrawal process, and counselling and ongoing treatment to help patients remain free of substance abuse.

Cardiology □ a diagnostic department that does testing of patients with confirmed or suspected heart disease.

Diagnostic Imaging □ provides X□ray, CT, MRI, ultrasound and other services to give clinicians a non□invasive look inside the patient.

Emergency Services □ care for patients suffering from severe trauma or critical illnesses, though the definitions of severe and critical may be open to interpretation.

Endocrinology and Diabetes Clinic □ testing, diagnosis, treatment and on□going counselling of patients with endocrine disorders such as Addison□s Disease, growth hormone abnormalities, and diabetes.

ENT (Ear, Nose & Throat) □ concerned with diseases and traumas involving the self□described systems.

Family Medicine □ a holistic approach to working with patients in the context of their family and community.

Gastroenterology □ concerned with the digestive system: esophagus, stomach, small and large intestines, and associated organs.

Geriatrics □provides care for elderly patients.

Intensive Care Units □ ICUs treat patients with severe illnesses or traumas, often after being stabilized in the ER, but also after major surgery or following a medical crisis. ICUs may be specialized depending on their specific type of patients.

Laboratory □ provides testing and analysis of tissue and fluid samples from patients.

Long Term Care □ care of patients with conditions that require hospitalization for extended periods of time, such as those recovering form devastating illnesses or traumas, or those with severe chronic diseases or conditions.

Maternity and Neonatal Care □ prenatal and perinatal care for expectant mothers and their infants.

Neurosciences □ concerned with diseases and conditions involving the brain and nervous system.

Oncology □ counselling, cancer diagnosis and treatment including radiation therapy and chemotherapy.

Operating Rooms □surgical suites.

Ophthalmology □ conditions of the eye. A large portion of many ophthalmology units may be involved with performing cataract removal and lens replacement surgery.

Orthopaedics □ diseases, injuries and conditions of bones and connective tissues, especially joints.

Outpatients □a unit that provides care for patients who need specific medical treatments but do not require overnight stays. This may include minor surgeries, administration of critical drugs, or procedures such as gastroscopies or colonoscopies.

Pediatrics □ dealing with children and their specific, unique needs and conditions. Various diseases are almost exclusively found in children, as well.

Palliative Care □ providing terminally ill patients and their families with counselling and support, and working to ensure the patient is as comfortable and pain□free as possible while respecting their wishes or those of their families should they not be able to respond themselves.

Physical Medicine □ also known as rehabilitation or physiotherapy and occupational therapy, helps to maximize patient function and comfort while reducing recovery time, through physical manipulation and exercise, and application of various therapies.

Psychiatry □ dealing with patients with mental illnesses, ensuring the optimal treatment and counselling while protecting the safety of patients and others.

Pulmonary Medicine & Respiratory Care □ diagnosis and rehabilitation of patients with suspected or known pulmonary or respiratory problems. Also may be involved with support and application of patient ventilators and anesthetic machines.

Renal Unit □ providing support and treatment for patients with temporary or permanent kidney function impairment or failure. Treatment may include hemodialysis or peritoneal dialysis.

Women's Health □ may also be known as gynecology, though units often now deal with health issues for women in a more holistic manner. Women□s Health units may include maternity.

Urology □ dealing with medical issues involving the urinary system, including the kidneys, bladder and prostate.

Appendix B – Surgery, Surgical Teams and Anesthesia

Some surgery can be performed by a single person, but anything more complex than a lesion removal usually requires a team of people. With more complex procedures, the team grows.

<u>The team</u>

A surgeon is the core of any surgical team, and there may be one or more other surgeons involved, though one person will be the lead. Some situations, such a live donor kidney transplant, mean that two teams are working in close proximity and coordination with one another. Surgeons might perform general, relatively simple procedures, or they may specialize in specific areas such as orthopaedic, cardiovascular, neurological, cosmetic, ophthalmic or thoracic surgery.

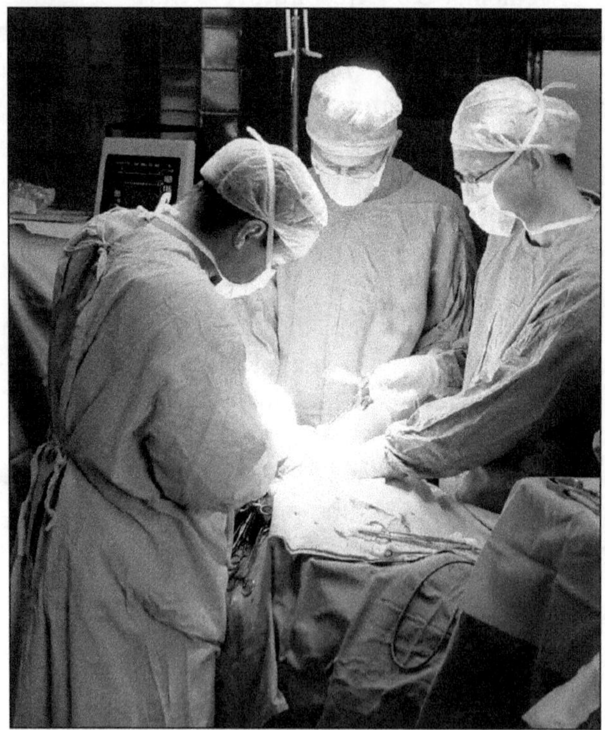

Surgeons at work.

(Modified from Shutterstock, Inc, www.shutterstock.com, with permission)

An anesthesiologist will usually be present to take care of **anesthetizing** and monitoring the patient. The anesthesiologist also often interviews the patient immediately before surgery to confirm any drug allergies, to try to allay any possible apprehensions and to ensure that the patient is aware of the surgery that is about to be performed. They may administer the initial sedative and later intubate the patient, select, administer and regulate gaseous agents, determine and monitor the level of consciousness and vital signs of the patient, bring them out of anesthesia at the end of the procedure, and then check on their recovery.

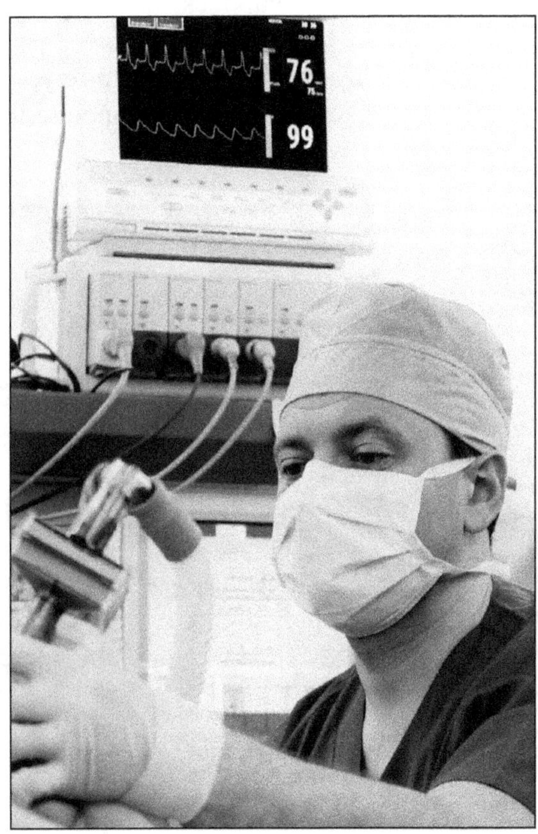

Anesthesiologist holding mask on patient.

(Modified from Shutterstock, Inc, www.shutterstock.com, with permission)

Operating Room nurses assist surgeons, providing instruments and supplies as needed, removing items from the surgical field as required, ensuring that fluids are removed as effectively as possible, and generally keeping things working smoothly. They may also do such mundane things as drying the surgeon's forehead or changing CDs for background music, but generally their functions are critical for the team. OR nurses may be directly assisting, or they may "float", moving about the OR as required. Nurses often set up the

OR before surgery, preparing any supplies and equipment and arranging everything in the OR to suit the particular procedure and surgeon.

Respiratory therapists/technologists may assist the anesthesiologist in intubating patients and in running the **anesthetic machines (47)**. They may perform functional tests of the machine before procedures, and check that anesthetic-related supplies and equipment are ready.

During open heart or heart transplant surgery, a specialized technologist or nurse will likely be present to operate the **heart–lung machine (57)**.

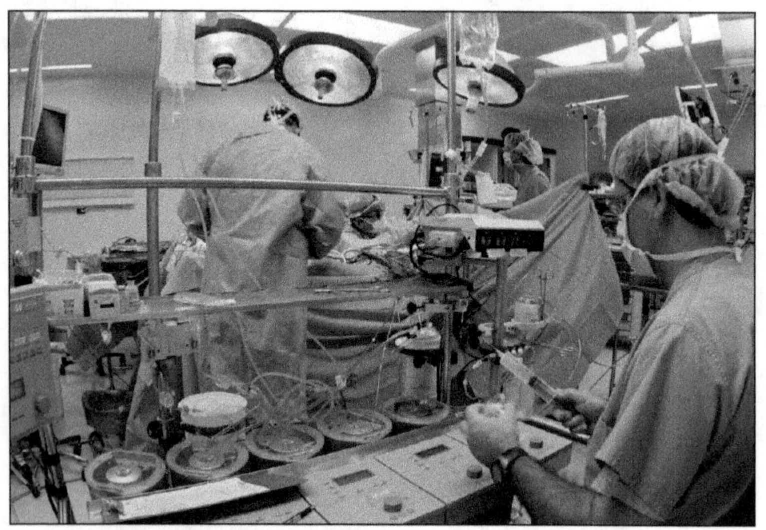

A perfusionist operating a heart–lung machine.

(Modified from Shutterstock, Inc, www.shutterstock.com, with permission)

Biomedical engineering technologists may be in the Operating Room or on close stand-by to provide advice and support regarding technical functions of the high-tech equipment being used.

Laboratory technologists may be stationed near the operating room to help in examining tissues and organs removed during surgery, so that determinations can be made regarding the need for further intervention.

Imaging technologists may be called into the OR to obtain **x–ray (212)** or **ultrasound (217)** images as part of the surgical process.

In a teaching hospital, students of any the surgical team disciplines may be present in the OR, as well as observing through viewing windows or video links.

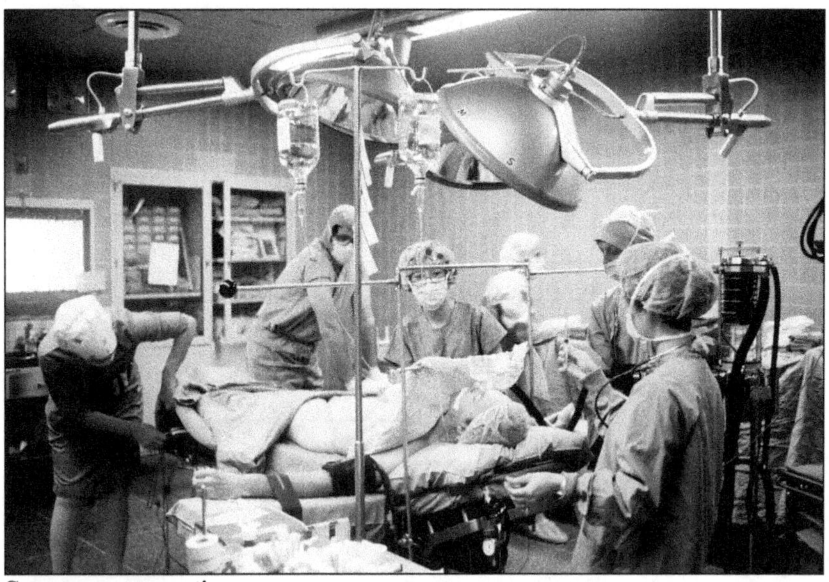

Surgery preparation.
Public domain image, from the National Cancer Institute Archives.

Equipment vendor representatives often come into the OR to assist in the use of a new device, providing advice and recommendations to hospital staff to help them get the most out of the device.

Housekeeping staff members are an integral part of the team, as they have the responsibility of cleaning up after each surgery (often a messy job that requires special training in biohazardous material handling) and ensuring that the room is clean and antiseptic before the next procedure.

An OR manager takes care of scheduling, staffing and equipment and supply ordering and control.

General type of surgery

Surgery can be divided into various categories depending on the overall goals of the procedures:

- Removal of diseased or damaged tissues or organs.
- Replacement of body parts, including joints, eye lenses, and heart valves, with artificial substitutes.
- Transplantation of organs and other body parts.
- Diagnostic or exploratory surgery. Such procedures may be combined with removal surgery depending on findings.
- Orthopaedic surgery, in which bones and cartilage are adjusted, removed, repaired or repositioned.
- Caesarean births.
- Cosmetic or □plastic□surgery.

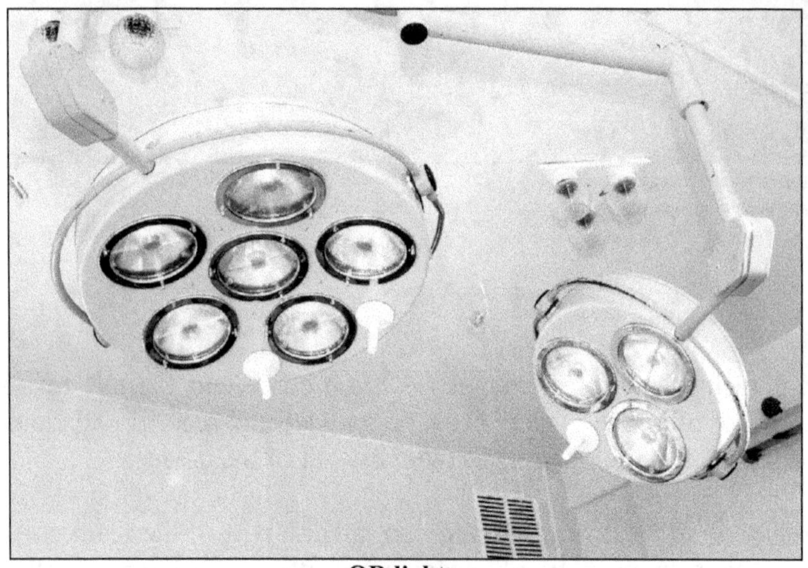

OR lights.

Modified from Shutterstock, Inc, www.shutterstock.com, with permission.

Minimally invasive surgery

Many surgical procedures can be done with minimally invasive or **endoscopic (130)** techniques, in which small incisions allow the insertion of one or more tubes into an area of the patient's body. The surgeon can visualize the specific site on which they are working, and thin instruments can be inserted within the tubes to provide cutting, cauterization, suctioning and suturing. A gas such as carbon dioxide is used to **inflate (148)** the area surrounding the surgical site, and illumination is provided by **fiber optics (142)** either integrated into the access tubes or built into the exploratory or operating instruments. Accessory tubes provide irrigation and suction.

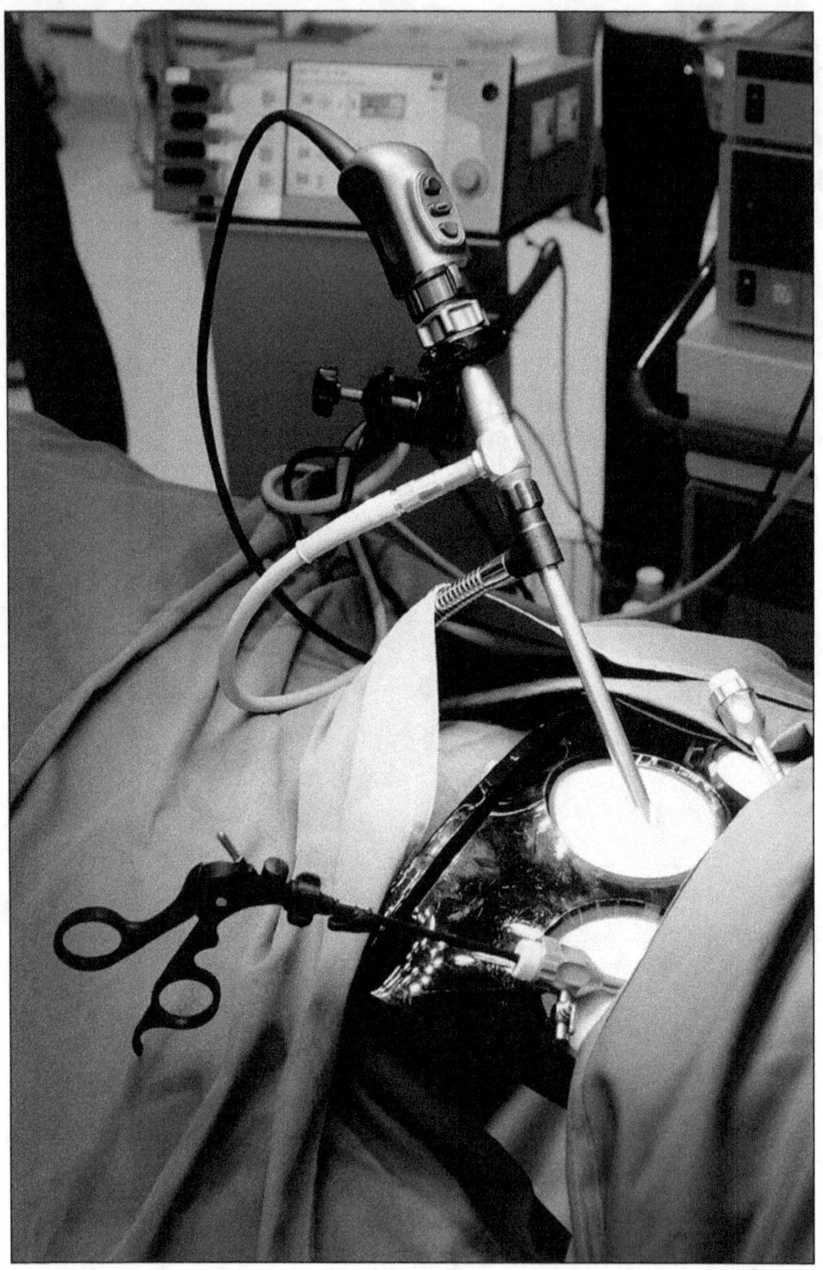

Instruments being used in a laparoscopic surgical procedure. The largest device has a camera head on top; the one in the lower left is used for grasping or cutting tissue.

(Modified from Shutterstock, Inc, www.shutterstock.com, with permission)

Post-surgery

After the surgery is completed and the patient has been brought back to consciousness (or has stabilized following conscious surgery), they must be **monitored (314)** carefully for some time before being returned to a general ward in the hospital or, in the case of day care surgery, before being allowed to go home. Vital signs are monitored and checked frequently, pain medication is administered as required and the surgical site is observed to make sure there is no excessive bleeding or other problems. Some catheters and IV lines may be removed as part of the post-operative care, and patients may be given ice chips or small sips of water depending on their condition. The length of post-operative stay depends on the condition of the individual patient and the degree of trauma produced during surgery. Post-op areas are in close proximity to the ORs so that surgical staff and facilities are readily available if they are needed.

Anesthesia

Surgery has been performed for thousands of years, as evidenced by ancient writings as well as physical signs such as prehistoric skulls with incised holes, some of which were healed over. But for most of the history of surgery, it was performed as a last resort, and the patient endured intense agony during the process, often to such a degree that they died of shock. Alcohol and opium were used to lessen the pain, but patients still remained conscious during surgery. It wasn't until the advent of ether that physicians and dentists were able to induce somewhat controlled unconsciousness in their patients so that surgery became more bearable —for both patient and surgeon! Ether was the first general anesthetic, William Morton being the first physician to use it successfully.

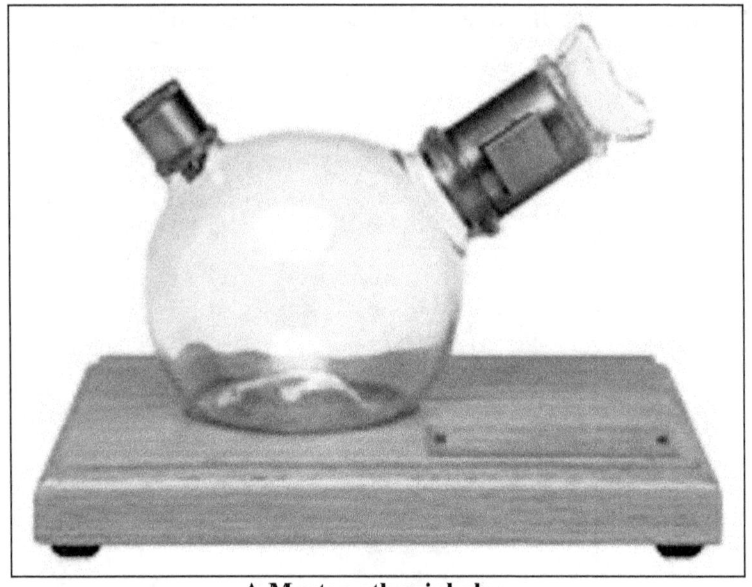

A Morton ether inhaler.

Courtesy of the National Institute of Diabetes and Digestive and Kidney Diseases, National Institutes of Health.

Anesthesia means, literally, "without sensation" and in medical practice can refer to several different processes.

Types of anesthesia

Various prescription and non-prescription medications are able to reduce pain when taken internally, either orally or by intravenous injection. These medications, also called analgesics, usually are non-specific; that is they relieve pain in whatever area of the body it is being experienced. Ideally the agents work without impairing other mental or physical functions, but more powerful drugs do have some such side effects. Examples of these agents include acetylsalicylic acid (Aspirin®), acetaminophen (Tylenol®), ibuprofen (Advil®), and opium derivatives such as heroin, codeine, oxycodone, methadone and morphine.

Local anesthetics are, as the name implies, agents that have a very localized effect. They may be administered topically or by injection. Ideally they affect only the area of the body near the administration site, and have only a temporary effect. Local anesthetic agents range from simple ice packs, to aloe vera juice, to cocaine and derivatives such as novocaine and benzocaine. Dentists use injected local anesthetics to help make their work more comfortable for patients, and an injection into the spinal canal can block some of the pain associated with labor and delivery or other abdominal or lower limb surgery.

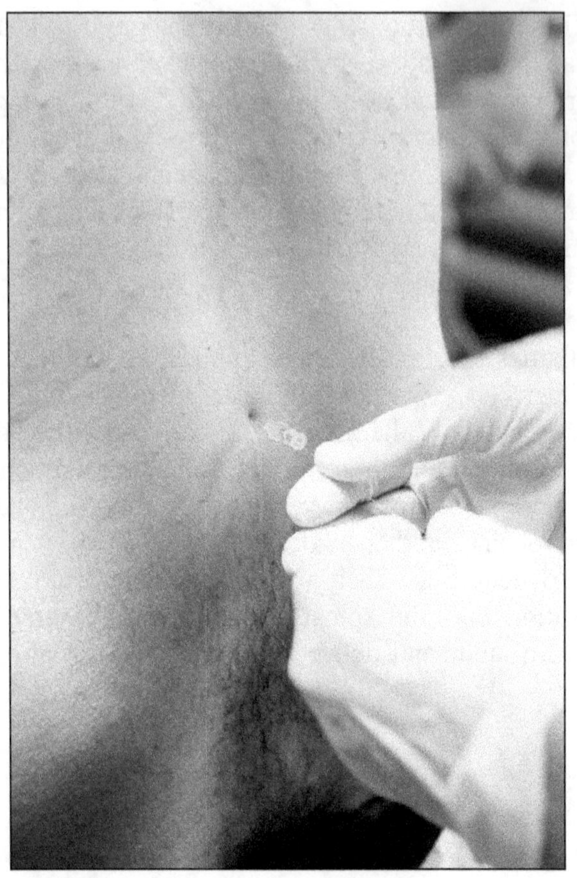

11244367 Needle inserted into the spinal canal for anesthesia.

(Modified from Shutterstock, Inc, www.shutterstock.com, with permission)

General anesthetics are those that produce unconsciousness. Hypnotic (allowing the patient to "ignore" pain) or amnesiac (causing the patient to not remember pain) medications may be included in this definition. Amnesiac drugs have the benefit of allowing the patient to be conscious during procedures so that they can respond to medical staff and cooperate with the procedures; for the patient, after the procedure is complete, not remembering pain or discomfort is effectively like not having that pain or discomfort at all. These drugs also tend to have fewer side affects than agents that produce unconsciousness do. Examples of amnesiac drugs include midazolam, Propofol and scopolamine.

Sedatives reduce the patient's level of consciousness to levels that are sufficient for a particular procedure. The level of sedation may be classified as deep, moderate or minimal. In deep sedation, patients can respond to clear, sharp instructions, but are generally unresponsive. They may require breathing assistance. With minimal sedation, patients can respond normally but are in a relaxed state, and do not require breathing assistance. The original sedative was alcohol, but its influence is widely variable and it produces a number of undesirable side effects. Current sedatives include barbiturates, benzodiazepines, Ketamine and Propofol. Some of these drugs may serve as both a sedative and an amnesiac.

One of the first general anesthetic agents that produced unconsciousness was ether, which was wondrous at the time as it allowed patients to undergo surgical procedures without being in agony. However, ether had undesirable features such as being difficult to control, having short acting effects and being extremely flammable. Newer substances were developed that reduced or eliminated these features, and the most common general anesthetic agents in use now are isoflurane, desflurane and sevoflurane.

Related to anesthetic drugs, though not actually producing anesthesia, are muscle relaxant substances. These drugs reduce or eliminate the contractions of skeletal muscles in order to make surgery easier and to prevent unwanted movement, especially in response to electrosurgery impulses. Intubation of a patient is much easier when their muscles are relaxed. Some of these drugs were derived from the curare used by South American Indians for their poisoned arrows or blowgun darts. Examples of muscle□relaxant agents are Succinylcholine, Mivacurium, Vecuronium and Gallamine.

Anesthesia in surgery

Most major surgery involves the use of multiple agents. A sedative is administered, usually intravenously, in advance of the surgery, to relax the patient. Once they are in position on the operating table, sedation is increased until the patient can be intubated and the general anesthetic agent is administered via the tracheal tube. After unconsciousness is achieved, muscle relaxants are given, and when all levels are sufficient, surgery can commence.

The condition of the patient must be monitored closely during surgery, both to ensure their vital signs remain stable and to maintain an adequate level of unconsciousness, neither too high nor too low. Vital signs can change due to the general condition of the patient and to the trauma of the surgery itself. Level of consciousness is important since, if too high, the patient can become aware of the surgery being performed, and if too low, cardiovascular function can be compromised or even halted.

Side note: In the US, a physician who administers anesthetics is referred to as an anesthesiologist, while a specialist nurse who does so is called an anesthetist. In Canada, the United Kingdom and Australia, the terms anesthetist and anesthesiologist are both used to refer to a physician who is trained in anesthetic administration. For the purposes of this book, the term anesthesiologist will be used to mean any person who is administering anesthesia.

Anesthetic machines

In the course of any major surgery, anesthesia must be monitored and maintained, and along with this, the patient must be monitored and maintained as well. **Anesthetic machines (47)**, handled by an anesthesiologist, provide these functions.

The primary function of an anesthetic machine is to regulate the flow of gases to the patient, including medical air, oxygen and anesthetic agents. Various mechanical and/or electronic components provide this regulation as well as giving readouts of the current values. Current systems record readings for later examination if necessary.

Anesthetic machines are usually operated electrically, and may have gas pressures provided by hospital distribution systems, by attached pressurized tanks, or by internal compressors, or a combination of these. Some units have internal batteries that can continue normal functions in case of a line power failure, though usually only for a limited time.

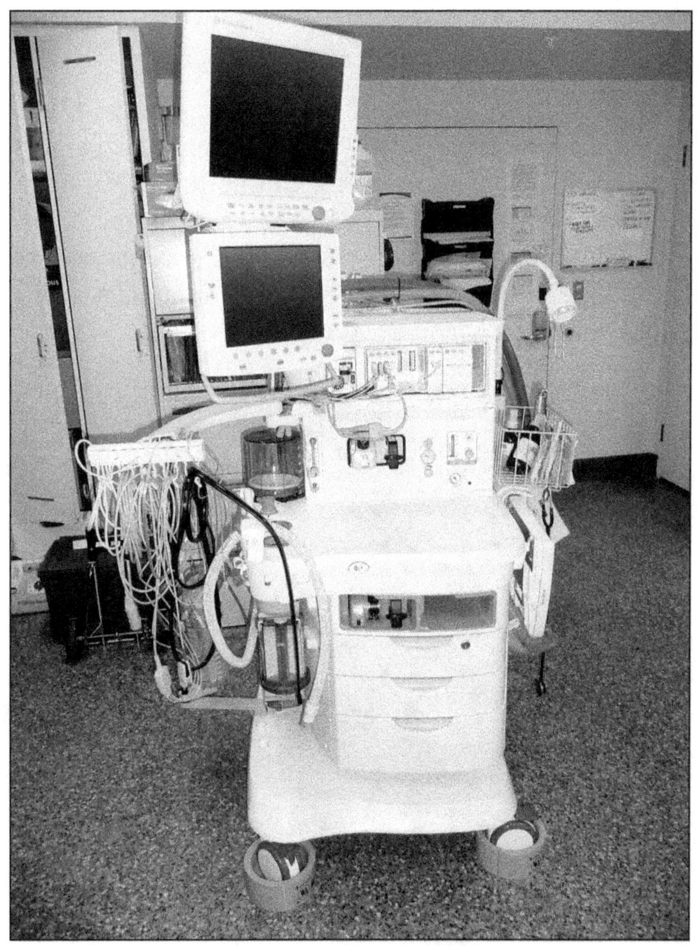

An anesthetic machine.

Anesthetic agents such as isoflurane, desflurane and sevoflurane are liquids at room temperature, and must be vaporized in a controlled manner before they can be mixed with air and/or oxygen. Special vaporizer units attached to the anesthetic machine both contain the agent and vaporize it as necessary. Because the agents each have different physical properties, the vaporizers are somewhat different for each.

Since patients undergoing surgery are often unable to breathe on their own, the machine provides a means of mechanical ventilation. The parameters of ventilation are controllable to various degrees depending on the model, but include rate, flow and volume as a minimum. These parameters and measurements are displayed and often logged.

In order to reduce the amount of anesthetic agent used, the exhaled breath of the patient is recycled, which means that carbon dioxide must be removed before the mixture can be returned to the patient. This is accomplished by passing the gas through a canister containing soda lime, which absorbs CO2. The canister is clear, and the soda lime changes color as it becomes saturated with CO2, so that the operators can change it when necessary.

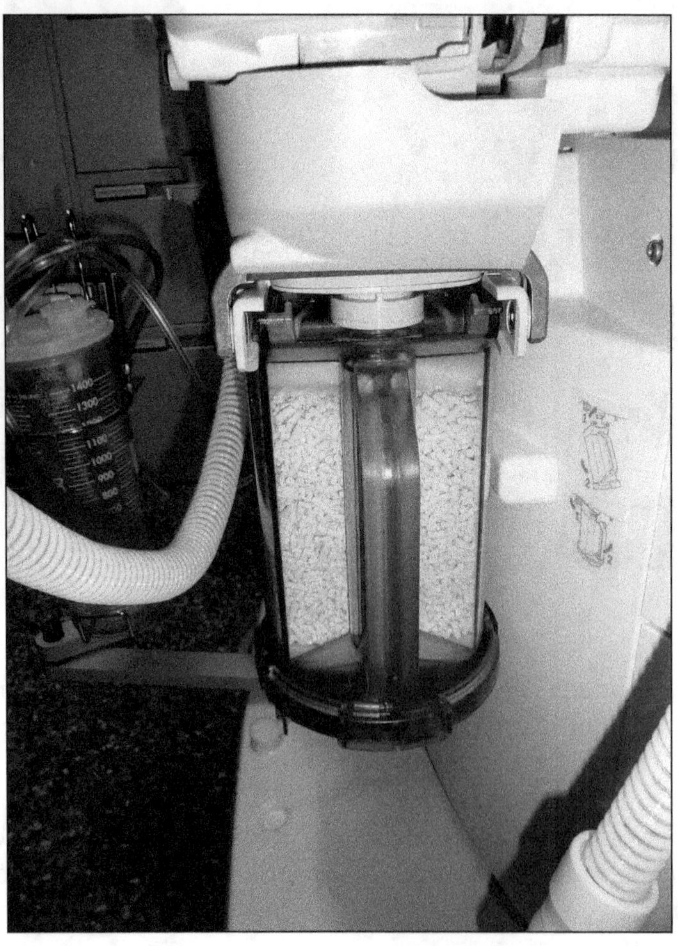

Anesthetic machine CO2 absorber

Since anesthetic agents can be harmful, there must be a system in place to remove any excess from the area.

Various physiological parameters must be monitored during surgery, and this may be done with a **stand–alone external system (314)**, or with one integrated into the anesthetic machine. In either case, ECG, respiration and blood pressure can be monitored, plus blood oxygen saturation (SpO2) and expired CO2 levels. The system records measurements and has settable alarms in case parameters go beyond specific limits.

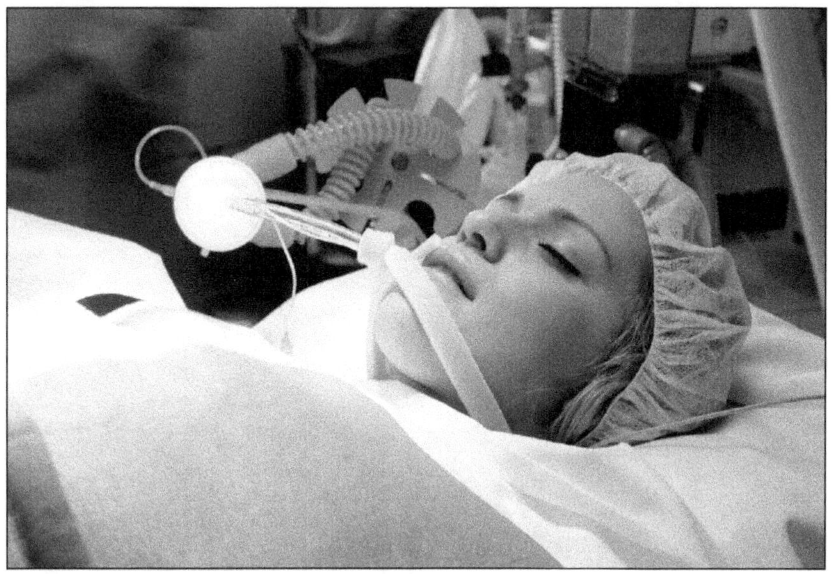

Patient undergoing surgery, with the anesthetic machine breathing circuit (corrugated hose) connected through their mouth into the trachea.

(Modified from Shutterstock, Inc, www.shutterstock.com, with permission)

Level of consciousness is an important factor during surgery, and various means have been used to try to determine this. **Nerve/muscle stimulators (63)** apply an electrical signal to a part of the patient's body such as the hand or foot, and the degree of muscle contraction elicited is a measure of depth of anesthesia, though not necessarily level of consciousness. Most manufacturers now offer a means of giving a quantitative value for the **depth of consciousness (276)**, usually by measuring and analyzing specific EEG waveforms. Some controversy exists as to the efficacy of these methods, however they do provide more information than was previously available.

Appendix C – Anatomy Illustrations

Basic anatomical drawings of major body systems are provided for reference.

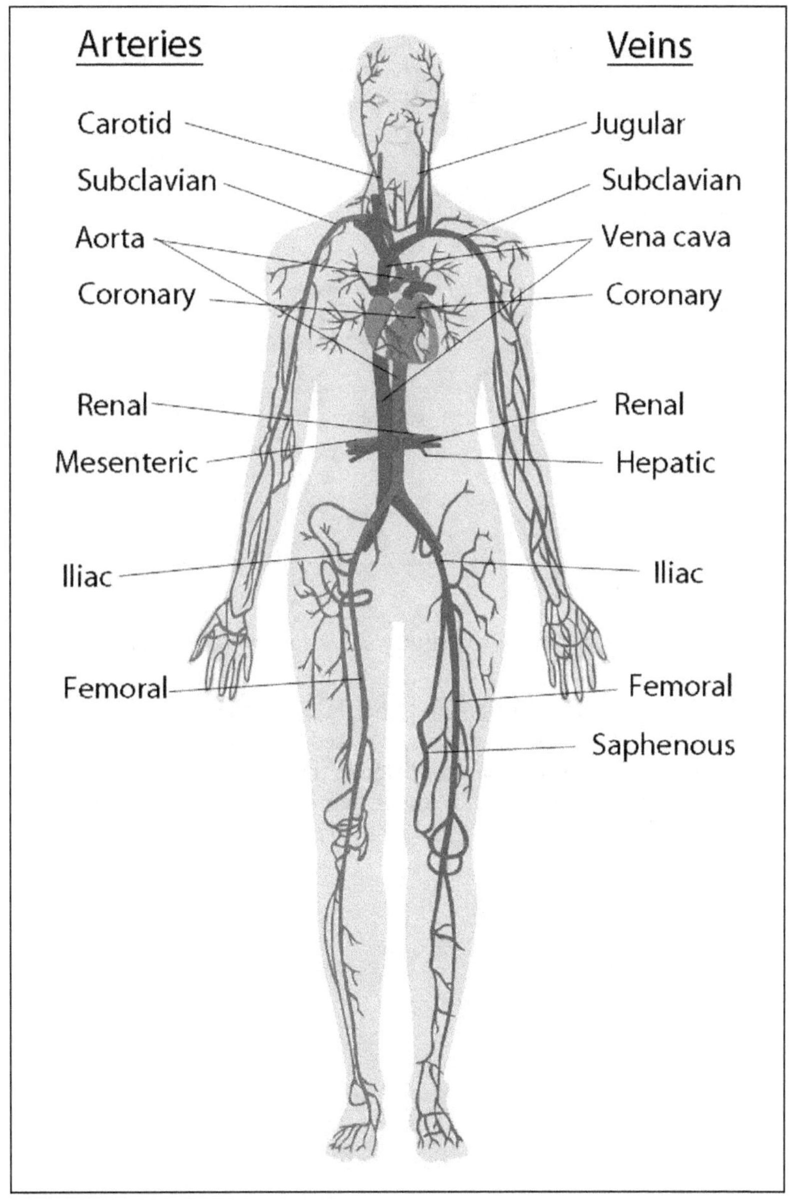

Circulatory System.

(Modified from Shutterstock, Inc, www.shutterstock.com, with permission)

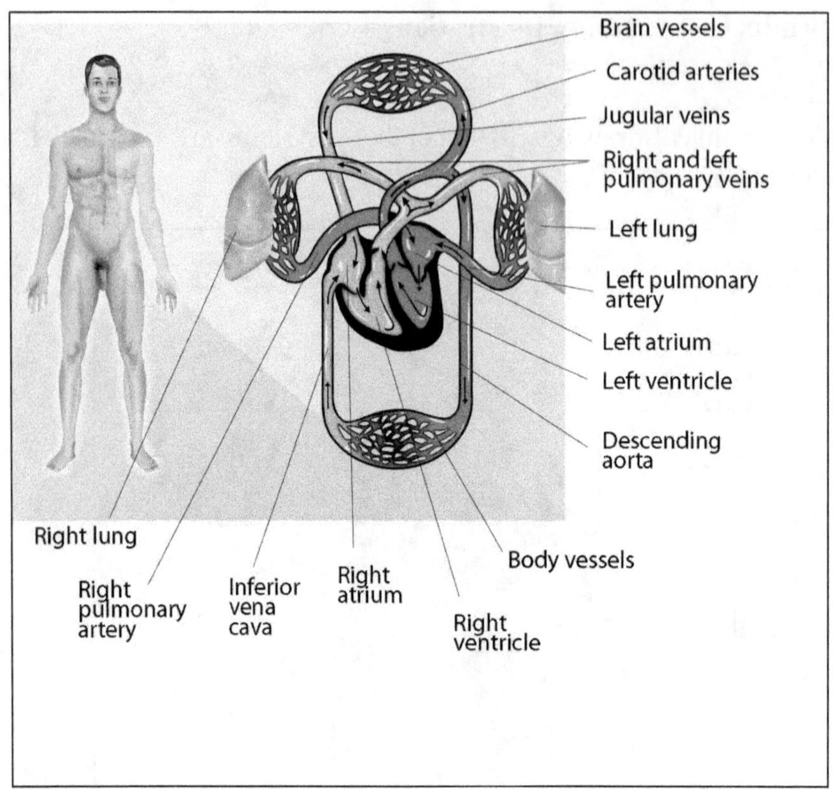

Circulatory System Schematic.

(Modified from Shutterstock, Inc, www.shutterstock.com, with permission)

Blood is pumped from the right atrium into the right ventricle, and from there to the lungs, where excess carbon dioxide is removed and fresh oxygen acquired. Returning from the lungs, the blood passes through the left atrium and then the left ventricle to be distributed to the rest of the body, including the heart itself. Returning from the body, blood is now back at the right atrium.

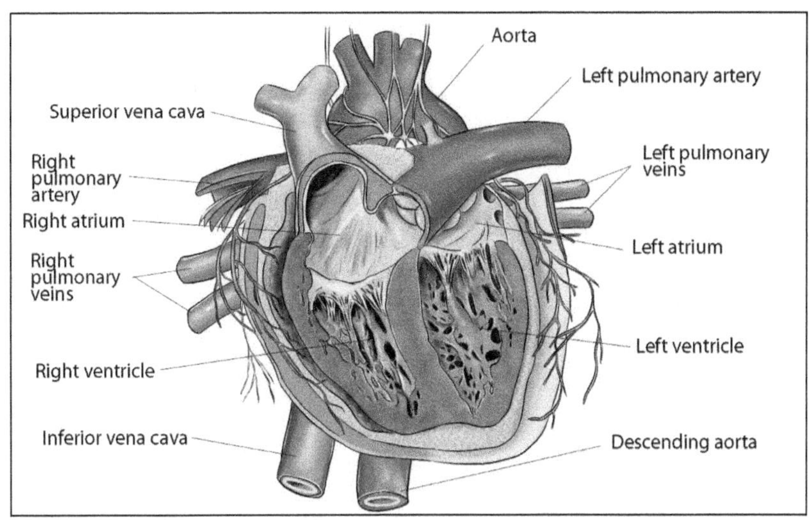

Heart Cross–section.

(Modified from Shutterstock, Inc, www.shutterstock.com, with permission)

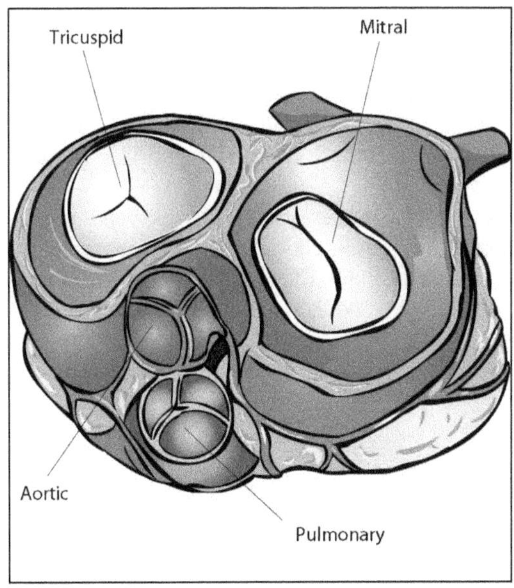

Heart Valves.

(Modified from Shutterstock, Inc, www.shutterstock.com, with permission)

The four heart valves prevent blood from flowing backwards in the heart during contractions.

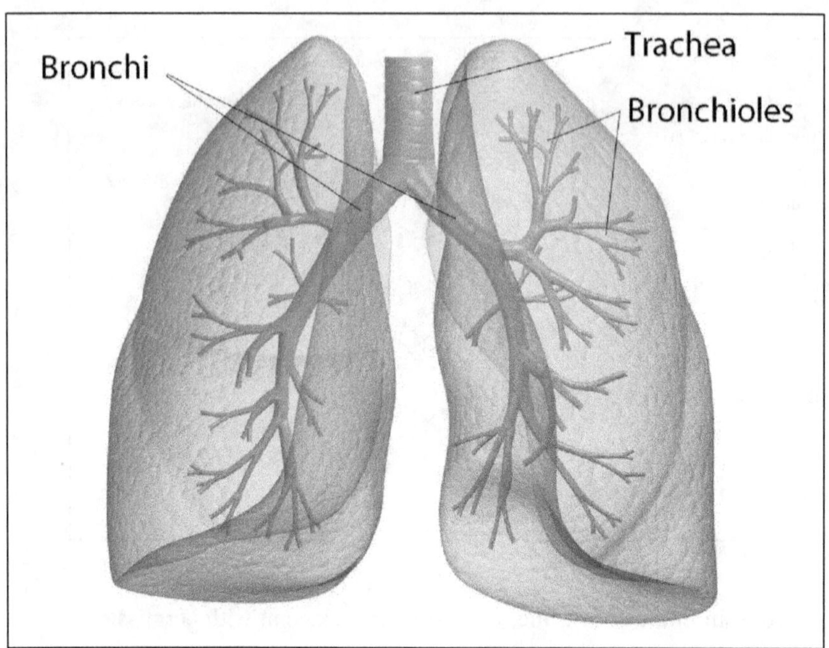

Respiratory System.

(Modified from Shutterstock, Inc, www.shutterstock.com, with permission)

Air is taken in through the mouth or nose and passed down the trachea, or windpipe. It then splits into the left and right bronchi going to each lung, and then divides further into bronchioles connecting to all of the lungs. The smallest bronchioles end in tiny sacs called alveoli.

Blood flowing from the heart moves through smaller and smaller branches until it reaches the capillary nets that surround the alveoli. Oxygen is taken into the blood from inhaled air within the alveoli, and carbon dioxide is released from the blood into the alveoli; it is then expelled from the body during exhalation.

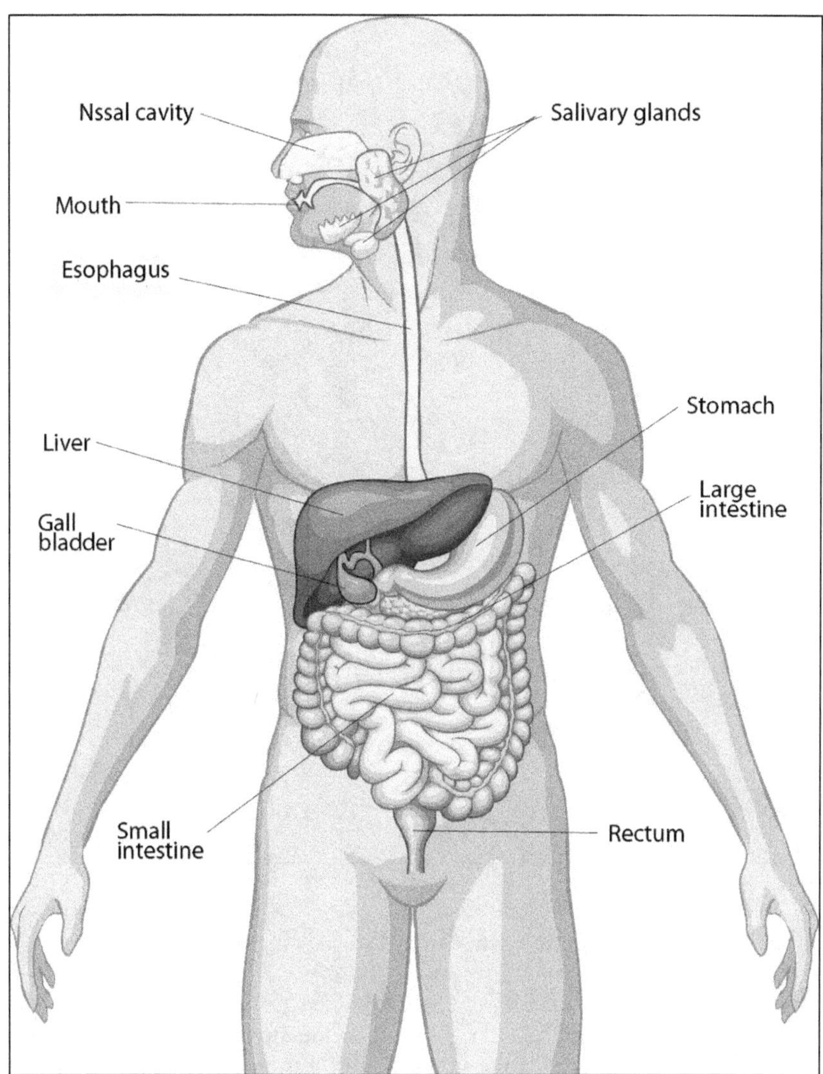

Digestive System.

(Modified from Shutterstock, Inc, www.shutterstock.com, with permission)

Food is mechanically broken down by chewing, and the salivary glands add saliva to start digesting starches and help lubricate the food for swallowing.
The small intestine is divided into three main parts, the duodenum, the jejunum and the ileum. The small intestine continues digestion and absorbs nutrients. The parts of the large intestine, or colon, are designated the ascending colon, the transverse colon and the descending colon. The main function of the colon is to remove water and salt from the digested material. The rectum holds wastes until they are passed from the body.

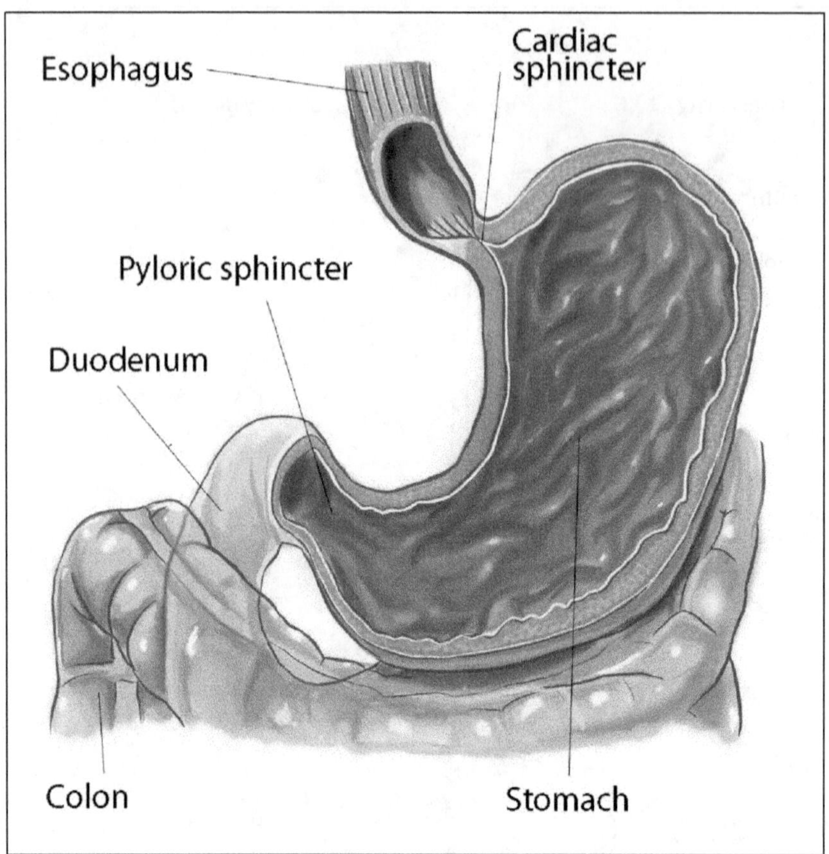

Stomach.

(Modified from Shutterstock, Inc, www.shutterstock.com, with permission)

Digestive enzymes and hydrochloric acid are added to food by the stomach to continue digestion, while muscles in the wall of the stomach help to churn the food. The sphincters keep food in the stomach until it is ready to be passed into the duodenum, the first part of the small intestine. If the cardiac sphincter allows some of the stomach contents to move back into the esophagus, acid reflux can result.

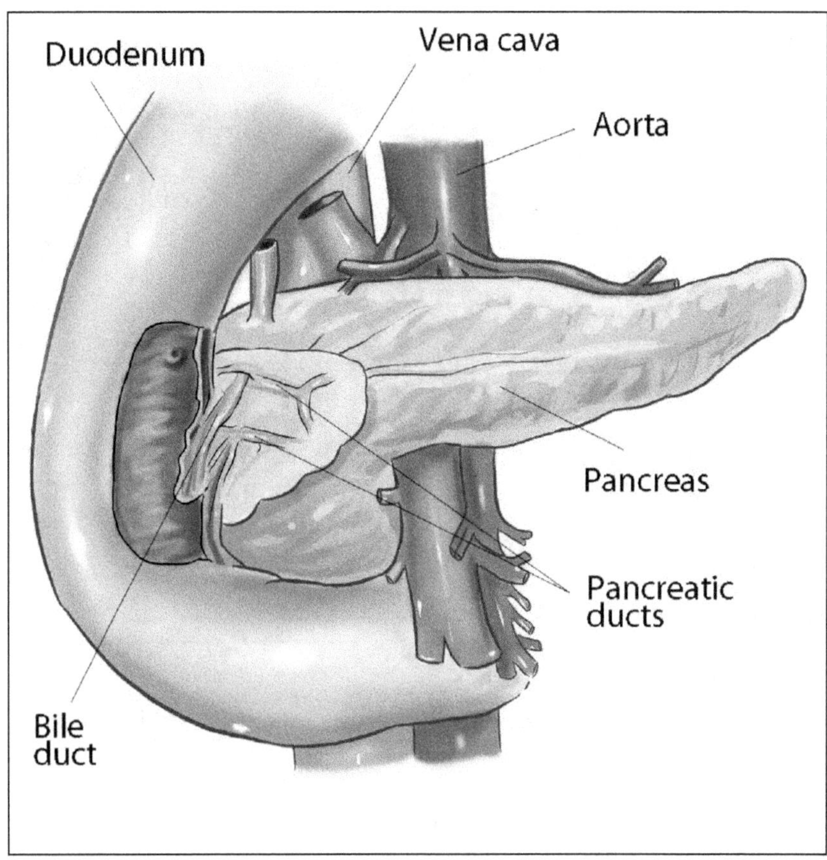

Pancreas.

(Modified from Shutterstock, Inc, www.shutterstock.com, with permission)

The pancreas adds digestive enzymes to the food in the duodenum, helping to digest carbohydrates and some fats and proteins. The pancreas also produces insulin, which is passed directly into the blood stream to regulate glucose levels in the body.

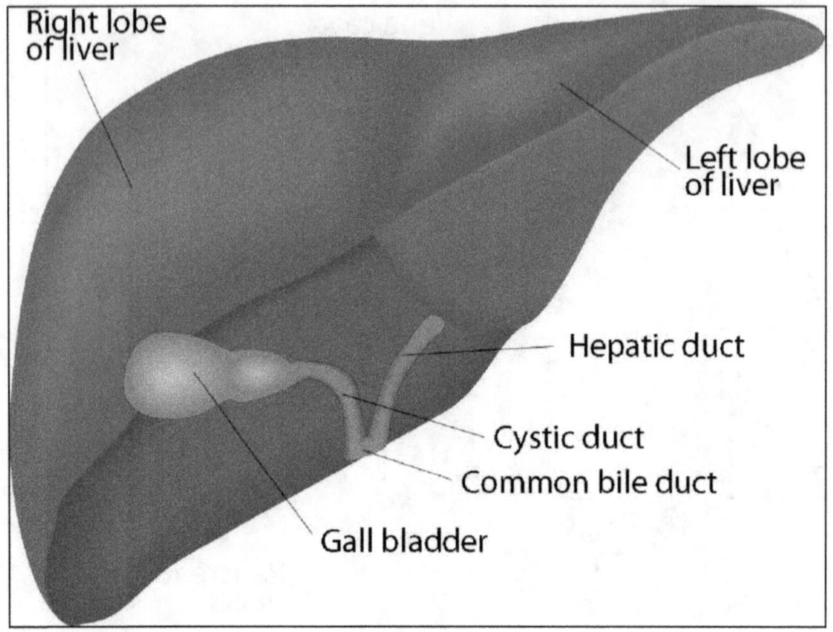

Liver and Gall Bladder.

(Modified from Shutterstock, Inc, www.shutterstock.com, with permission)

The liver produces bile, which emulsifies fats in the food so they can be absorbed more easily by the intestines. Bile is collected from throughout the liver via the main hepatic duct and its smaller branches, and then either moved via the cystic duct and stored in the gall bladder until needed or passed directly into the duodenum via the common bile duct. The liver also functions to break down toxins in the blood, rendering them harmless or passing the results out into the digestive system for elimination. Bile can become over‑concentrated in the bile dusts or more commonly in the gall bladder, producing gall stones.

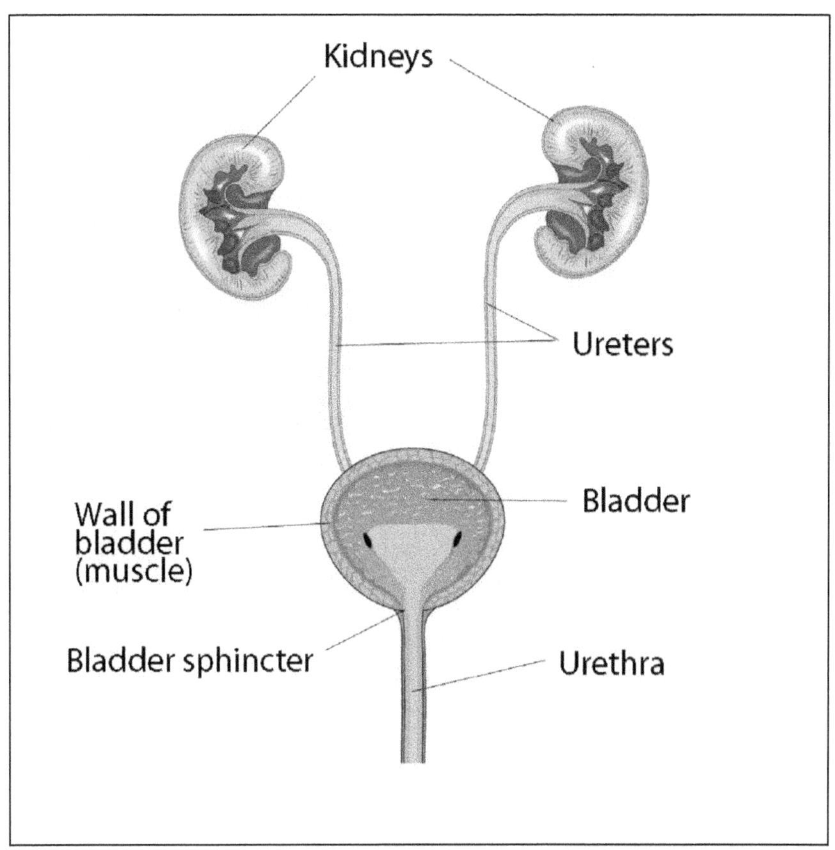

Urinary System.

(Modified from Shutterstock, Inc, www.shutterstock.com, with permission)

The kidneys filter impurities such as excess salt, urea and ammonium, and are also vitally involved in maintaining proper fluid balances within the body by regulating the amount of water removed from the bloodstream. Kidney stones or renal calculi are formed in the calyx, pelvis, ureters or urinary bladder. The stones can be formed from calcium compounds, struvite (an ammonium magnesium compound), or uric acid. The bladder collects urine from the kidneys via the ureters and contains urine until it can be released via the urethra, with the bladder sphincter controlling the flow.

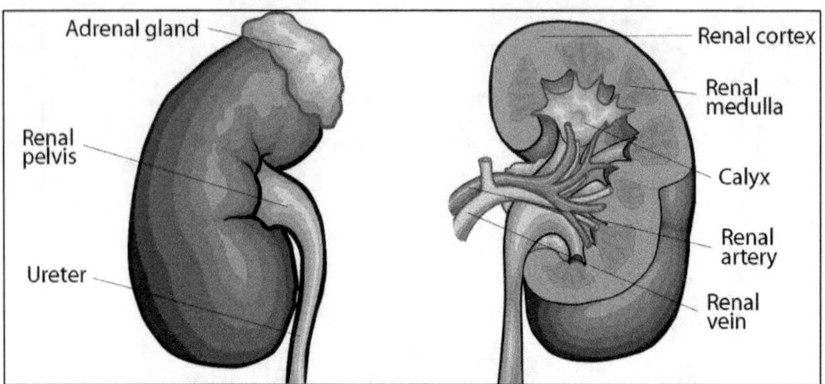

Kidneys.

(Modified from Shutterstock, Inc, www.shutterstock.com, with permission)

The kidneys and adrenal (or suprarenal) glands, including a cross section of one kidney. The adrenal glands produce a variety of endocrine hormones involved in metabolism, most notably adrenaline, also called epinephrine.

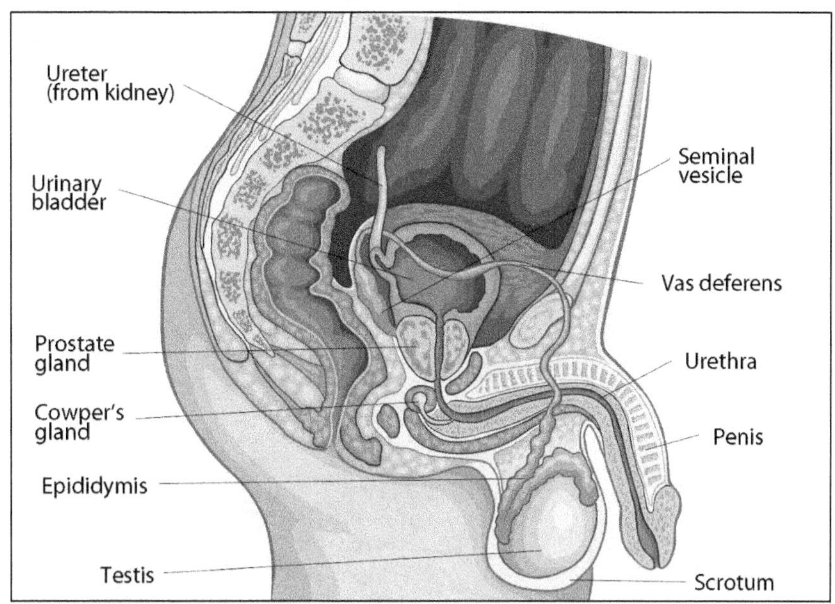

Male Reproductive System.

(Modified from Shutterstock, Inc, www.shutterstock.com, with permission)

Sperm cells are produced by the testes (testicles) and stored temporarily in the epididymis During ejaculation, fluids are added to the sperm by the Cowper's gland and the prostate to form semen. These fluids are a medium for the sperm to be carried in and also provide nutrients to the cells. The prostate often becomes enlarged, especially in older males, causing problems with both sexual function and urination. The enlarged gland can press on the bladder, reducing its capacity, and compress the urethra, restricting urine flow.

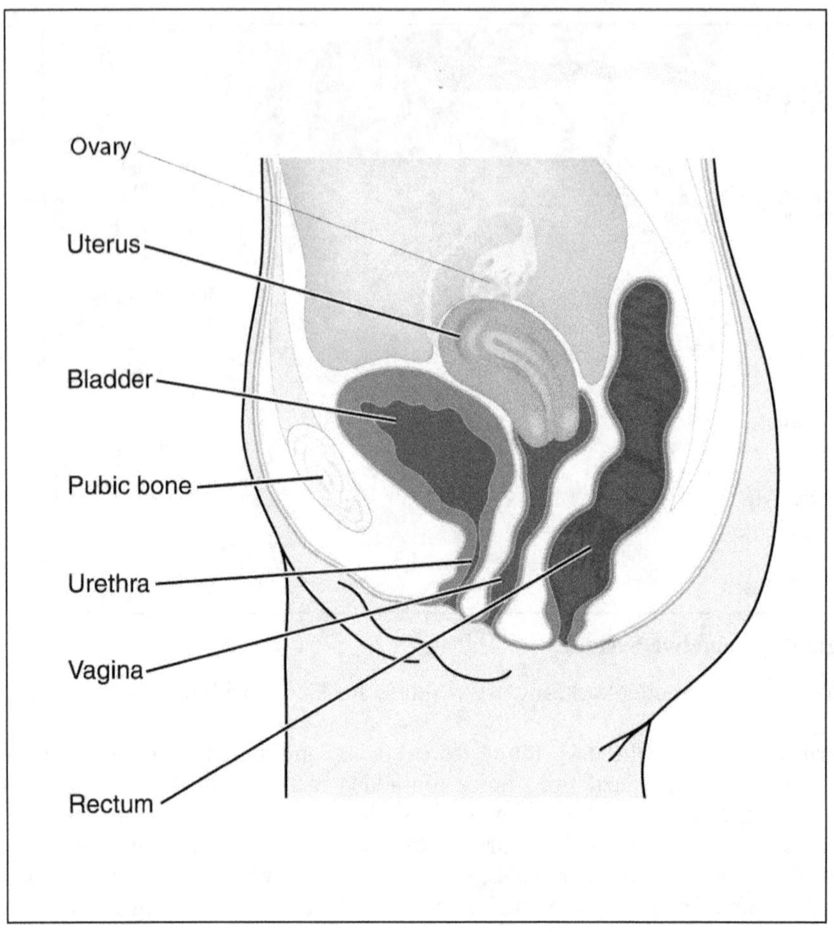

Female Reproductive System.

(Modified from Shutterstock, Inc, www.shutterstock.com, with permission)

Ova (egg cells) are produced by the ovaries and are released, usually one at a time, on a monthly cycle. They move through the fallopian tubes to the uterus. If the ovum is fertilized by a sperm cell during this time, it can implant in the wall of the uterus, which has been prepared with extra tissues with lots of blood supply. This fertilized ovum then develops into a fetus. If the ovum isn't fertilized, or if it fails to implant, it, along with the extra lining of the uterus, is released as the menstrual flow.

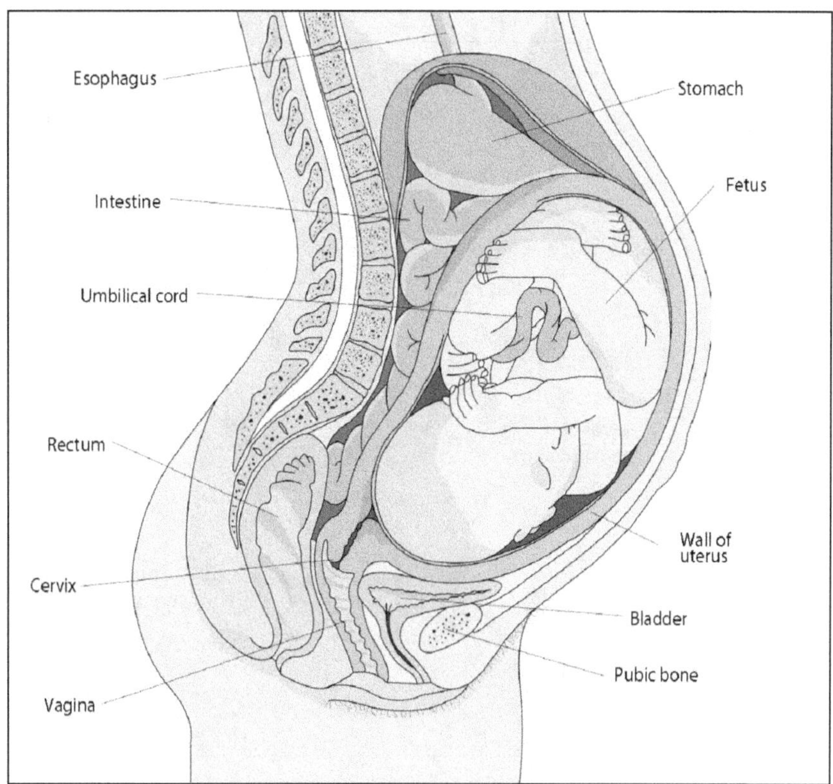

Pregnant Anatomy.

(Modified from Shutterstock, Inc, www.shutterstock.com, with permission)

The fetus grows and develops within the mother's uterus (womb), surrounded by a thin membrane called the amniotic sac, which also contains amniotic fluid that helps support and protect the fetus. The umbilical cord carries blood to and from the fetus and connects to the placenta, where nutrients and oxygen from the mother's blood supply is exchanged for wastes and carbon dioxide from the fetus. At a time determined by various hormones, the cervix (opening of the uterus) begins to dilate (enlarge) and the muscles of the wall of the uterus begin to contract in cycles in the process of labor. At some point, the amniotic sac bursts, releasing the remaining amniotic fluid. Further cervical dilation and uterine contractions push the fetus out of the uterus, through the cervix and vagina, and into the outside world. The umbilical cord is tied off and cut, and some time later, the placenta is expelled from the uterus (the afterbirth.)

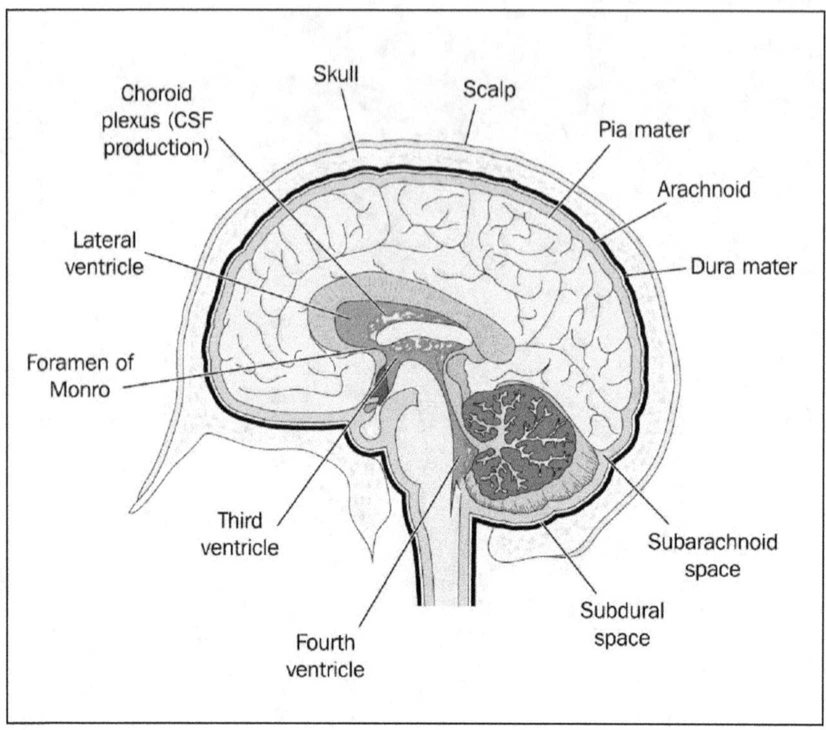

Brain Cross–section.

(Modified from Shutterstock, Inc, www.shutterstock.com, with permission)

The pia mater, arachnoid and dura mater are three membranes that surround and protect the brain within the skull. Cerebrospinal fluid circulates within the subarachnoid space and the ventricles of the brain, providing further cushioning. The main, folded part of the brain is the cerebrum and is mainly involved in perception and thought processes. The lower portion is the cerebrum, which coordinates balance and coordination. The brain stem, at the top of the spinal cord, controls basic functions such as breathing and heart rate.

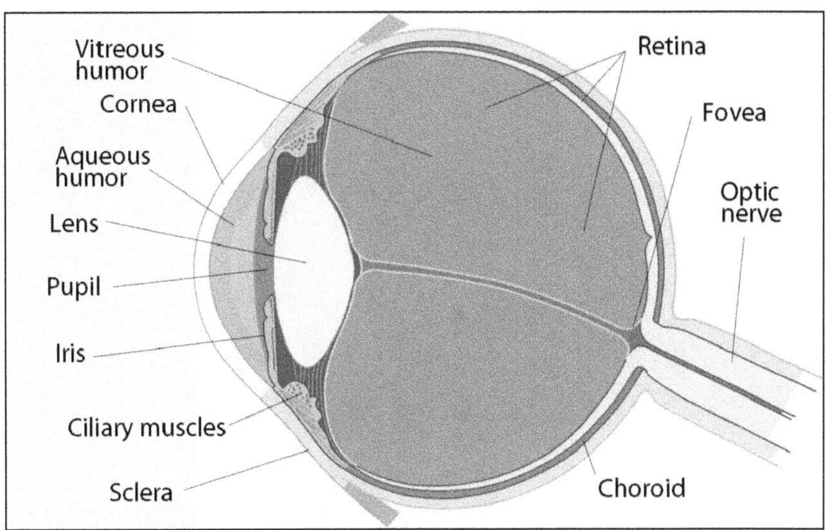

Eye cross–section.

(Modified from Shutterstock, Inc, www.shutterstock.com, with permission)

Light passes through the cornea, which provides both structure to the eye and some initial focussing. The amount of light entering the inside of the eye is controlled by the iris, which contracts or expands in order to change the pupil opening. Further focussing is done by the lens, whose shape and therefore focal distance can be modified by the ciliary muscles. The focussed light falls on the retina, where rod and cone cells convert the light into nerve signals corresponding to color and intensity. These signals are collected into the optic nerve and passed to the brain. The sclera, aqueous humor and vitreous humor provide the physical structure of the eye.

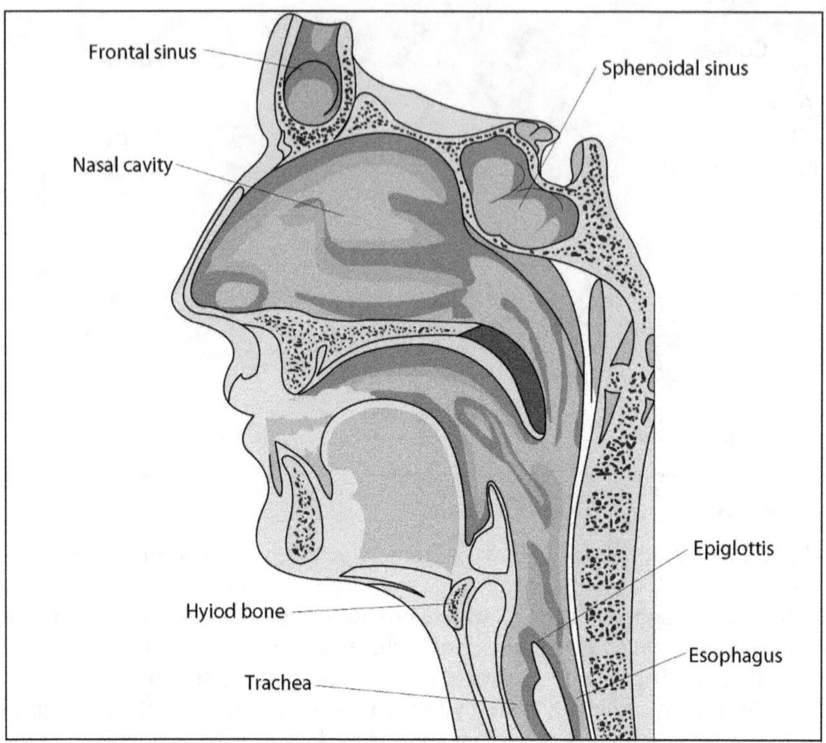

Nose, mouth and throat cross–section.

(Modified from Shutterstock, Inc, www.shutterstock.com, with permission)

The mouth serves multiple purposes, including tasting, chewing and swallowing food, breathing, vocalizing and social signalling. The nose provides breathing and the sense of smell, as well as filtering and warming of incoming air. The epiglottis blocks the opening of the trachea (windpipe) when swallowing.

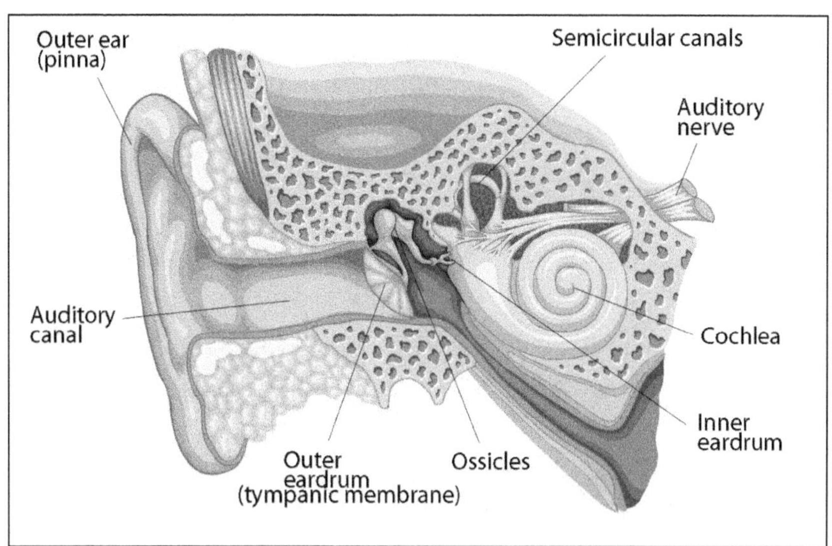

Ear cross–section.

(Modified from Shutterstock, Inc, www.shutterstock.com, with permission)

Sound is focussed by the outer ear and carried inside by the auditory canal. It then causes vibration of the outer eardrum. These vibrations are amplified and modified by the ossicles (three bones called the incus, or anvil, the malleus, or hammer, and the stapes, or stirrup), and then transferred to the inner eardrum. The sound vibrations then pass into the cochlea where they are converted into nerve signals that correspond to different frequencies and amplitudes of sound. The semicircular canals, though part of the inner ear structure, are involved in balance and spatial orientation rather than hearing.

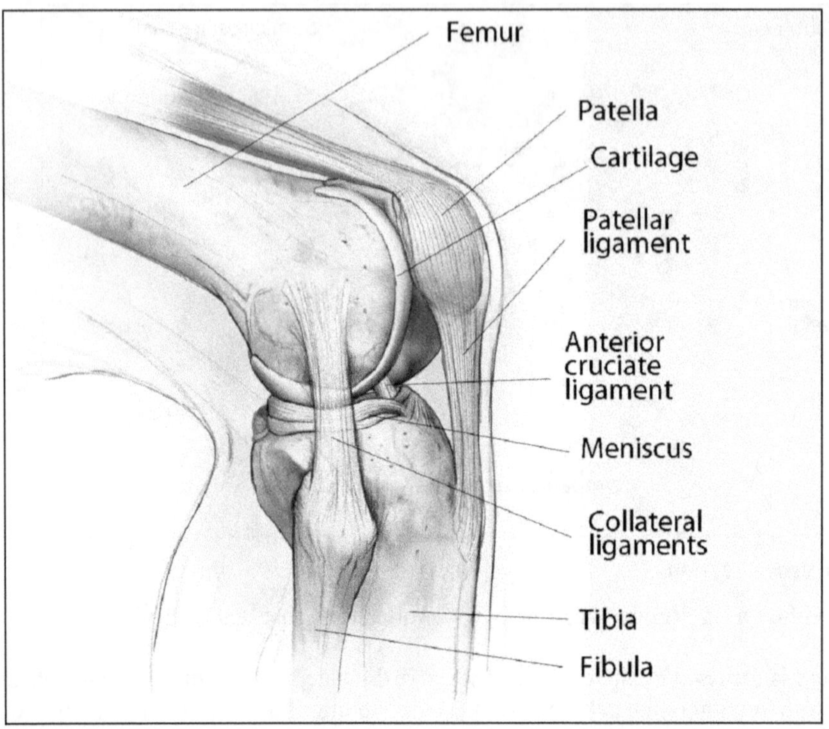

Knee joint.

(Modified from Shutterstock, Inc, www.shutterstock.com, with permission)

The knee joint moves on the cartilage surfaces at the ends of the femur and tibia, lubricated by an oil‑like substance called synovial fluid. The various tendons either hold the joint together or transmit muscle contractions through the joint. The patella, or kneecap, slide over the top of the joint to allow the thigh muscles to pull the knee straight. If the cartilage is damaged or worn, there can be bone‑on‑bone contact, which can be very painful. This can be treated temporarily by the injection of artificial lubricating fluids, or more permanently by performing total knee replacement surgery, in which the ends of the femur and tibia are removed and steel and plastic replacements are attached. A plastic surface is attached to the underside of the patella, as well. Progress is being made on growing cartilage cells from the patient in the lab, which may some day be able to be transplanted into the knee, avoiding the need for knee replacement surgery.

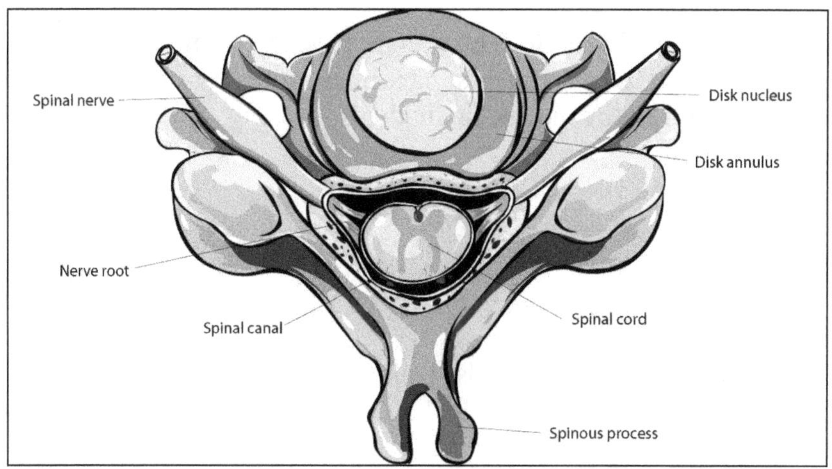

Spinal column lateral section.

(Modified from Shutterstock, Inc, www.shutterstock.com, with permission)

The spinal cord carries nerve signals between the brain and the body. The bony spine, made up of 24 vertebrae, serves both to support the body and to protect the spinal cord. Spinal disks act as bearing surfaces and shock absorbers between the vertebrae. Disease or trauma can cause the disks to rupture, allowing some of the softer nucleus to protrude out of the disk. If this material presses on one or more spinal nerves, it can cause excruciating pain.

Appendix D – Normal Values

This section is included to give perspective on some of the more common medical measurements. □Normal values□ is the range of values found in healthy, normal individuals.

Hematology □Red Blood Cells (erythrocytes)	
RBC (Male)	4.2 □5.6 M/µL (million cells/µL)
RBC (Female)	3.8 □5.1 M/µL
RBC (Child)	3.5 □5.0 M/µL

Hematology □White Blood Cells (leukocytes)	
WBC (Male)	3.8 □ 11.0 K/mm^3 (thousand cells/mm^3)
WBC (Female)	3.8 □11.0 K/mm^3
WBC (Child)	5.0 □10.0 K/mm^3

Hemoglobin	
Hgb (Male)	14 □18 g/dL
Hgb (Female)	11 □16 g/dL
Hgb (Child)	10 □14 g/dL
Hgb (Newborn)	15 □25 g/dL

Hematocrit	
Hct (Male)	39 □54%
Hct (Female)	34 □47%
Hct (Child)	30 □42%

General Chemistry	
Bilirubin, total	0.2 □1.4 mg/dL
BUN	6 □23 mg/dL
Calcium (total)	8 □11 mg/dL
Carbon dioxide	21 □34 mEq/L (milliequivalents/L)
Carbon monoxide	symptoms at >= 10% saturation
Chloride	96 □112 mEq/L
Ethanol	0 mg%; Coma at >= 400 □500 mg%
Glucose	65 □99 mg/dL
HDL (Male)	25 □65 mg/dL
HDL (Female)	38 □94 mg/dL
Potassium	3.5 □5.5 mEq/L
Sodium	135 □148 mEq/L

Urea nitrogen	8 □25 mg/dL

Lipid Panel (Adult)	
Cholesterol (total)	< 200 mg/dL desirable
Cholesterol (HDL)	30 □75 mg/dL
Cholesterol (LDL)	< 130 mg/dL desirable
Triglycerides (M)	> 40 □170 mg/dL
Triglycerides (F)	> 35 □135 mg/dL

Urine	
Specific gravity	1.003 □1.040
pH	4.6 □8.0
Na	10 □40 mEq/L
K	< 8 mEq/L
Cl	< 8 mEq/L
Osmolality	80 □1300 mOsm/L
Glucose	>= 180 mg/dL)

Cerebrospinal Fluid	
Osmolality	290 □298 mOsm/L
Pressure	70 □180 mm H_2O

Hemodynamic Parameters	
Cardiac index	2.5 □4.2 L/min/m^2
Cardiac output	4 □8 L/min
Stroke volume	60 □100 mL/beat
Systolic arterial pressure	90 □140 mm Hg
Diastolic arterial pressure	60 □90 mm Hg
Central venous pressure	2 □6 mm Hg
Ejection fraction	60 □75%
Left atrial pressure	4 □12 mm Hg
Right atrial pressure	4 □6 mm Hg
Pulmonary artery (PA) systolic pressure	15 □30 mm Hg
PA diastolic pressure	5 □15 mm Hg
PA mean pressure	10 □20 mm Hg
PA wedge pressure	4 □12 mm Hg
PA end diastolic pressure	8 □10 mm Hg
Right ventricular end diastolic pressure	0 □8 mm Hg

Neurological Values

Intracranial pressure	5 □15 mm Hg

<u>Blood Gases □Arterial Values</u>

pH	7.35 □7.45
$PaCO_2$	35 □45 mm Hg
HCO_3	22 □26 mEq/L
O_2 saturation	96 □100%
PaO_2	85 □100 mm Hg

<u>Blood Gases □Venous Values</u>

pH	7.31 □7.41
$PaCO_2$	41 □51 mm Hg
HCO_3	22 □29 mEq/L
O_2 saturation	60 □85%
PaO_2	30 □40 mm Hg

Basic Vital Signs

- Cuff blood pressure □ as measured by automatic or manual cuff□inflation methods at the arm. Normal for adults is considered to be 120 mm Hg systolic and 80 mm Hg diastolic, expressed as □120 over 80□ or 120/80. Adult pressure is usually considered to be borderline high when pressure is above 140/90, and treatment is suggested for pressures over 160/100. Extreme hypertension (high blood pressure) can produce pressures as high as 230/135. Low□ normal adult blood pressure is 100/65, though some athletes may have pressure in this range as a normal condition. Children tend to have pressures in this range as well. Hypotension (low blood pressure) is below about 90/60, and patients are likely to enter a coma state if pressures fall below about 50/30. Note that different methods of measuring cuff pressure, or even different people using the same method, can produce somewhat different values. Automatic **non–invasive blood pressure machines (296)** usually give repeatable results, but these may not agree perfectly with results obtained manually. Values from both ways of measuring cuff pressure should be taken as approximate and used more to detect trends than to represent true, high□accuracy pressures.

- Pulse rate □pulse rate varies over a large range depending on the individual, their state of health, and amount of exercise being performed. Normal resting rates for healthy adults can range from 60 to 100 beats per minute (bpm) with athletes generally having lower rates, in the 45 to 55 range. Children have higher resting rates than adults, and in utero, a fetus might have a normal pulse rate of around 200 bpm. Exercise increases pulse rates, as high as 150 or even 200 bpm, while rates often drop during sleep. A normal, non□athlete adult resting rate of below about 60 bpm is called bradycardia, while such a rate above about 100 bpm is called tachycardia.

- Respiration rate □ like pulse rate, respiration rate can vary over a wide range, with exercise increasing rates and rates for children being generally higher than those for adults. Normal resting rates for adults are between 10 and 20 breaths per minute, while for infants rates may be between 20 and 40 breaths per minute. During exercise, rates may increase to about 45, with athletes reaching up to 70 breaths per minute.

- Temperature — body temperature can be measured at a variety of points in the body, including the temporal area of the head, under the tongue, in the rectum or vagina, at the outer eardrum, or at internal organs during tests or surgery. Normal oral temperature is considered to be 36.8 degrees C, plus or minus 0.7 degrees, although some individuals may have healthy temperatures somewhat outside of this range. Core body temperature is usually about 1 degree higher than oral temperature. Body temperature follows a daily or diurnal rhythm, with lowest temperatures occurring during deep sleep. A temperature of over about 38 degrees is called hyperthermia and can result in a severe medical crisis, while temperatures below about 34 degrees is called hypothermia and can again cause major problems. Exercise, emotional state, ambient temperature, various disease processes and some drugs can all affect body temperature.

- Blood oxygen saturation — this parameter is measured with a device called a **pulse oximeter (320)**, which passes different wavelengths of light through a well-perfused (good blood flow) body part, such as a finger or earlobe. Analysis of the transmitted light provides a reasonably accurate measure of the percentage ratio of oxygen in the patient's blood, with 100% being the maximum possible.

Glossary for Normal Values

Bilirubin □ A by□product of the breakdown of red blood cells, it is normally destroyed by the liver. High levels can indicate liver problems. High concentrations of bilirubin in the body can cause the skin to turn yellow (jaundice).

BUN □Blood Urea Nitrogen.

Cardiac index □The amount of blood pumped by the heart per unit of time divided by body surface area, usually expressed in $L/min/m^2$.

Cardiac output □ A measurement of blood flow through the heart, expressed in L/min.

Central venous pressure □The blood pressure in the right atrium or veins near the heart, mainly the vena cava.

Cerebrospinal fluid □ A clear, colorless fluid containing small amounts of glucose and protein. Cerebrospinal fluid fills the ventricles of the brain, spaces between the brain and the cerebral membranes, and the central canal of the spinal cord. It acts as a shock absorber as well as carrying some nutrients and materials involved in immune response.

Cholesterol □A fatlike steroid alcohol found in animal fats and oils, in bile, blood, brain tissue, milk, yolk of egg, myelin sheaths of nerve fibres, the liver, kidneys and adrenal glands. It is the main component of most gallstones and is involved in atherosclerosis (hardening of the arteries.)

Diastolic arterial pressure □The peak pressure reached in arteries close to the heart (such as the ascending and descending aorta,) corresponding to the maximal contraction of the ventricles.

Ejection fraction □ A measure of the ability of the ventricles to contract.

HCO_3 □ Bicarbonate. A chemical produced in red blood cells, liberated through exchange with chloride. The kidneys may then excrete it.

HDL □High Density Lipoprotein (□good cholesterol□).

Hemoglobin (Hgb) □A molecule involved in carrying oxygen in the blood; an Iron atom forms part of the molecule.

Hematocrit (Hct) □The relative volume of blood occupied by red blood cells.

Intracranial pressure □The pressure exerted by cerebrospinal fluid within the skull.

Mole □A mole is the quantity of anything that has the same number of particles as are found in exactly 12 grams of carbon□12. That number of particles is referred to as Avogadro's Number, which is $6.02 x 10^{23}$.

O_2 saturation □A measure of the amount of oxygen carried by the blood compared to the maximum theoretically possible, expressed as a percentage.

Osmolality □The concentration of osmotically active particles in solution expressed in terms of osmoles of solute per kilogram of solvent.

Osmole □a unit indicating the number of moles of a chemical compound that contribute to a solution's osmotic pressure.

$PaCO_2$ □Partial pressure of carbon dioxide in the blood.

PaO_2 □Partial pressure of oxygen in the blood.

pH □A logarithmic measure of the activity of hydrogen ions in a solution, which also indicated relative acidity/alkalinity. pH 7 is neutral, pH 0 is extremely acidic, pH 14 is extremely alkaline.

Pulmonary artery wedge pressure □The pressure measured in the pulmonary artery when blood flow in the artery is occluded, usually by a small balloon on the tip of a catheter. This catheter also contains a pressure transducer.

Specific gravity □The density of a liquid compared to water, pure water having a specific gravity of 1.

Stroke volume The amount of blood pumped out of one ventricle of the heart as the result of a single contraction.

Systolic arterial pressure The low reached in the cycle of pressure in arteries close to the heart (such as the ascending and descending aorta,) corresponding to the maximal relaxation of the ventricles.

Triglycerides Glycerides in which the glycerol has three fatty acid molcules attached. They are the main constituent of vegetable oil and animal fats.

Appendix E – ECG Measurements and Arrhythmias

ECG Signals

The electrical signals within the heart can give important information concerning the state of that vital organ. These signals can be detected on the skin of the patient's chest, where they can be recorded and measured via an **electrocardiogram (ECG) machine** or **monitor**. The waveform has a typical shape, and the parts of the waveform have been given labels, P, Q, R, S and T. As muscles go through a cycle of contraction and relaxation, they develop an electrical signal that is either positive (polarization) or negative (depolarization).

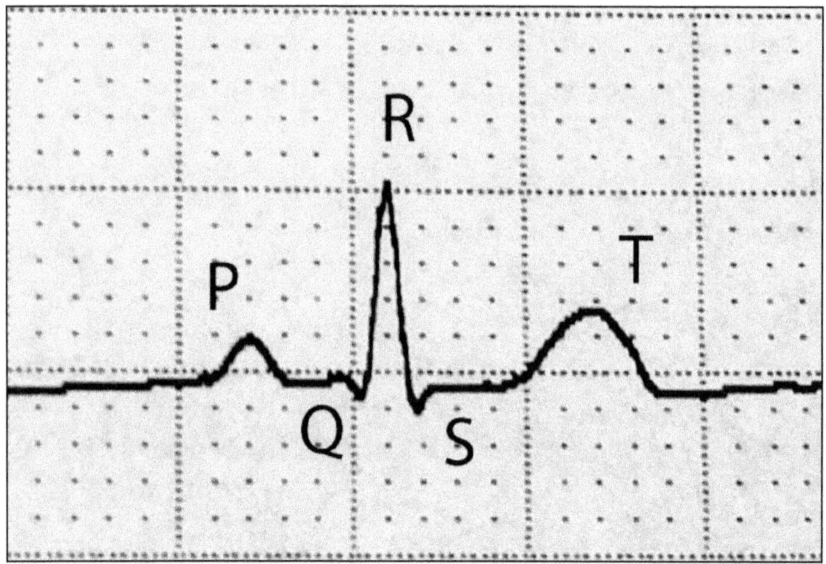

ECG QRS complex waveform.

The P wave is caused by the atria depolarizing. It is usually smooth and positive and has a short duration, less than 0.12 sec.

The time between the P wave and QRS portion is called the PR interval and is normally about 0.12 □0.20 seconds long.

The QRS complex is a result of depolarization of the ventricles. It normally is about 0.04 sec □0.12 seconds long.

The ST segment is the time during which the ventricles contract. The length and shape of this segment of the waveform in particular is often measured to give further information regarding cardiac health.

The QT interval begins at the onset of the QRS complex and to the end of the T wave. It indicates the time from which the ventricles depolarize until they start to repolarize.

The T wave is a result of ventricular repolarization. It is normally rounded and positive.

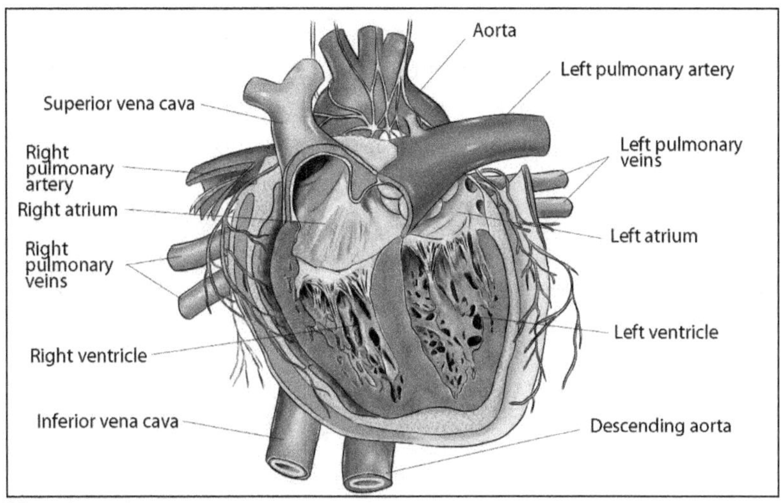

Heart anatomy.
Modified from Shutterstock, Inc, www.shutterstock.com, with permission.

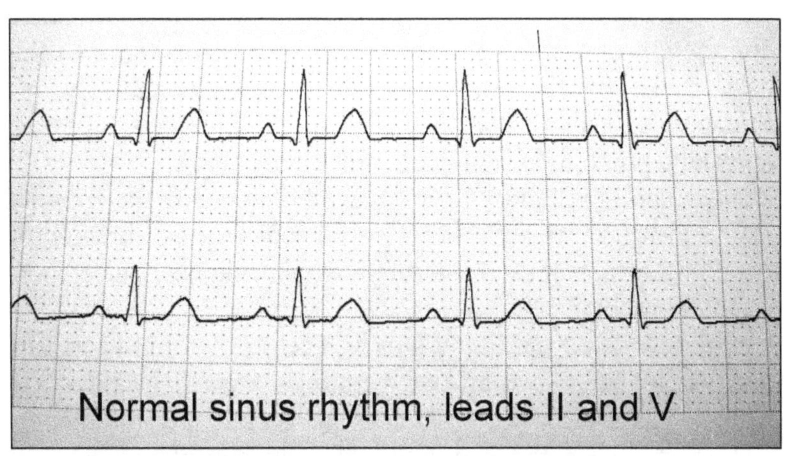

ECG waveform recording with traces from two different leads.

Arrhythmias

Any variation from a normal ECG rhythm (or normal sinus rhythm) is called an arrhythmia. Arrhythmias range from occasional odd beats that don't affect the well-being of the patient and can be present for years, to critical patterns that, if not corrected immediately, will result in death.

Arrhythmias may also simply be a normally shaped waveform that, in a patient at rest, is too fast (tachycardia) or too slow (bradycardia).

Arrhythmias can arise from a variety of causes: an imbalance in the chemicals that are involved in cardiac function; damage or interruption to the signal pathways in the heart; faults in the systems that control heart activity; or damage to the heart muscle, either through inadequate blood flow (ischemia) or complete loss of blood supply to a particular area of the heart, which results in muscle tissue death (necrosis), called a cardiac infarction.

Some of the more common arrhythmias include:

- Asystole – This is not really an "arrhythmia" as there is no rhythm at all. Asystole means the complete cessation of any contractions – the patient is "flat lined." There is no blood flow, so obviously it is a critical situation and must be treated immediately to prevent death, usually by using a defibrillator.
- Atrial Fibrillation (A Fib) – Fibrillation is an uncoordinated contraction of various groups of muscles in the heart, in this case those of the atria. A Fib is not immediately life threatening, since the ventricles continue to contract normally, pumping a significant amount of blood.
- Ventricular Fibrillation (V Fib) – Fibrillation of the muscles of the heart ventricles. This is an immediately life threatening condition which must be treated within minutes, since there is almost no blood flow.
- Ventricular Tachycardia (VT or V Tach) – A rapid heart rate that is initiated within the ventricles, usually caused by serious heart disease. V Tach is potentially life threatening and must be treated promptly. Usually considered as 5 or more consecutive PVCs (see below).

- Premature Ventricular Contractions (PVCs) □ These extra beats originate spontaneously within the ventricles and can give the sensation of the heart □skipping□ a beat. PVCs are relatively common, especially in younger people, and often disappear with time.
- Bigeminy □ This rhythm consists of alternating normal beats and PVCs.

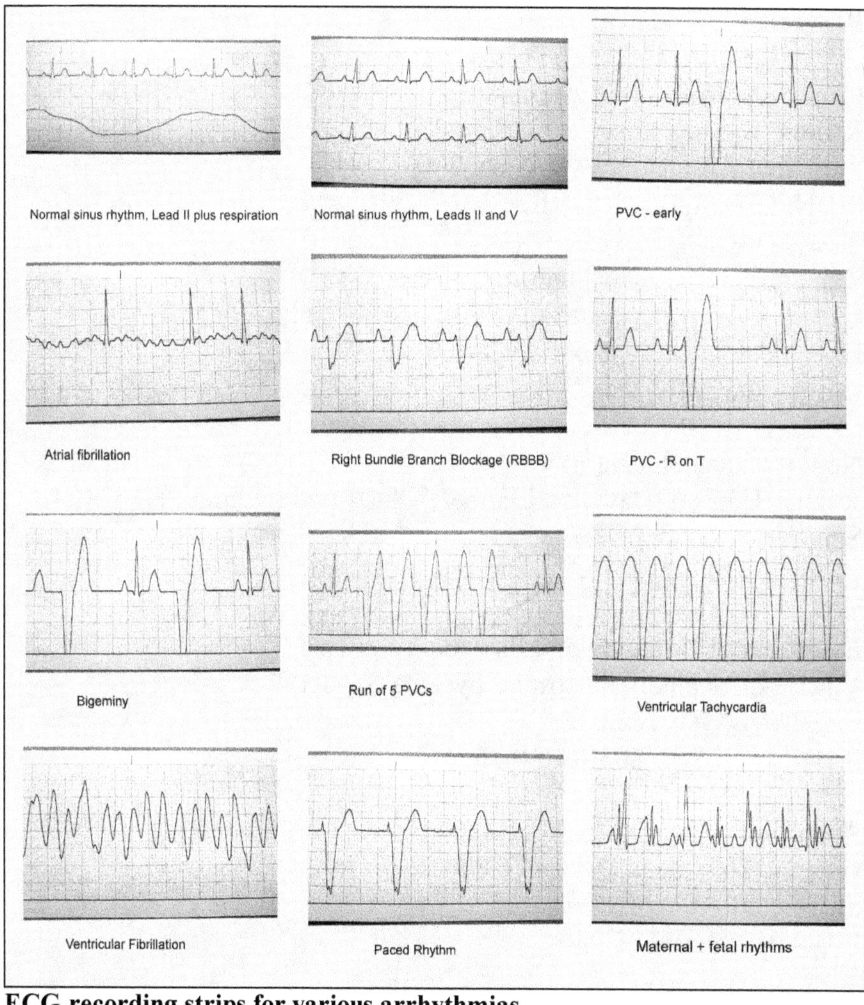

ECG recording strips for various arrhythmias.

Appendix F – Bibliography

Selected texts for reference.

Basic Anatomy for the Allied Health Professions
Royce L. Montgomery
Urban & Schwarzenberg, 1981
ISBN 0□8067□1231□7

Clinical Anatomy by Systems
Richard S. Snell
Lippincott, Williams & Wilkins, 2007
ISBN□13 978□0□7817□9164□9

Principles of Human Anatomy, 5th Ed.
Gerard J. Tortora, illustrated by Leonard Dank
Biological Sciences Textbooks, Inc. 1989
ISBN 0□06□046685□5

Netter□s Clinical Anatomy
John T. Hansen, David R. Lambert, illustrated by Frank H. Netter
Saunders, 2005
ISBN 1□929007□71□X

Essentials of Anatomy and Physiology, 5th Ed.
Valerie C. Scanlon, illustrated by Tina Sanders
F.A. Davis Co., 2003
ISBN□13 978□0□8036□1546□5

Anatomy & Physiology, 5th Ed.
Gary A. Thibodeau, Kevin T. Patton
Mosby, 2003
ISBN 0□323□01628□6

Anatomy & Physiology in Health and Illness, 9th Ed.
Anne Waugh, Allison Grant, illustrated by Graeme Chambers
Churchill Livingstone, 2001
ISBN 0□443□06468□7

Surgical Technology for the Surgical Technologist, 2nd Ed.
Kevin Frey, Teri L. Junge, Senior Editors
Thomson Delmar Learning, 2004
ISBN 1□4018□3848□0

Essential Surgery □Problems, Diagnosis and Management, 4th Ed.
H. George Burkitt, Clive R.G. Quick, Joanna B. Reed, illustrated by Philip J. Deakin
Churchill Livingstone Elsevier, 2007
ISBN 9780443103469

Appendix G – Internet Resources

Selected web sites for reference, with a brief description of the site from it□s introductory section, unless self□explanatory.

http://www.americanheart.org/
The mission of the American Heart Association is to build healthier lives, free of cardiovascular diseases and stroke.

http://www.ctc.nhs.uk/
Liverpool Heart and Chest Hospital

http://www.prk.com/cataracts/history_of_lens_implants.html

http://www.medscape.com/
Medscape offers specialists, primary care physicians and other health professionals the Web's most robust and integrated medical information and educational tools.

http://www.fmc□ag.com/internet/fmc/fmcag/neu/fmcpub.nsf/Content/Product_Portfolio
Fresenius Medical Care provides a complete line of dialysis services and products.

http://www.meditec.com/normal□lab□values.html

http://www.lasersurgeryforeyes.com/cataracthistory.html

http://www.virtual□anesthesia□textbook.com/index.shtml
The Virtual Anesthesia Textbook is sponsored by GE Healthcare's Clinical Window information service.
The goal of the Virtual Anesthesia Textbook is to organize all Internet resources on anesthesia into one concise, textbook style website.

http://www.courseweb.uottawa.ca/medicine□histology/English/Renal/Default.htm
Information on the renal system plus links to other body systems.

http://medlineplus.gov/
MedlinePlus will direct you to information to help answer health questions. MedlinePlus brings together authoritative information from NLM, the National Institutes of Health (NIH), and other government agencies and health□related organizations.

http://emedicine.medscape.com/
eMedicine is the most authoritative and accessible point of care medical reference available to physicians and other healthcare professionals on the Internet. The evidence□based content, updated regularly by nearly 10,000 attributed physician authors and editors, provides the latest practice guidelines in 59 medical specialties. The eMedicine Clinical Knowledge Base contains articles on nearly 7,000 diseases and disorders and is richly illustrated with some 30,000 multimedia files.
http://www.acc.org/
The mission of the American College of Cardiology is to advocate for quality cardiovascular care□ through education, research promotion, development and application of standards and guidelines□ and to influence health care policy.

http://health.allrefer.com/
Welcome to AllRefer Health, a medical and health information resource containing outstanding database of health articles and reference materials. Consumers and health professionals alike can depend on it for information that is authoritative and up□to□date. AllRefer Health has extensive information from trusted sources on over 4,000 topics including diseases, tests, symptoms, injuries, surgeries, nutrition, poisons, and special topics.

http://www.adam.com/
We are A.D.A.M.
We create online information and technology solutions for employers, benefits brokers, healthcare organizations and Internet companies. Our Employer and Broker Solutions help employers and benefits brokers provide employees a better benefits experience while helping to manage workflow and cut costs. Our customizable Health Solutions help hospitals, managed care organizations, and

consumer web sites become an integral part of the online consumer healthcare experience.

We create the content and tools that help companies help people. Our award-winning health content and technology solutions are an integral part of helping employees and healthcare consumers manage important aspects of their health and make important benefits and health decisions. Whether they're looking for information about health coverage, a healthcare provider, or searching for credible health information, we help our clients connect them to the right information.

Index

www.ingramcontent.com/pod-product-compliance
Lightning Source LLC
Chambersburg PA
CBHW051438170526
45166CB00001B/30

* 9 7 8 1 4 7 0 1 9 5 0 2 1 *